THE ECONOMICS OF
HEALTH CARE

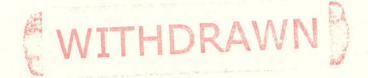

The Economics of Health Care

A REFERENCE HANDBOOK

Michael D. Rosko
&
Robert W. Broyles

Foreword by Sylvester E. Berki

Greenwood Press
New York • Westport, Connecticut • London

Library of Congress Cataloging-in-Publication Data

Rosko, Michael D.
    The economics of health care : a reference handbook / Michael D.
  Rosko and Robert W. Broyles.
        p. cm.
    Bibliography: p.
    Includes index.
    ISBN 0–313–25416–8 (lib. bdg. : alk. paper)
    1. Medical economics—United States—Handbooks, manuals, etc.
  I. Broyles, Robert W. II. Title.
  RA410.53.R67 1988
  338.4′33621′0973—dc19   87–36101

British Library Cataloguing in Publication Data is available.

Library of Congress Catalog Card Number: 87–36101
ISBN: 0–313–25416–8

First published in 1988

Greenwood Press, Inc.
88 Post Road West, Westport, Connecticut 06881

Printed in the United States of America

The paper used in this book complies with the
Permanent Paper Standard issued by the National
Information Standards Organization (Z39.48–1984).

10 9 8 7 6 5 4 3 2 1

CONTENTS

FIGURES

TABLES

FOREWORD

Health economics comprises a body of thought, a set of concepts, an approach to analysis that emphasizes explicit modelling, and certain skills in applying these to empirical phenomena. The body of economic thought and applications is vast and the complexity of the health care sector immense. The student and the analyst are challenged by the need to select, develop and apply models that help to reveal the often hidden dynamics of individual and organizational behaviors in the markets that constitute the health care sector. Understanding market behavior, whether it be pricing strategy or the role of economies of scale, is never easy. The task is further complicated in markets that are continually buffeted by rapid technological change, swings in government policies, and changes in the basic relationships between providers of care, institutional managers, third-party payers, and patients. These structural transformations, ranging from the rapid development of various types of health maintenance and preferred provider organizations and hospital chains, to the introduction of new incentives exemplified by the prospective payment system, manifest themselves in altered behaviors and performance. The health care industry is undergoing fundamental change. Yet its functions remain constant.

Improvement in health, amelioration of disease, prevention of illness remain the fundamental rationale of the health care sector. The achievement of these objectives with the lowest resource expenditures, at the best levels of efficiency, remains the major challenge of health economics, the age-old challenge of efficiency in resource allocation. But distributional equity, guaranteeing access to prevention and care on a reasonably equal basis to all Americans, is not less of a challenge or a less important social goal. Current proposals in Congress to expand Medicare by implementing catastrophic health insurance, initiatives to mandate health insurance for the unemployed and the working poor, developing public mechanisms to fund care for victims of AIDS, devising insurance schemes to cover the costs of nursing home care all are examples of a wavering but nonetheless strong social commitment to distributional equity based on need. Health economics is the science and art of identifying the ways by which distributional equity can be achieved in an efficient manner. Professors Rosko and Broyles show us how.

This comprehensive, analytic, and up-to-date exploration of applied health economics provides a superb introduction to the challenges of understanding the workings of the health care system. Broad in its scope, fair and critical in its assessment of the state of the art, logical and lucid in its exposition, it is an excellent text. It integrates the literature in almost all of the major areas of health economics and relates it to current developments and data and does so in a policy framework. Taking a balanced approach to major policy issues, ranging from prospective payment for Medicare beneficiaries in HMOs to improvements in the prospective payment system for hospital care, Professors Rosko and Broyles dissect the economics of health care policy and illuminate alternatives for improved effectiveness and efficiency.

The dominant trends of integration, diversification, corporatization, technological change, and expansion of health benefits are occurring in an environment of increasing resource constraints. Society may be willing to help everyone have lunch, but the lunch is never free. Both the invisible hand of competition and the visible hands of regulation may be necessary to attain efficiency in resource use while achieving the social goal of improved health care for all. The daunting challenge for future policy makers and managers is to devise the most appropriate combinations of economic structures and incentives to achieve those goals. This book will help them make a good beginning.

Sylvester E. Berki

Professor
Department of Health Services,
Management and Policy
School of Public Health
The University of Michigan
Ann Arbor, Michigan

PREFACE

In recent years, the literature in the field of health economics has grown exponentially and currently addresses a broad spectrum of theoretical and policy issues. A satisfactory treatment of the totality of health economics in a single book is a difficult, if not impossible task, a consideration that limits the scope of this effort. Recognizing the problems of biting off more than we can chew and having a desire to keep our forests green, we adopted the conventional but restrictive view of the health services industry as a market consisting of hospitals, physicians, long-term care facilities, home health agencies, health maintenance organizations, and other alternate delivery systems. Although important, neither public health programs nor the techniques, such as cost-benefit analysis, commonly used to evaluate these efforts have been examined here.

The scope of the text is limited further by our focus on the multivariate analyses that appear in the literature; however, we include case studies and tabular analyses in those areas that have not been examined more rigorously. For example, the paucity of available evidence has prevented multivariate analyses of the effects exerted by recently emerging phenomena such as the rapid growth in alternate delivery systems, the impending surplus of physicians, and the decline in participation rates of nurses. In addition, the effect of recent cost-containment initiatives on access to care has not been the subject of extensive empirical examination, an outcome that also limits our review.

This book might be designed for several audiences, to include administrators, students of economics or health administration, planners, policy analysts, regulators, and medical educators. Rather than attempting to satisfy all of these groups, and serving none well, we learned early that compromises were required and that it was necessary to impose an additional limitation on our focus. This book is designed to supplement texts that are used by those who are responsible for courses in health economics. Although our analysis assumes a background in microeconomic theory, we review basic concepts prior to our discussions of empirical findings. The book is also designed as a source of recent references that are of value to researchers and policy analysts. We hope that the review presented here will serve as a source of information for these two groups, improve policy analysis, and stimulate new or improved avenues of inquiry. Finally, it is hoped that the book will provide a frame of reference that will enhance the administrator's understanding of economic forces that are external to the health institution but influence internal operations.

The book is divided into four major components. For several reasons, Part I is devoted to a discussion of the growth in health expenditures. First, inflationary pressures in the health care industry and the resulting reduction in access have been the dominant concerns of policy analysts. Further, given the interrelationships between the health care sector and other components of the economy, the growth in health care costs exerts profound effects on other industries. For example, the need to compete with international enterprises on the basis of price and quality has accelerated the need of employers to control all costs, including expenditures for employee health care benefits. Finally, our discussion of health care expenditures allows us to integrate an overview of the health care sector with a unified framework of analysis. Accordingly, Chapter 1 includes descriptive statistics about expenditures for health care, as well as a discussion of economic theories which have attempted to explain the rapid growth in health care expenditures.

In Part II we turn to an examination of demand-side issues. Recognizing the profound effects that third-party payments exert on the health care industry, we analyze the demand for health insurance in Chapter 2. Included in this chapter are analyses of employer and employee choices of health insurance, as well as an assessment of issues that are germane to the elderly and the uninsured. In Chapter 3 we examine not only the determinants of demand but also various theories of the demand for health services.

Part III is devoted to supply-side analyses. Chapter 4 examines behavioral models of health care organizations and, unlike the other chapters of the book, this discussion is devoted primarily to conceptual issues rather than to a critique of empirical studies. Although a number of early behavioral models are discussed, the chapter emphasizes models that can be used to explain hospital responses to prospective payment and the preferential admission policies used by nursing homes.

In Chapters 5 and 6 we discuss attempts to define the output of hospitals, nursing homes and other health care providers with greater precision. Our analysis is devoted to conceptual issues that are likely to be of interest to researchers and policy analysts who are responsible for the development of efficacious payment mechanisms.

Analyses of the production and cost functions are the subjects of Chapters 7 and 8, respectively. Since cost functions of health care organizations have been examined more extensively than production functions, Chapter 7 emphasizes the dual nature of production and cost function analysis. Chapter 8 is devoted not only to a discussion of the technical problems of estimating cost functions but also to a review of the findings pertinent to the determinants of the costs of hospitals and other organizations.

In Chapters 9 and 10 our focus turns to the supply and distribution of physicians. Chapter 9 includes a critique of the methods used to calculate physician requirements as well as a review of the determinants of specialty choice. Chapter 10 includes a discussion of the geographic distribution of physicians and concludes with a review of policy options that might reduce the maldistribution of physicians.

In Part IV our emphasis turns to cost-containment initiatives. Chapter 11 examines the competitive approaches with an emphasis on health maintenance organizations, while in Chapter 12 we focus on the regulatory approaches with an emphasis on rate regulation. In the epilogue we summarize our review and suggest future directions for policy and research.

ACKNOWLEDGMENTS

Clearly this book would not have been possible without the assistance of a large number of people. Tom Getzen, Jay Halpern, Dave Salkever, and Helen Smits read preliminary drafts of some chapters and made valuable comments that improved the quality of the book. We appreciate the efforts of the authors and journal editors who have improved the conceptual and empirical content of the recent literature. Inevitably, we missed some important studies; we apologize to the researchers who conducted them and hope that the number of these omissions is few.

This work would not have been possible without the support of Widener University and the assistance of many friends and colleagues. Our department chair, Larry Walker, has succeeded in creating an environment conducive to our scholarly efforts. Our graduate research assistant, Carolyn Reid, was an invaluable jack-of-all-trades who served as researcher, organizer, copyeditor, and liaison with libraries and journals. Our sincere gratitude is expressed to Ann Marie Kasarsky, who deciphered our handwriting and prepared numerous drafts of the manuscript. We thank Scott Chain and Peggy Frick for the long hours they spent on the art work. We are grateful to the colleagues in our department who lent us resources; and to Michael George and Louise Ciccarelli, who helped proof the final version of the manuscript. Michael Rosko is grateful for the sabbatical grant from Widener University, which supported much of his efforts. We are, of course, indebted to those from whom we have learned; in order to avoid errors of omission, we shall not attempt to name them.

We are certainly grateful to S.E. Berki for contributing the foreword to this book. Sy Berki's work inspired us to undertake this effort, and we were honored when he agreed to comment on our manuscript.

Finally, for their encouragement and understanding, a special word of gratitude is expressed to our families, Rita and Erin Broyles, and Joan Rosko. Without their support and patience, this effort would not have been possible.

Recognizing the contributions of others, we must accept the responsibility for errors and omissions.

Part I

Introduction

1

RISING HEALTH CARE EXPENDITURES: AN OVERVIEW OF THE HEALTH CARE INDUSTRY

We begin this book with a discussion of the rising costs of health care services. Given the public concern about this issue, an analysis of the growth of health services expenditures is an appropriate place to start. An examination of this problem is a convenient and logical way not only to present an overview of the health care industry but also to identify the topics covered in later chapters. In the first part of this chapter, we summarize a set of background statistics that describe changes in spending on health care. This is followed by a review of theories of hospital cost inflation. In the final section, we provide a linkage between the demand-pull and cost-push theories of inflation.

OVERVIEW OF HEALTH CARE EXPENDITURES

Expenditures for health services in the United States have grown dramatically during the last three decades. As shown in Table 1.1, total health care expenditures increased from $42 billion in 1965 to an estimated $497 billion in 1987, an average annual increase of 11.3 percent. During the same period, the Gross National Product (GNP) of the United States grew from $691 billion to $4,433 billion, an average annual increase of 8.4 percent. Besides growing dramatically in aggregate terms, national health expenditures have risen rapidly on a per capita basis and as a percentage of GNP. Per capita health care expenditures increased from $207 in 1965 to $1,974 in 1987. During the same period the percentage of GNP spent on health care almost doubled from 6.1 to 11.2. These trends underscore concerns of policy analysts that the cost of procuring health services may preclude the purchase or provision of other goods and services and that many individuals may be unable to afford needed health services.

The distribution of expenditures by type of health service for selected years during the period from 1965 to 1985 is presented in Table 1.2. As this table

Table 1.1

National Health Expenditures, Selected Years, 1965–1987: Aggregate, Per Capita, and Percent of Gross National Product (GNP)

Year	Gross National Product (Billions)	Total National Health Expenditures		
		Amount in Billions	Per Capita	Percent of GNP
1965	691	42	207	6.1
1970	993	75	350	7.6
1975	1,549	133	591	8.6
1980	2,632	248	1,048	9.4
1981	2,958	285	1,197	9.6
1982	3,069	321	1,334	10.5
1983	3,305	355	1,461	10.7
1984	3,663	387	1,580	10.6
1985	3,989	425	1,721	10.7
1986[a]	4,207	454	1,820	10.8
1987[b]	4,433	497	1,974	11.2

Sources: Arnett, R., D. McKusick, S.Sonnefeld, and C. Cowell. 1986. Projections of health care spending to 1990. Health Care Financing Review 7 (3): 6.

Waldo, D., K. Levit, and H. Lazenby. 1986. National health expenditures, 1985. Health Care Financing Review 8 (1): 13.

Arnett, R., M. Freeland, D. McKusick, and D. Waldo. 1987. National health expenditures, 1986-2000. Health Care Financing Review 8 (4): 24.

[a] Projection by Arnett et al. (1986).

[b] Projection by Arnett et al. (1987).

shows, the allocation of the health services dollar changed over the period. In 1985, over half of all health care dollars were spent for hospital services (39.3 percent) or physician services (19.5 percent). Reflecting the graying of America, the proportion of resources allocated to nursing home services increased during the last two decades from 4.8 percent in 1965 to 8.2 percent in 1985.

Analysts from the Health Care Financing Administration (HCFA) decomposed changes in health care expenditures that occurred from 1974 to 1984 into five broad categories: general inflation, aggregate population growth (including changes in population composition), increases in per capita visits or per capita patient days, increases in intensity of health care services (''real'' services per visit or per patient day), and health care price increases in excess of general price inflation (Arnett, McKusick, Sonnefeld et al. 1986). As shown in Table 1.3, the analysis focused on total health expenditures, as well as on specific types of health services. An inspection of Table 1.3 reveals that about 55 percent of the increase in total national health expenditures was due to general inflation in the economy. From another perspective, we see that almost 50 percent of

Table 1.2
National Health Expenditures, Selected Years, 1965–1985, by Type of
Expenditure ($ billions) and by Percent of Total (in parentheses)

Type of Expenditure	1965	1970	1975	1980	1985	Average Annual Percent Change
Total health expenditures	42	75	133	248	425	11.7
Hospital services	14	28	52	102	167	12.5
	(33.3)	(37.3)	(39.1)	(41.1)	(39.3)	
Physician services	9	14	25	47	83	11.2
	(21.4)	(18.7)	(18.8)	(18.9)	(19.5)	
Dentist services	3	5	8	15	27	11.0
	(7.1)	(6.7)	(6.0)	(6.0)	(6.3)	
Nursing home services	2	5	10	20	35	14.6
	(4.8)	(6.7)	(7.5)	(8.0)	(8.2)	
Drugs and medical services	5	8	12	19	29	8.7
	(11.9)	(10.7)	(9.0)	(7.7)	(6.8)	
All other services	9	15	26	45	84	11.2
	(21.5)	(20.0)	(19.5)	(18.1)	(19.8)	

Source: Waldo, D., K. Levit, and H. Lazenby. 1986. National health expenditures, 1985. Health Care Financing Review 8(1): 14.

health care cost inflation was due to factors other than those that affected the general economy. Indeed, the health care industry has been the focus of intensive scrutiny because its rate of inflation has consistently exceeded that of most other industries. Table 1.3 also shows that among health sector specific factors, changes in the intensity of medical treatment (i.e., real services per visit or per patient day) has been the single most important source of expenditure growth. Further examination of Table 1.3 suggests that most of the health care sectors have followed a similar pattern with respect to growth in expenditures. The most notable exception is nursing home services, which, relative to other health services, experienced much more growth in patient days per capita and lower price increases. Although not as extreme as nursing homes, outpatient facilities enjoyed a greater than average increase in per capita visits. Further, outpatient care was the only health care service for which less than 50 percent of expenditure increases was attributed to economy-wide factors.

Expenditures for Hospital Services

In recognition of the dominant position hospitals occupy in the health care industry, it is appropriate to emphasize this sector in our discussion of health

Table 1.3
Factors Accounting for Growth in Expenditures from 1974 to 1984 in Selected Categories of Health Care Services

Factor	Community Hospital Care			Physicians Services	Nursing Home Care	Total Health Expenditures
	Inpatient Expenses		Outpatient Expenses			
	Inpatient Days	Admissions				
Economy - wide factors						
General inflation	51.2	51.5	40.8	52.8	53.2	55.6
Population growth	7.3	7.5	5.8	7.5	7.6	7.9
Health - sector factors						
Growth in per capita visits or patient days	-8.5	-.8	10.9	-7.5	15.0	-
Growth in real services per visit or per day (intensity)	33.4	25.4	29.3	27.5	15.4	22.9
Medical care price increases in excess of general inflation	16.6	16.4	13.2	19.7	8.8	13.6

Source: Arnett, R., et al.. 1986. Projections of health care spending to 1990. Health Care Financing Review 7(3): 4.

Table 1.4

Inpatient Hospital Utilization in Nonfederal, Short-Term General, and Other Special Hospitals, Selected Years, 1965–1986

Year	Admissions (in Thousands)	Average Length of Stay (in Days)	Patient Days (Per Thousand Population)
1965	26,463	7.8	1058
1970	29,252	8.2	1163
1975	33,519	7.7	1188
1980	36,198	7.6	1206
1981	36,494	7.6	1212
1982	36,429	7.6	1198
1983	36,201	7.6	1166
1984	35,202	7.3	1048
1985	33,501	7.1	992
1986	32,410	7.1	923

Source: Hospital Statistics, 1987 edition, published by the American Hospital Association, copyright 1987.

care expenditures. The increases in aggregate spending for hospital care have been due to both increased utilization and increased charges. Table 1.4 presents a summary of utilization statistics. The number of hospital admissions has increased from 26,463,000 in 1965 to 32,410,000 in 1986, an increase of 22.4 percent. During this period, population growth was less than 23 percent. In contrast to increases in the number of hospital admissions, the average length of stay decreased from 7.8 days in 1965 to 7.1 days in 1986. Part of this decline is attributed to utilization review programs and the influence of case-based prospective payment systems. Similar reductions in the rate of admissions occurred during the period from 1980 to 1986. When combined with shorter hospital stays, the decline in the admission rate precipitated a reduction in the number of patient days during the period 1980–1986.

In the hospital industry, the most commonly used measures of costs per unit of output are total cost per day and total cost per admission. As Table 1.5 indicates, the average cost of a patient day rose from $45 in 1965 to $551 in 1985, an average annual increase of 12.7 percent. Increases in cost per admission have risen at a slightly lower pace due to the decreased length of stay. From 1965 to 1985, the cost per admission increased at an average annual rate of 12.2 percent or from $346 to $3,901. These drastic increases in the cost of hospitalization can be placed in perspective by comparing them with the rise in the price of other consumer goods and services. As shown in Table 1.5, the value of the consumer price index for all items except medical care rose by an average annual rate of 5.9 percent between 1965 and 1985. During this same period, the medical

Table 1.5
Trends of Hospital Unit Costs and the Consumer Price Index, Selected Years, 1965–1985

	1965	1970	1975	1980	1985	Average Annual Percent Change
[a]Average cost per patient day ($)	45	81	151	281	551	12.7
[b]Average cost per admission	346	669	1167	2126	3901	12.2
[c]Consumer Price Index (all items, less medical care, 1967=100)	95	116	161	258	318	5.9
[d]Medical Care Price Index (1967=100)	90	121	169	276	403	7.4
[e]Semi-private Room Hospital Charges Index (1967=100)	76	145	236	450	711	11.2

Sources: [a-b]Hospital Statistics, 1986 edition, published by the American Hospital Association, copyright 1986.
[c-e]U.S. Department of Health and Human Services. 1986. Social Security Bulletin 49 (12):58,60.

services index rose annually by 7.4 percent and the hospital semiprivate room index increased by 11.2 percent. Thus, hospital charges increased relative to the price of nonmedical consumer goods and services as well as with respect to other components of medical care. Although hospital cost increases have exceeded the rate of inflation in the general economy, it is not valid to use these statistics to conclude that hospitals are grossly inefficient since the data are not adjusted adequately for product changes. Improvements in medical technology tend to increase costs, improve quality and induce consumers to pay more for hospital care. Hence, the observed increase in the cost of care might be attributable more to improvements in quality than inefficient operations, suggesting that an assessment of efficiency and a valid comparison of costs require more homogenous measures of output.

Martin Feldstein (1971) decomposed changes in per diem costs into four components: (1) more personnel per patient day, (2) higher wage rates, (3) increased use of nonlabor inputs per patient day, and (4) higher prices for nonlabor inputs. This disaggregation is a useful framework for illustrating how

Table 1.6
Components of Increases in Hospital Costs, Selected Years, 1965–1985

	1965	1970	1975	1980	1985	Average Annual Percent Change
[a] Average cost per patient day ($)	45	81	151	280	551	12.7
[b] Labor cost per patient day ($)	27	47	90	158	304	12.2
[c] Personnel per 100 census	246	265	300	335	386	2.2
[d] Average annual salary ($)	4072	5921	8649	13,010	20,140	7.9
[e] Nonlabor cost per patient day	17	34	62	123	247	13.6
[f] Nonlabor inputs per patient day, in 1967 dollars	18	31	35	46	80	7.4
[g] Producer Price Index (1967=100)	97	110	175	269	310	5.7
[h] Labor costs as percentage of total costs	62	58	59	56	55	-

Sources: [a-f, h] Hospital Statistics, 1986 edition, published by the American Hospital Association, copyright 1986.

[g] U.S. Bureau of the Census. 1986. Statistical Abstract of the United States: 1987 (107th edition). Washington, D.C..

hospital cost inflation occurred, but not why. The following discussion uses the approach developed by Feldstein and explores the factors that combined to increase the costs per day of care.

Table 1.6 presents data for selected years in the period from 1965 to 1985. During this period, per diem costs rose from $45 to $551 or about 12.7 percent per year. Labor costs per patient day increased at a slightly lower annual rate of 12.2 percent, or from $27 to $304. The increase in labor cost is attributed to higher wages and the use of more personnel. The average annual income of full-time equivalent employees increased from $4,072 to $20,140, an annual increase of 7.9 percent. The number of full-time equivalent personnel per 100 average daily census grew from 246 to 386, an annual increase of 2.2 percent.

Nonlabor costs per patient day increased from $17 to $247, or about 13.6 percent per year. Since no natural unit measures nonlabor inputs, it is difficult to allocate changes in spending on these factors of production between higher costs or increases in quantity. Feldstein (1971) suggests that the producer price index can be used as a deflator to hold prices constant. After this correction, the change in cost over time can be attributed to increased quantities of ''real'' nonlabor inputs. As shown in Table 1.6 (Line f), expenditures were adjusted by dividing the nominal value of nonlabor inputs per patient day by the value of the relevant year's producer price index. These data indicate that the use of real nonlabor inputs increased at an annual rate of 7.4 percent, an amount exceeding average annual increases in the producer price index, which rose by about 5.7 percent per year.

THEORIES OF HOSPITAL COST INFLATION

In the previous section, we saw how hospital costs increased over the last three decades. In this section, different theories that attempt to explain hospital cost inflation are presented. Rising costs have been attributed by economists to *demand-pull inflation*, as well as *cost-push inflation*. However, there is no consensus among economists about a unified theory of hospital inflation. Although it is likely that the rapid rise in hospital costs has been caused by both demand-side and supply-side factors, as well as interaction between the two, it is convenient to analyze the two types of theories separately.

Before turning to the theories of inflation, it is appropriate to mention that the development of a realistic hospital model is complicated by the multiproduct nature of this industry. As is well known, the standard economic analysis of equilibrium price and output determination examines the relationship between market supply and demand. As shown in Figure 1.1, normative theory predicts that equilibrium price and output will occur at point E, the intersection of the market supply and demand curves. Market forces will result in an equilibrium price and output of P_1 and Q_1 respectively. If price is greater than P_1, quantity supplied will exceed quantity demanded and a surplus will occur. Further, price will fall until equilibrium is restored at point E. Conversely, if price is less than P_1, a shortage will occur and consumers will bid prices up until P_1 is reached. It is important to note that the market supply curve is usually based on the assumption that the products or services it reflects are homogeneous; however, the homogeneity assumption is violated in the health care industry. For example, the federal prospective pricing mechanism assumes that the output of hospitals corresponds to 471 Diagnosis Related Groups (DRGs). Although we will discuss the incorporation of the multiproduct nature of the hospital in production function models (Chapter 7) and cost function models (Chapter 8) in subsequent chapters, a complex model is not appropriate for an introductory chapter. Thus in our

Figure 1.1
Market Equilibrium

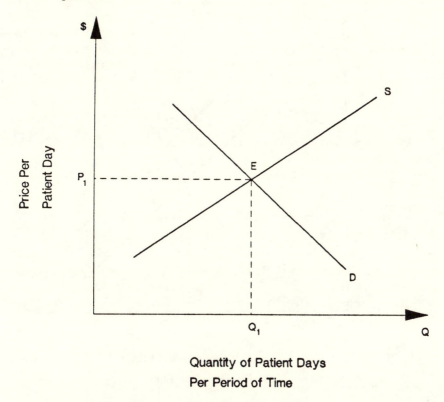

Quantity of Patient Days
Per Period of Time

analysis of hospital inflation, we assume that our simple expository model pertains to a broadly defined abstract product which we call hospital care. In this
model, we accommodate product variations that result in the use of more resources per unit or a more expensive input mix as an upward and left shift of
the supply curve. An example of this is the diffusion of equipment-embodied
medical technology, such as magnetic resonance equipment, which entails more
expensive equipment and requires more highly skilled personnel to operate it.

Demand-Pull Inflation

Executives of the American Hospital Association concluded "that the prices
of hospital services have traditionally been susceptible to *demand-pull inflation*,
that is, the demand for health care services grows more quickly than the industry's
ability to accumulate, without bidding up prices, the resources necessary to
produce the quantity and types of services demanded" (McMahon and Drake
1978).

Figure 1.2
A Demand-Pull Model of Hospital Cost Inflation

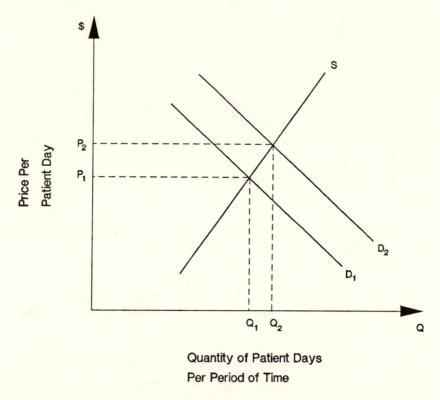

Quantity of Patient Days
Per Period of Time

What are the determinants of market demand for hospital care and how have they caused an increase in demand for hospital care over the last 20 years? In its broadest sense the quantity of hospital care demanded per unit of time is a function of the price of hospital care; the price of complements; the price and availability of substitutes; income; the number of consumers in the marketplace; and tastes and preferences. Figure 1.2 illustrates the effect of a change in demand on equilibrium price and output. With the exception of the price of hospital care, the price of complements or the availability of substitutes, an increase in any of the determinants of demand will shift the market demand curve upward from D_1 to D_2. This implies that, at the same price level, consumers are willing to purchase more hospital care. Furthermore, if the supply curve does not shift, normative economic theory predicts that an increase in demand will cause the equilibrium market price to increase from P_1 to P_2. This phenomenon is termed *demand-pull inflation*.

A brief examination of the determinants of market demand for hospital services offers several insights into the phenomenon of demand-pull inflation in this sector of the economy. As described in Chapter 3, economic theory suggests that the quantity demanded is inversely related to the price of the item. A number of studies that used either admissions or patient days as the measure of output have found hospital care to be a normal good and one whose demand is relatively insensitive to price. Thus, *ceteris paribus*, if the price of hospital care increased we would expect demand to decrease; however, during the period from 1965 to 1980, hospital costs and patient days both increased. What can explain this apparent contradiction in economic theory? The most obvious explanation is that the *ceteris paribus* assumption has been violated. That is, a shift in the demand curve from D_1 to D_2, due to changes in income, tastes and other demand determinants, has neutralized the impact that price alone might have exerted. However, and more fundamentally, we must ascertain whether the price of hospital care, faced by the consumer, really increased during this period.

Given the prevalence of insurance and other third-party payments, the best measure of price for hospital care may be out-of-pocket payments. As Table 1.7 shows, the percentage of hospital care expenditures paid by consumers decreased from 16.8 percent in 1965 to 7.8 percent in 1980. Thus, although the nominal cost per admission increased from $346 to $2,126 during this period (see Table 1.5), direct patient payments (expressed in 1967 constant dollars) rose by less than $3, or from $61.25 to $64.17. Given changes in other determinants of demand, it is not surprising that patient days per thousand population rose by about 14 percent during this period (see Table 1.4), resulting in an increase in expenditures for hospital services.

Increased expenditures for hospital care have caused hospital insurance premiums to rise. One might expect that an increase in premiums would result in less extensive (or less intensive) insurance coverage as price (premiums) rationed the quantity of insurance demanded. Using the direct patient payment data in Table 1.7 as a crude measure of the extent of insurance coverage, this did not occur until the 1980s. As discussed in Chapter 2, an increase in the price of hospital care may cause a substantial increase in the demand for health insurance. Feldstein (1971) argues that there is mutually reinforcing behavior between the purchase of insurance and the demand for hospital care. It is suggested that a growth in health insurance coverage reduces the effective price of care, an outcome that increases demand, the quantity of care supplied, and the costs of care. Further, higher costs are believed to stimulate additional demand for health insurance, which, in turn, results in a growth in demand for care and rising costs. Furthermore, consumers are insulated from increases in health insurance premiums. Most private health insurance coverage is obtained through employers, and, until recently, most employers' contributions to health benefit plans were excluded from employees' taxable income. Thus, a sizable tax subsidy encouraged the substitution of employer-paid health insurance for other forms of compensation, resulting in a greater demand for coverage.

The trend toward more extensive employer-sponsored insurance coverage was reversed during the 1980s as corporations responded to the rising costs of employee benefits and other threats to their profits by increasing cost-sharing pro-

visions in employee health insurance plans. Undoubtedly, employee concerns about job security during the "Reagan recession" reduced employee resistance to benefit "give-backs." Thus, changes in employer policies with respect to health insurance benefits were one reason why direct patient payments for hospital services increased from 7.8 percent in 1980, to 9.3 percent in 1985. Although other factors were at work (e.g., HMOs and utilization review), it is not coincidental that patient days per thousand population declined by almost 18 percent during a period in which the patient's responsibility for the payment of hospital costs increased.

The growth of HMO enrollment in the 1980s has reduced the out-of-pocket cost of ambulatory services, in some cases a substitute for inpatient care, to those who were previously insured under indemnity plans that traditionally offered more extensive inpatient benefits. Developments in medical technology and the expansion of the scope of insurance benefits to cover the more cost-effective ambulatory services also reduced the demand for hospital services. Ironically, although this downward shift in demand may have reduced pressures on demand-pull inflation, it resulted in increases in the traditional measures of hospital costs (i.e., cost per day, cost per case), as more of the less costly patients were treated outside of the inpatient setting, leaving a more severely ill patient population for the hospital.

In addition to the expansion of third party payments, changes in *tastes and preferences* have undoubtedly caused an increase in demand for hospital care during the last three decades. *Tastes and preferences* is a catchall term that reflects noneconomic factors affecting demand. Joseph (1971) identified health status, education level, family size, marital status, and standards of physician practice as factors that influence tastes for hospital care.

Perhaps the most important of these factors are health status and standards of physician practice. The former is determined by age, heredity, health habits, and environmental factors. The strains that an aging population have placed on the Medicare Program have caused many analysts to emphasize changes in population composition as an important cause of increased health expenditures in the United States. In 1960, 9.2 percent of the U.S. population was 65 years of age or over (U.S. Bureau of the Census 1986). By 1985, that age group represented 11.9 percent of the population, having an annual growth since 1960 of almost twice that of the general population, 2.1 percent compared with 1.1 percent. The differential growth rate for the population group 75 years and older was even more striking, averaging 2.8 percent per year during the period. Given the pronounced increase in the rate of hospital utilization that begins at about 60 years of age (Arnett et al. 1986), it is clear that changes in population composition have had a greater impact on the demand for hospital services than aggregate population growth. As Table 1.3 showed, however, the combined effects of these changes accounted for less than 8 percent of the increase in national health expenditures during the period from 1974 to 1984. Although not inconsequential, the graying of America has more severe implications for financing care from the limited resources of a population living on a fixed income or from the financially strapped Medicare Trust Fund than it does for the overall impact on demand-pull inflation.

Standards of physician practice, another taste factor, has affected the volume and mix of services demanded. Physician practice patterns have been influenced by: the level of medical science, economic factors, and legal considerations. The effect of advances in medical science is discussed in the cost-push section of this chapter. Regarding the economic factors, it is commonly thought (see Chapter 3) that physicians induce demand for their services in order to achieve a target income. Many analysts are concerned that the increases in the supply of physicians will rise faster than the population, resulting in more supplier-induced demand.

Finally, the malpractice crisis of the 1960s, which provoked the practice of defensive medicine, undoubtedly has caused physicians to add otherwise unnecessary diagnostic and treatment procedures and referrals to a patient's care. Although difficult to estimate, the practice of defensive medicine may have added as much as $40 billion to the annual national health expenditures (American Medical Association 1984). A 1983 survey of 1,240 physicians, randomly selected by the American Medical Association, provides more insight about physician responses to the epidemic of malpractice litigation (Zuckerman 1984). Physicians reported (with percentage of respondents in parenthesis) that they responded to increases in professional liability insurance premiums by: prescribing additional diagnostic tests (40.8) and providing additional treatment procedures (27.2). Both responses shift the demand curve outward and to the right. In addition to changes in prescribing patterns, increases in insurance premiums induced physicians to maintain more detailed patient records (56.7 percent), hire additional support staff (11.1 percent), and increase fees (31.4 percent), outcomes that affect costs and spending on health care.

A final noteworthy change related to tastes and preferences for hospital care is the emergence of hospital marketing during the 1980s. As part of their competitive strategies, hospitals have increased marketing activities in recent years in order to change the shape and location of their demand curves to more favorable positions. It is unclear, however, whether increased marketing efforts have given certain hospitals a larger slice of the same pie or have resulted in increasing industry demand, thereby creating a larger pie for all hospitals to share.

In summary, since 1965, increases in third-party payments and changes in population composition and standards of medical practice have had the most profound effects on the demand for health services. Among these, the growth of third-party payments has been cited by many as a leading cause of hospital cost inflation.

Joseph Califano (1977), Secretary of the U.S. Department of Health, Education, and Welfare (DHEW) stated:

This retrospective payment method has proven to be highly inflationary because reimbursement simply covers rising hospital costs, however unnecessary or wasteful those

Figure 1.3
A Cost-Push Model of Hospital Inflation

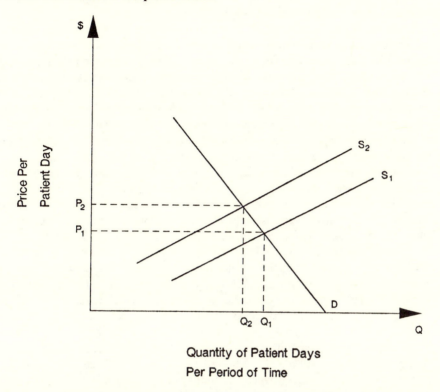

Quantity of Patient Days
Per Period of Time

costs may be. By reimbursing hospitals for most insured costs, this method provides virtually no incentives for efficiency . . . This method of reimbursement—which also applies in other health programs (besides Medicare and Medicaid)—has contributed to rampaging inflation in the hospital industry.

It is clear that the growth of private and public insurance in the United States has contributed to demand-pull inflation by inducing more consumer demand; and to cost-push inflation, now to be discussed, by reducing incentives for hospitals to perform efficiently.

Cost-Push Inflation

A simple model of cost-push inflation is shown in Figure 1.3. The upward sloping market supply curve, S_1, indicates that as market price increases, *ceteris paribus*, an increased quantity of services will be supplied. The supply curve implicitly holds factor input prices and technology (productivity) constant. If factor prices increase or inputs become less productive, the supply curve will shift up and to the left from S_1 to S_2. If demand remains constant, the shift in the supply curve will increase the equilibrium price from P_1 to P_2. This type of inflationary pressure is termed *cost-push*.

The *catching-up hypothesis* of hospital wage rates has been a very popular explanation for cost-push hospital inflation. Proponents of this theory state that hospital workers, relative to other occupations, have been underpaid for a long period of time. This perceived inequity motivated hospital workers to demand greater wage increases during the last 25 years. The growth in retrospective reimbursement during the 1960s allowed hospitals to generate more revenue which, in turn, allowed them to pay their workers more (Davis 1974).

Salkever (1979) developed a variant of this theory, which suggested that secular changes in the market for unskilled labor during the 1960s caused wages of all unskilled workers to increase relative to skilled workers. He argued that increases in welfare payments made leisure more attractive; and a reduction in racial discrimination diminished the *crowding* of nonwhites into the unskilled market. Thus, both of these secular changes probably reduced the supply of labor and, consequently, caused wages of unskilled labor to rise faster than those in other labor markets. Salkever's empirical analysis of hospitals in 20 large Standard Metropolitan Statistical Areas (SMSAs) suggests that unskilled hospital workers benefited from these secular changes; however, multicollinearity among the independent variables reduced the reliability of his estimates.

Martin Feldstein (1971) criticized the catching-up hypothesis on the grounds that, at some point, hospital wages would achieve parity with other industries, and a source of cost-push pressure would be eliminated. Indeed, he suggested that hospital wages had already achieved parity because, in certain situations, hospital wages now exceed wages in similar occupations. Feldstein presented evidence to support a variant of this theory in which he hypothesized that hospitals might have engaged in philanthropic behavior by paying employees more than would be necessary to attract the necessary labor force. Fuchs (1976) corroborated Feldstein's findings. Using a different data base, he concluded that the wages of health workers, starting at a relatively low level in 1954, had risen by 1969 almost to a point of parity with other industries.

Another cost-push theory cites lagging labor productivity as a cause of hospital cost increases (Klarman 1965). If labor productivity matched wage increases, *catching up* with other industries would not be inflationary. Payroll expenditures would remain constant as fewer, highly paid, but more productive workers would replace the lower paid, less productive workers. However, the hospital industry is very labor intensive and it has been difficult to increase labor productivity by substituting capital for labor. A report prepared by the Bureau of Industrial Economics (1983) suggests that, during the period from 1973 to 1981, the productivity of health care workers not only lagged behind their wage increases but also actually declined by an average of 0.6 percent per year. Given the absence of a commonly accepted measure of hospital output, however, it is as difficult to evaluate this theory as it is to assess changes in labor productivity.

Although our perceptions may be colored by the increased emphasis to operate hospitals as a "business," it is hard to accept Feldstein's contention that hospitals voluntarily compensated workers more than the going rate. Similarly, Klarman's view of lagging labor productivity is also tenuous if it does not consider outside pressures. A more plausible hypothesis is that hospitals increased wage rates in response to employee pressures, which may have been manifested in the form of union demands or the threat of employees to unionize. Indeed, as we shall discuss in Chapter 8, Adamache and Sloan (1982) estimate that union activity has increased hospital costs by at least 10 percent.

McMahon and Drake (1978) broadened the labor cost-push theory to include virtually all inputs. They contend that hospital inflation in the post-ESP (Economic Stabilization Program) (i.e., after 1974) environment has been of the cost-push variety; that is, the inflationary pressure stems from increases in the prices hospitals must pay for the resources needed to produce services. McMahon and Drake supported their argument by citing statistics from the American Hospital Association (AHA) Nonlabor Input Price Index which showed that the prices of products purchased by hospitals grew at a faster rate from 1967 to 1975 than did either the Consumer Price Index or the Wholesale Price Index. This pattern has persisted into the 1980s. From 1975 to 1983, the National Hospital Input Price Index, which reflects price level changes for inputs purchased by hospitals, increased annually by 9.6 percent. In contrast, during the same period, the implicit price deflator for GNP, a widely used indicator for the overall economy, increased by an average of 7.2 percent per year (Freeland and Schendler 1984).

It has been argued by many health economists that advances in medical technology have added fuel to the inflationary fires. Although some changes in technology can reduce costs (Romeo, Wagner, and Lee 1984) it is commonly agreed that the acquisition of expensive equipment in which new technology is embodied leads to higher costs. Unlike firms in other industries that can reduce costs by substituting capital for labor, the acquisition of new capital equipment by hospitals often requires that they employ more skilled personnel to operate the new devices. The net result is an increase not only in the average cost of capital equipment and labor but also in the number of full-time equivalent employees per patient day. Although patients have benefited from improvements in technology, newer and more sophisticated equipment is expensive. Indeed, many are concerned that the marginal costs of new technology exceeds its marginal benefits (Romeo, Wagner, and Lee 1984; Garrison and Wilensky 1986).

Recognizing the impact of changing technology on the mix of inputs employed by hospitals, we have included technological advances as a cost-push factor; however, the development of new technology also has induced a demand for new services. Several economists (Waldman 1972; Feldstein and Taylor 1977; Freeland and Schendler 1984) have used "intensity of care" (i.e., services per patient day or services per admission) to measure the effects of technologically induced demand on hospital expenditures.

The most recent analysis suggests that 33.4 percent of the growth in community hospital expenses during the period from 1974 to 1984 was attributed to growth in intensity of care per inpatient day (Arnett et al. 1986). Although the intensity of care approach is not entirely satisfactory because changes in intensity may be due to nontechnological factors (e.g., defensive medicine and third party coverage provisions), the intensity statistics suggest that technology has been an important, albeit not precisely measured, source of increased expenditures. In some cases, scientific advances simultaneously led to both cost-push inflation (e.g., more expensive inputs) and demand-pull inflation (e.g., new sources of demand). Renal dialysis machines provide a good example. These machines are expensive, but instead of providing a cure, they merely help the patient to stay alive. Thus, a new source of demand for medical services is created. Typical renal dialysis patients must return for treatment at least two times per week for the rest of their lives.

Similar to advances in technology, the malpractice crisis of the 1970s generated inflationary pressures on both the supply and demand sides. As mentioned earlier, physicians responded to the threat of litigation by ordering more services. However, regarding liability insurance as a factor input (i.e., an operational requirement), increases in malpractice premiums have shifted the hospital supply curve up and to the left.

Despite extensive attention by the media, the impact of malpractice on hospital input costs has been relatively small. According to the Task Force on Medical Liability and Malpractice (1987), hospitals spent an estimated $1.3 billion on self-insurance, premiums and uninsured losses in 1985, a 57 percent increase from 1983 when malpractice insurance and losses cost hospitals $849 million. Although large in aggregate terms, expenditures related to malpractice represented only 1.2 percent of total hospital costs in 1985.

SYNTHESIS OF DEMAND- AND SUPPLY-SIDE HOSPITAL INFLATION THEORIES

A number of theories of hospital cost inflation have been introduced. The major ones are: demand-pull, catching-up hypothesis, general cost-push, lagging productivity, and technological changes. None of these theories is accepted by a consensus of health economists. Berry (1976) has developed a simple conceptual model, illustrated in Figure 1.4, that integrates most of these theories. In this simplified model, Berry postulates that an increase in demand leads to increased prices, which, in turn, leads to an increased operating surplus. The increased operating surplus is used to hire more inputs per unit of output (or pay inputs more), which then raises costs. In other markets, we would expect an increase in price to reduce demand which would serve to reduce inflationary pressures; however, the widespread insurance coverage for hospital expenses and consumer insensitivity to price changes for many hospital services insulates demand responses from price changes. If anything, price increases can be expected to increase insurance coverage, which then removes utilization consid-

Figure 1.4
Berry's Model of Hospital Cost Inflation

Δ↑ Demand → Δ↑ Price → Δ↑ Surplus → Δ↑ Inputs/Output → Δ↑ Cost

Source: Berry, R. 1976. Prospective rate reimbursement and cost
containment: Formula reimbursement in New York. Inquiry
13 (Sept.): 291.

erations even further from price changes (Feldstein 1979). This model was developed for expositional purposes and not for prediction. Its premises do have a high level of face validity, and it suggests the need for a complex model that reflects in more detail the effects of supply-side, demand-side and reimbursement interactions.

Berry's model hinted at the linkage between increased demand for health services and increased expenditures for inputs used by producers of these services. A better understanding of this linkage is provided by an examination of the accounting identity, which equates total expenses for health services with incomes of inputs employed by health service producers. Total expenditures for medical care services can be expressed:

$$TE = \sum_{i=1}^{n} P_i Q_i \qquad (1.1)$$

where TE represents total expenditures; P_i represents the average price per unit of the ith type of health service; and Q_i represents the quantity of the ith type of health service supplied. However, applying the national income accounting approach, total expenditures also equal the total incomes of those supplying resources (i.e., capital, labor, raw materials, supplies, etc.) to be used in the production of health care.

Thus, equation 1.1 can be rewritten:

$$TE = \sum_{j=1}^{n} Y_j N_j \qquad (1.2)$$

where Y_j represents the average level of income earned by supplying the jth type of factor input; and N_j represents the quantity of input j supplied. Equation 1.3, which follows from equations 1.1 and 1.2, shows the identity between income and expenditures:

$$\sum_{i=1}^{n} P_i Q_i = \sum_{j=1}^{n} Y_j N_j \qquad (1.3)$$

The supply and demand interactions between factor and product markets were illustrated by Paul Feldstein (1979). Our adaptation of his model, shown in Figure 1.5, posits that demand for health care services is jointly determined by

Figure 1.5
An Overview of the Medical Care Sector

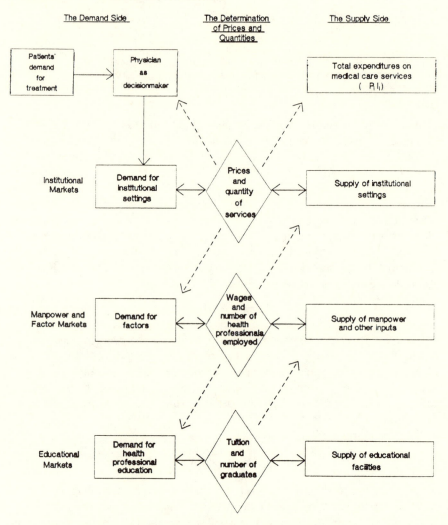

Source: Feldstein, P. 1979. Health Care Economics. New York, NY:
John Wiley & Sons, p. 35.

Reprinted by permission of John Wiley & Sons, Inc. Copyright © 1979 by
John Wiley & Sons, Inc.

the patient, who initiates a demand for treatment, and the physician who decides the course of treatment (if any) for the patient. Assuming an agency relationship between the doctor and patient, the physician's demand (on behalf of the patient) for health services in institutional product markets is influenced by supply-side factors such as relative costs and availability of services. Demand-side factors, such as the patient's willingness and ability to pay, also affect the physician's decisions. The literature on *moral hazard* suggests that insurance provisions affect the type of care ordered. For example, given that a health problem can be treated efficaciously on either an inpatient or an ambulatory basis, it is often argued that physicians will tend to hospitalize the patient if insurance will not cover outpatient services.

Proceeding down the left-hand side of the model, we see that demand for factor inputs is derived from the demand in the product markets. An increase in hospital insurance, *ceteris paribus*, will induce greater demand for hospital services. In turn, hospitals will exert a greater demand for factor inputs. For example, if the labor complement is working at full capacity, the hospital is forced to hire more factor inputs to satisfy the increased demand for services; however, the demand for factors of production will be influenced by the relative productivity and costs of acquiring resources. An increase in the demand for hospital personnel may cause wages to rise. The magnitude of the wage increase will be influenced by supply-side factors, such as the extent of unemployment in the labor market.

Finally, if the compensation of health care personnel should increase relative to other occupations, the demand for education in the health professions should increase as more people are attracted by the more lucrative opportunities in these occupations. The demand for education, however, also is influenced by tuition levels, which are determined in part by the interaction between the demand and supply for education.

Moving up the supply-side of Feldstein's model, we see that the number of graduates, along with the existing stock constitute the supply of health personnel. The supply of personnel in each category interacts with the demand for personnel in each category to determine income as well as the participation rate. This, in turn, affects the supply and costs of services in the product markets. For simplicity, assuming that all providers are nonprofit with a break-even goal, prices will be adjusted to cover the costs of operation.

The price and availability of services will interact with the demand for services to determine the price and utilization of health care services, the two components of health care expenditures. Thus, this model demonstrates that in order to explain (or forecast) total health expenditures, we must be able to understand the supply and demand interactions among product markets, factor markets, and education markets.

Predictions and policy recommendations might be derived from an application of a model depicting market interactions to the emerging shortage of registered nurses. In the mid–1960s the American Nurses Association made a decision that

RNs should receive baccalaureate training. Subsequently, the locus of nursing education has moved away from hospital diploma schools. This shift has caused the cost of nursing education to increase, depressing the demand for nursing education and eventually the supply of RNs. Moving up Figure 1.5, we see that a reduction in the supply of RNs may eventually cause their wages to increase. This will cause the costs of hospital care to increase, which, in turn, may deter access of low-income individuals who do not have hospital insurance and who are not eligible for public assistance. Further, anecdotal evidence also indicates that the shortage of RNs has caused some hospitals to close down units. Those who are concerned about increases in hospital costs or barriers to access might recommend public actions, such as tuition subsidies or changing the locus of nursing education, to address these problems.

SUMMARY

In the first part of this chapter we examined five factors—general inflation, changes in the size and composition of the population, intensity of care, utilization, and medical care price increases in excess of general price inflation—which accounted for the growth in national health expenditures. Next, our focus turned from how expenditures increased to why these changes occurred as we examined theories of hospital inflation. We emphasized the hospital sector because it is the largest part of the health care industry. Further, although there are important differences in both degree and kind, most of the factors affecting increases in hospital expenditures also affect the other parts of the industry. Consequently, a sector-by-sector analysis would tend to be redundant.

In our analysis of increased hospital costs, we examined the major theories of inflation using an arbitrary distinction between demand-side and supply-side factors. However, in order to depict the causes of rising health expenditures more realistically, we presented a model that illustrated the interactions between supply, demand, product markets, and factor markets.

In the remainder of this book, we will examine in more detail the causes and potential solutions to the problem of rising health care expenditures. These influences and the chapters in which they are discussed are summarized in Table 1.8. In brief, the book is organized as follows. Following our conceptual distinction of the causes of rising costs, we provide a demand-side analysis in Part II, where we examine various theories of demand, and pay particular attention to the influence of health care insurance on utilization. In Part III, we perform supply-side analysis, focusing on defining and measuring the output of hospitals and other health care organizations, examining models of the behavior of health care organizations, and examining production and cost functions of health care organizations and physician supply issues. In Part IV, we examine the dominant cost containment strategies: regulation and the cultivation of market-like incentives.

Table 1.8
A Summary of Demand-Side and Supply-Side Influences on National Health Expenditures

Demand-Side Influences	(Chapters in which topic is discussed)	Supply-Side Influences	(Chapters in which topic is discussed)
Insurance	(1,2,3)	Unions	(1,4,8,12)
Population increase	(1)	Productivity	(1,5,7,8,11,12)
Composition of population	(1,3)	Input prices	(1,4,12)
Defensive medicine	(1)	Cost-based retrospective reimbursement	(1,12)
Supplier-induced demand	(1,2,3,4,9)	General inflation	(1)
Availability of new services	(1)	New technology	(1,12)
Physician practice style	(1,3,11)	Teaching	(5,7,8,9,12)
Consumer income	(1,3)	Organization and delivery systems	(4,7,11)

REFERENCES

Adamache, K. W., and F. A. Sloan. 1982. Unions and hospitals: Some unresolved issues. *Journal of Health Economics* 1(1):81–108.

American Hospital Association. 1987. *Hospital Statistics, 1987 edition*. Chicago, IL: AHA.

American Medical Association. 1984. *Professional Liability in the 80's, Report 1*. Chicago, IL: AMA.

Arnett, R. H., D. R. McKusick, S. T. Sonnefeld et al. 1986. Projections of health care spending to 1990. *Health Care Financing Review* 7(3):1–36.

Arnett, R. H., M. Freeland, D. McKusick, and D. Waldo. 1987. National health expenditures, 1986–2000. *Health Care Financing Review* 8(4):1–36.

Berry, R. 1976. Prospective rate reimbursement and cost containment: Formula reimbursement in New York. *Inquiry* 13 (3):288–301.

Bureau of Industrial Economics. 1983. *1983 U.S. Industrial Outlook for 250 Industries with Projections for 1987*. Washington, DC: U.S. Department of Commerce, January.

Califano, J. A. 1977. Department of Health, Education, and Welfare, statement before the Subcommittee on Health of the Senate Subcommittee on Finance, June 7, 1977. Quote in Abt Associates, *Evaluation of Nine Prospective Rate Setting Programs, Vol. I: Technical Proposal*, Cambridge, MA: Abt Associates, 1978, 1–8.

Davis, K. 1974. The role of technology, demand and labor markets in the determination of hospital costs. In M. Perlman, ed., *The Economics of Health and Medical Care*, New York, Halsted Press, 283.–301.

Feldstein, M. S. 1971. *The Rising Cost of Hospital Care*. Washington, DC: Information Resource Press, pp. 16–20.

Feldstein, M. S., and A. Taylor. 1977. *The Rapid Rise of Hospital Costs*. GPO stock No. 052–003–003.03.1. Washington, DC: U.S. Government Printing Office, January.

Feldstein, P. 1979. *Health Care Economics*. New York: John Wiley & Sons, 107–16.

Freeland, M. A., and C. E. Schendler. 1984. Health spending in the 1980's: Integration of clinical practice patterns with management. *Health Care Financing Review* 5(3):1–68.

Fuchs, V. 1976. The earnings of allied health personnel—Are health workers underpaid? *Explorations in Economic Research* 3:408–31.

Garrison, L. P., and G. R. Wilensky. 1986. Cost containment and technology. *Health Affairs* 5(2):46–58.

Joseph, H. 1971. Empirical research on the demand for health care. *Inquiry* 8(1):61–71.

Klarman, H. 1965. *The Economics of Health*. New York: Columbia University Press.

McMahon, J., and D. Drake. 1978. The American Hospital Association perspective. In M. Zubkoff, I. Raskin, and R. Hanft, eds., *Hospital Cost Containment: Selected Notes for Future Policy*. New York: Prodist, 78.

Romeo, A., J. Wagner, and H. Lee. 1984. Prospective reimbursement and the diffusion of new technologies in hospitals. *Journal of Health Economics* 3(1):1–28.

Salkever, D. 1979. *Hospital Sector Inflation*. Lexington, MA: D. C. Heath and Company.

Task Force on Medical Liability and Malpractice. 1987. *Report of the Task Force on Medical Liability and Malpractice*. Washington, DC: Department of Health and Human Services, August.

U.S. Bureau of the Census. 1986. *Statistical Abstract of the United States: 1987*. 107th edition. Washington, DC.

Waldman, S. 1972. The effect of changing technology on hospital costs. *Research and Statistics Note*. U.S. Department of Health, Education, and Welfare, Publication No. (OS) 76–502. Washington, DC:DHEW, February 28.

Waldo, D., K. Levit, and H. Lazenby. 1986. National health expenditures, 1985. *Health Care Financing Review* 8(1):13.

Zuckerman, S. 1984. The costs of medical malpractice. *Health Affairs* 3(3):128–34.

Part II

Demand-Side Analysis

2

THE DEMAND FOR HEALTH INSURANCE

Recently, public policy has focused on increased competition as a mechanism for controlling the rising costs of health care. Many analysts contend that health insurance coverage represents an economic buffer between consumers and providers, which reduces market pressures that induce consumers to select less expensive care and motivate providers to engage in price competition, improve efficiency, or control costs. Accordingly, it is possible that decisions in the health industry have focused more on the premiums and attributes of health insurance than on the prices, mix, and costs of health services.

It is possible to argue that the favorable tax treatment of insurance coverage sponsored by employers has contributed to the proliferation of policies characterized not only by relatively low coinsurance rates and deductibles but also by generous benefit provisions. That increases in the breadth and depth of insurance coverage reduce the user's price or out-of-pocket expenditures is well recognized. Consistent with traditional economic theory, a reduction in the effective price of care is expected to increase consumer demand, resulting in greater consumption and, other things remaining constant, higher costs. Further, since insurance is intended to protect the individual from unpredictable fiscal risks, it is possible that an increase in cost generates demand for additional insurance coverage, an outcome that fuels inflationary pressures in the health industry.

It is common to argue that the exclusion of the employer's contribution to the payment of premiums from the employee's taxable income leads to excessive insurance coverage. Recently, Chernick, Holmer, and Weinberg (1987) examined the linkage between overinsurance, the demand for medical care, and expenditures on health services. Employing midrange estimates of the elasticities of demand for health insurance and medical care, the study suggested that an elimination of the tax subsidy would reduce the demand for health insurance by 16 to 27 percent and the demand for medical care by 4 to

6 percent. These results are consistent with conventional expectations but fail to support the conclusion that the linkage between overinsurance and the demand for medical care is an adequate explanation of the rapid increases in expenditures on health care.

Even though it is unlikely that the linkage assessed by Chernick et al. constitutes a complete explanation of the rising cost of medical care, many analysts contend that the reliance on the insurance mechanism to finance the use of service has contributed to the inflationary pressures in the health industry. For example, recent estimates suggest that approximately 50 percent of the expenditures on physician services and 80 percent of the costs of hospital care are financed through the insurance mechanism (Pauly 1980; Gibson and Waldo 1982; Wilensky, Farley, and Taylor 1984).

Perhaps the most important aspect of the private insurance market is the dependence of coverage on employment status. Among the nonelderly, most private insurance coverage is provided through employment-related group policies. In 1980, premiums on individual or nongroup policies represented approximately 10 percent of the total payments to Blue Cross and commercial insurers. The balance was comprised of premium payments on group insurance offered at the workplace (Blue Cross and Blue Shield Association 1981; Arnett and Trapnell 1984).

Further, the employer rather than the insured employee financed most of the premium payments on group insurance. For example, Chollet (1984) indicates that 97 percent of employees enrolled in a group plan benefited from employer contributions, which represented more than 50 percent of the policy costs. Employers also contributed an amount equal to the full cost of coverage extended to not only 84 percent of their employees but also the dependents of 60 percent of the participants. Accordingly, the dependence of coverage on employment status suggests that the demand for health insurance involves the employer, the employee, and suppliers of insurance.

Appearing in Figure 2.1 is a schematic representation of the interrelation among insurers, employers, and employees. In this figure, it is assumed that suppliers of insurance (i.e., commercial insurance firms, Blue Cross/Blue Shield, Health Maintenance Organizations, and other independent plans) offer a mix of policies the employer might adopt and include as an option(s) in the employee benefit package. After evaluating the full set of options and eliminating a portion of these from potential inclusion in the benefit package, it is assumed that the employer offers one or more of the plans to employees. Thus, when examining the demand for group insurance, it is useful first to assess the factors that influence the choices implemented by employers, a topic considered in the first section of this chapter. Following this discussion is an examination of the traditional theory of demand for health insurance and the influence exerted by the effective price of coverage on the individual choices of those who are offered multiple plans for selection. In addition, this section also focuses on the demand for coverage that protects the elderly

Figure 2.1
Overview of the Relation Among Suppliers of Insurance, the Employer, and Employee

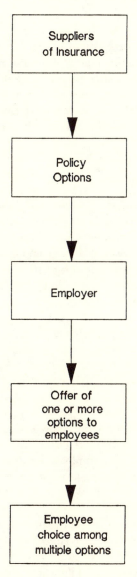

from the fiscal risks that are attributable to the exclusion of various components of care and the cost sharing arrangements that characterize the Medicare program. The final section addresses the problem of uncompensated care, to include not only the costs of treating high risk and uninsurable groups, but also the mechanisms that might be adopted to finance these expenses.

EMPLOYER CHOICE

When viewed from the perspective of the employer, contributions to the payment of insurance premiums represent a labor-related expense. To explore the choices implemented by the employer, consider a profit maximizing firm that secures the services of labor in a competitive market. In such an environment, the employer equates the value of labor's marginal product with average compensation to include fringe benefits. Hence, in equilibrium, economic theory suggests:

$$VMP = W + P \tag{2.1}$$

where VMP represents the value of employees' marginal product; W represents the wage or market rate of compensation; and P corresponds to the employer's contribution to the worker's health insurance premium. The contribution of the employer, P, is usually expressed as a fixed amount or a percentage of the health insurance premium. Consistent with normative theory, an increase in P is expected to lower W and/or employment. Similarly, in order to maximize profits, it is expected that an employer will respond to excessive values of P, which may result from high premiums relative to a given set of characteristics, by lowering rates of compensation and/or the level of employment.

It is possible to argue that the insurance package offered to employees influences productivity in several ways. First, marginal productivity is probably influenced by the health status of employees. Hence, to the extent that the benefit structure induces utilization behavior that contributes to the maintenance of a healthy work force, the selection of the plan or plans offered to employees may contribute to: (1) an improvement in labor productivity; (2) the avoidance of disruptions in the production process due to preventable illnesses; and (3) a reduction in the costs of replacing employees who are absent from the workplace due to illness. These observations suggest that the selection of the benefit package may influence the health status of the work force and thereby contribute indirectly to the profitability of the firm.

Second, in addition to the objectives of maintaining a healthy work force, limiting the turnover rate and minimizing the costs of replacing absent employees, it is reasonable to expect a profit maximizing firm to select plans that control the use of health services, costs, premiums and, hence, the total wage bill. For example, as suggested by the Trident Industrial Health Coalition (Palmetto-Lowcountry Health Systems Agency, Inc. 1984), the benefit package offered to employees might be designed to control or reduce the level of health benefits financed by the employer. The use and costs of hospital care might be controlled by provisions that require employees to secure a second opinion prior to surgery.

Further, the inclusion of ambulatory surgery or home health care as an insured benefit and of provisions that require preadmission testing and the concurrent review of the employee's need to remain hospitalized are designed not only to reduce use, costs, and premiums but also the time employees commit to the use of health services rather than market activity. Also consistent with the goal of maintaining the health status of the work force, maximizing productivity, and increasing the hours employees are available for work-related activities are policies that include stay-well programs, alcoholism treatment, and drug rehabilitation as insured benefits.

In addition to the potential effects of altering the benefit structure, employers might control or reduce the cost of labor by increasing the employee's responsibility for financing health insurance premiums. In particular, employers contribute approximately 67 percent of premium payments, a practice that reduces the employee's incentive to select a more cost effective plan if it were offered. However, as suggested by Pauly (1986), many employers not only offer a single plan to their employees but also finance 100 percent of the premium payments for approximately 50 percent of the work force. For others, the arrangements by which premiums are financed differ. Among firms who finance less than 100 percent of the premiums, most employers pay a specific fraction of the insurance cost rather than requiring the employee to finance an increasing portion as the premium rises (Wilensky, Farley, and Taylor 1984). When combined with a favorable tax treatment, which is described later, these attributes induce employees to select plans offering extensive coverage that reduces the cost consciousness of the health consumer, stimulates use, and increases expenses, outcomes that also result in higher premiums.

A closely related issue involves the influence of unionization on (1) the decision to offer employment-related insurance; (2) the extent of coverage offered by the firm; and (3) the amount or percent of the premium financed by the employer. Results reported by Rice (1966) indicate that union activity failed to increase the level of fringe benefits or improve the insurance coverage of their members. Freeman (1981) and Woodbury (1980) report findings that are consistent with the conclusion that unions not only exerted a significant and positive influence on fringe benefits but also increased the proportion of total compensation committed to life, accident and health insurance, pensions, holiday pay and vacations. After controlling for region, industry, size, and characteristics of the work force, results reported by Rossiter and Taylor (1982) suggest that unions failed to increase the likelihood that coverage is offered by the employer; however, this study revealed that the amount and the percentage of premium payments financed by the employer and premium benefits were higher among union than nonunion firms.

Recognizing that health insurance coverage influences utilization behavior, recent policy deliberations have focused on proposals that increase competition among providers and insurers, enhance the cost consciousness of consumers, and, in general, magnify the effects of market forces as interrelated devices that might control costs. Perhaps the most widely discussed proposal is the Consumer Choice Plan advanced by Enthoven (1978). The primary focus of the approach is on the health insurance coverage of those who participate in the labor force and their dependents. Given the importance of employment status as a factor that influences the insurance coverage of the nonelderly, the proposal requires the employer to abandon the traditional practice of including a single policy in the benefit package and to offer each employee an opportunity to select coverage from mul'iple policies in which premiums, benefit provisions and cost sharing arrangements (e.g., deductibles, coinsurance rates, and maximum liability) differ. Depending on the proportion or amount of the premium financed by the employer, such an approach might induce the employee to select a policy characterized by lower premiums and higher deductibles or coinsurance rates, outcomes that are expected to increase the cost consciousness of the consumer of health services and reduce not only the quantity of care demanded but also expenditures on medical care.

A potentially undesirable outcome of increased competition involves the potential for instability in the insurance market place. As suggested by Rothschild and Stiglitz (1976), the adoption of a strategy in which employees are offered multiple choices may result in a biased selection. It is reasonable to expect employees to select the plan with the highest value, resulting in the enrollment of groups with disparate risks in different plans. In such a situation, biased selection may result in an increase in the premiums of high-option alternatives and thereby threaten the solvency of some plans (Buchanan and Cretin 1986; Wilensky and Rossiter 1986).

Perhaps the most obvious example of the competitive approach is the Federal Employees Health Benefits Program (FEHBP) which offers in excess of 120 different plans and allows employees to change their coverage each year. The options provide comprehensive benefits and differ in terms of cost-sharing provisions. In addition, the responsibility for the cost of each plan is shared by the enrollee and the federal government. The government's share is 75 percent of the premium, subject to a relatively low maximum. As a result, the government contributes a fixed amount for most plans.

Price and Mays (1985) examined the extent of biased selection in the FEHBP. After adjusting for the influence of moral hazard, the study indicated that, relative to the premiums that would be charged in the absence of adverse selection, biased decisions increased the premium of the high option offered by Blue Cross by 21 percent and favorable selection reduced the premium of the low option by 29 percent. The analysis also suggested that selection effects are not transient. Rather, the high-option coverage consistently attracted high-risk enrollees and lost healthier members to other less comprehensive plans.

Price, Mays, and Trapnell (1983) examined the responses of employees to rapid increases in their premium contributions during 1982 and 1983. In addition, the Office of Personnel Management ordered a reduction in benefits that, when combined with the rise in premiums, motivated one-third of all subscribers to change plans. Price et al. suggested that employees altered their coverage so as to maximize the effective employer contribution, which was defined:

$$ECON_x = [(1 - c_x) \, e \, (cost_i)] - ESP_x \qquad\qquad (2.2)$$

where, c_x is the average coinsurance rate of plan x; e (cost$_i$) represents the expected cost of medical care consumed by individual i, and ESP_x corresponds to the employees' share of the premium for policy x. The results indicated that, in general, plans characterized by a high $ECON_x$ attracted new subscribers and that those with a low $ECON_x$ experienced a decline in enrollment. Hence, these results indicate that instability in the FEHBP resulted from differences in the effective employer contributions and that "similar problems should be expected with any procompetition proposal which includes a multiple-insurer requirement" (Price et al. 1983, p. 213).

On the other hand, conflicting evidence has been reported by Neipp and Zeckhauser (1985), who surveyed two employers in Boston that offered employees multiple options in 1985. The results of the study indicated that 97 percent of these employees ($n = 19,757$) retained the coverage of the previous year. The reluctance of employees to alter coverage was attributed to the high transition costs of changing plans.

In addition to offering employees multiple choices, proponents of the competitive solution also contend that the contribution of employers to premium payments should be limited to a fixed amount, thus forcing those who select more expensive plans to assume responsibility for the additional cost. The transfer of the additional costs of more expensive plans to workers may force employees to increase the importance assigned to the premium and other attributes of each policy offered by the employer.

Suppose the employer adopts a policy in which the contribution of employees is positively related to the gross premium of the plan. Under a partial contribution scheme in which the employer pays either a fixed amount or a percentage of the premium, workers are motivated to select cost-effective plans, since, other things being constant, these policies require lower out-of-pocket expenditures.

Further, insurers who offer inefficient or less cost-effective plans are expected to lose their market shares in firms that offer their employees multiple choices. The decline in the market share motivates the insurer to offer more efficient policies or to withdraw from the market. Relative to employers who offer multiple choices and pay the full premium, proposals to increase competition in the insurance market should result in lower premiums for firms offering multiple choices and adopting a partial contribution policy.

Similarly, firms that offer multiple choices and adopt a partial contribution policy are expected to encounter lower premiums than employers who offer a single policy to their employees. Among firms that adopt a policy of offering a single policy, the insurer is guaranteed a 100 percent market share. In such an environment, there is no incentive for the insurer to become more efficient to lower premiums. It is also expected that employers who offer multiple choices and adopt a partial contribution policy will experience lower gross premiums than their counterparts who either offer a single policy or offer employees multiple options and pay the full premium.

Focusing on firms located in the Minneapolis–St. Paul area, Jensen, Feldman, and Dowd (1984) evaluated the effects of competition on the monthly premiums for single and family coverage provided to employees during 1981 and 1982. The effects of alternate policies related to insurance benefits were measured by four dummy variables. The reference category consisted of employee groups to which multiple plans were offered and employers contributed a fixed amount to the payment of the monthly premium. The dummy variables represented alternate strategies of (1) offering multiple choices and paying a fixed percentage of the premium, (2) offering multiple choices and paying the full premium, (3) offering multiple policies and using alternate methods to finance premiums, and (4) offering employees a single plan. In addition, the specification included variables depicting the demographic characteristics of the employee group, benefit provisions of the policy such as the coinsurance rate, deductible provisions, the generosity of coverage, and loading factors, which represented differences in expenses that are related to the size of the plan's enrollment.

Focusing on the premium rates for individual and family coverage as dependent variables, regression analysis was performed on the set of pooled data and separately on information assembled in 1981 and 1982. Relative to the reference category (i.e., employee groups offered multiple choices and the employer's contribution as a fixed amount), premium rates for individual coverage were higher among the multiplan groups for which the employers paid the full premium or adopted a policy of contributing a fixed percentage less than 100 percent to the premium payment. Coefficients depicting the effects of offering multiple plans and paying the full premium were significant in all specifications, while those relating premium rates to the practice of offering multiple choices and paying a fixed percentage were significant when the analysis was based on the 1981 data and the pooled set. Also supporting expectations were findings that indicated that, relative to the reference group, premium rates for family coverage were higher among employees who were offered multiple choices and for whom the employer paid the full premium or contributed a percentage of the premium to the cost of insurance. Similar to the results pertaining to individual coverage, these coefficients were significant in equations based on the 1981 data and the set of pooled data.

On the other hand, contradictory evidence was also reported in the study. In particular, the premium rates for both individual and family coverage were lower among employees who were offered a single plan, a finding that is not consistent with the competitive hypothesis. Hence, results reported by Jensen et al. (1984) indicate that the amount or percentage of the insurance cost paid by the employer clearly influences premium payments, but the expectations regarding the desirability of offering employees multiple choices were not confirmed by the study.

Findings that were inconsistent with expectations may be attributable to self-selection among employees who were offered an HMO option. If those who expected to use medical care extensively selected an indemnity plan rather than the HMO alternative, the issue of self-selection may explain the unexpected differences between the premium rates of single and multiple plan groups. In the sample examined by Jensen et al. (1984), indemnity coverage was provided to single plan groups, while an HMO alternative was available to those offered multiple choices. In such an environment, the premium rates of single plan groups would exceed the premiums of multiplan groups if healthier employees selected the HMO option. In addition, as the market share of the HMO increases, the proportion of high-risk enrollees in the indemnity plan also rises, an outcome that increases the premiums of indemnity coverage and the costs of offering a single plan.

Similarly, biased-selection might have contributed to findings that support the competitive hypothesis. Feldman and Dowd (1982) suggest that favorable selection enables an HMO to maximize profits at less than a 100 percent share of the market. The analysis also indicated that the premiums charged by the HMO were greater than an experience-rated premium that is based on fair actuarial costs; hence, given a favorable employee selection, the premium per employee is expected to be greater in firms offering an HMO option and an indemnity, fee-for-service plan than in firms offering a single experience-rated plan. In a comparison of alternate methods of determining the employer's contribution, Feldman and Dowd also concluded that, among those who offer indemnity and HMO coverage, employers who financed the full premium of the lowest cost plan (i.e., a fixed amount equal to the lowest premium) experienced lower average premiums than those who contributed a percentage of the premium cost of each plan. These factors may have contributed to findings reported by Jensen et al. (1984) and supported the expectation that adopting a strategy of offering multiple choices and paying a fixed amount lowers the premium rate relative to a situation in which employees are offered several options and the employer contributes a partial percentage to the payment of premium costs.

Given the paucity of empirical evidence that demonstrates a causal relation between increased competition in the insurance market and lower premium rates, additional research is clearly required prior to an endorsement of the competitive proposal. Future studies might attempt to disentangle the effects exerted on premium rates by increased competition in the insurance market, differences in the method of determining the employer's contribution to the payment of premiums, self-selection among employees, and the asymmetric knowledge of the insurer, the insured, and the employer. Further, the set of factors that influences the employer's selection of policies and the mix of benefits that are offered to workers might be productively investigated. For example, our understanding of employer behavior might be improved by an examination of differences in the mix of policies and benefit provisions that are attributable to labor market conditions, to include such factors as the de-

Figure 2.2
The Demand for Health Insurance: The Magnitude of Loss

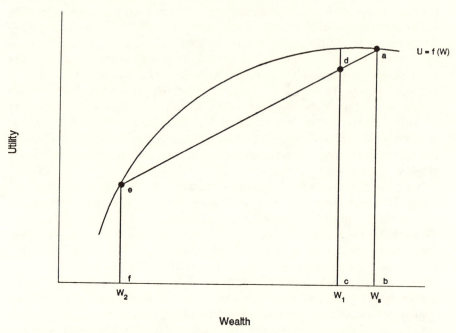

gree of unionization, the mix of employees, the costs of recruitment, and the product market.

THE INDIVIDUAL'S DEMAND FOR HEALTH INSURANCE

The traditional model of the demand for health insurance postulates that the risk-averse individual seeks to maximize expected utility. Ignoring employment-related coverage, the individual might adopt one of essentially two alternatives when faced with the uncertainty of illness and the resulting loss. The first option is to purchase insurance and accept a small but known expense amounting to the insurance premium. Alternatively, the individual might self-insure, a decision that requires an assessment of the probability that illness will occur and the magnitude of the resulting financial loss.

A Theoretical Framework

The traditional theory of demand for health insurance focuses on an individual and assumes that the probability of illness is low and that, if illness occurs, the magnitude of the resulting loss is large. Also, as shown in Figure 2.2, suppose that the marginal utility of wealth declines. If the premium is determined by the actuarial value of the expected loss, the purchase of insurance coverage results in a reduction in the wealth of the individual from W_s to, W_1 and a decline in utility represented by *ab-cd*. Conversely, assume the individual decides to self-insure and that, if illness occurs, the resulting financial loss reduces wealth from W_s to W_2 and utility from *ab* to *ef*. Letting $P(I_1)$ represent the probability that illness will occur, the expected utility resulting from the decision to self-insure might be expressed in the form:

$$P(I_1) \ (fe) + [1 - P \ (I_1)] \ [ab] \ = \ m \qquad\qquad (2.3)$$

where the magnitudes of *fe* and *ab* are defined by the heights of the corresponding line segments in Figure 2.2. If *m* exceeds the height of line segment *cd*, the individual is expected to purchase insurance coverage. Also note that a reduction (increase) in $P(I)$ increases (reduces) the complement, $1 - P(I)$; hence, holding the loss in wealth resulting from illness constant, the expected utility function is linear, connecting points *a* and *e* appearing on the actual utility function. If $P(I)$ is zero, actual and expected utility are represented by the height of line segment *ab*. As $P(I)$ increases and approaches one, expected utility declines along the linear function and approaches the height of line segment *ef*.

As just described, the function $U = f(W)$ is based on the assumption that actual marginal utility declines with rising wealth and lies above the linear function, which relates expected utility to wealth. Hence, if premiums are determined by the actuarial value of the anticipated loss, the individual is expected to purchase insurance coverage. Insurance premiums, however, consist of actuarial estimates of probable losses, which represent the pure premium, and a set of additional costs that are related to the performance of administrative functions, processing claims, marketing, and, for some insurers, a profit margin. As indicated below, excessive loading, represented by the portion of the premium in excess of the actuarial value of probable loss, may induce the individual to self-insure.

The amount in excess of the pure premium that the individual is willing to pay might be investigated by referring to Figure 2.3. As before, line segment $W_s - W_1$ represents the actuarial value of the probable loss resulting from the onset of illness. Also observe that the height of line segment *cg* represents the expected utility without insurance. Since line segment *gh* is parallel to the horizontal axis, the heights of line segments *cg* and *hi* are identical, indicating that actual utility is equal to expected utility. Accordingly, the maximum loading the individual is willing to pay for insurance is represented by $W_1 - W_3$, given $P(I_1)$ and loss $W_s - W_2$.

Consider next the effects on the decision to purchase health insurance that result from a change in the likelihood that illness will occur. Holding the cost of medical care constant and equal to $W_s - W_2$, suppose that $P(I_2) > P(I_1)$ and recall that each point on the expected utility function represents a different probability that illness will occur. As indicated previously, an increase in the probability that illness will occur is represented graphically by a movement down

Figure 2.3
The Demand for Health Insurance: The Influence of Likelihood

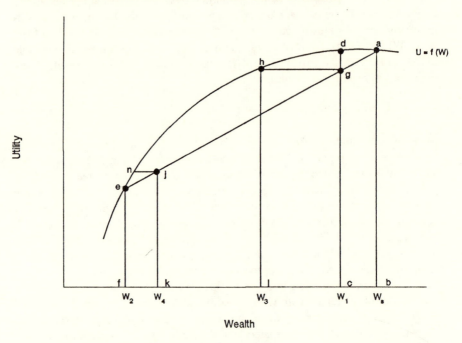

Wealth

the expected utility line. Referring to Figure 2.3, suppose that the higher probability $P(I_2)$ results in an expected utility represented by the height of jk. In this
case, the pure premium is defined by line segment $W_s - W_4$, and the maximum
loading the individual is willing to pay is defined by the length of nj. Hence,
as the event precipitating the loss becomes more probable, the individual is likely
to finance only a smaller additional amount and more willing to self-insure.
These observations indicate that, as $P(I)$ approaches zero or one, the individual
is willing to pay a smaller loading fee than all intermediate levels of likelihood.
For example, as the occurrence of the event becomes more certain, the individual
might avoid the portion of the premium that exceeds potential losses by deciding
to self-insure and accumulate savings required to finance the costs of care.

Another factor that influences the decision to purchase insurance results from
differences in the losses that are precipitated by the onset of illness. Previously,
we assumed that the potential loss was relatively large, as represented by the
length of line $W_s - W_2$. Suppose next, that the onset of illness precipitates a
smaller potential loss, as represented by $W_s - W_3$ in Figure 2.4. An inspection
of the figure reveals that the area between the actual utility function and the
expected utility line ac is greater than the area between the actual utility function
and expected utility line ab. As a consequence, holding the probability of the

Figure 2.4
The Demand for Health Insurance: The Effects of Loss and Likelihood

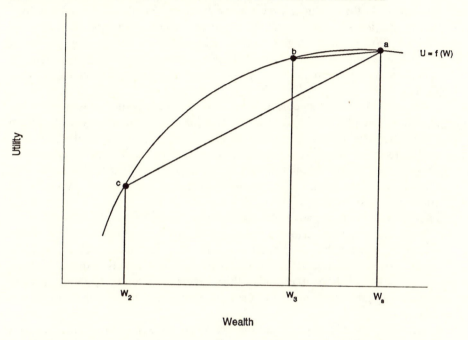

event occurring constant and equal, these observations suggest that the individual
is willing to pay a higher pure price for a larger than a smaller loss.

At this point, it is possible to combine the loading fee, the probability that
illness will occur and the magnitude of the potential loss to examine the demand
for insurance. As the probability of illness occurring increases, it is reasonable
to expect administrative costs to rise, suggesting that the probability $P(I)$ is
positively related to price. Accordingly, as the price rises, the individual is less
likely to purchase insurance coverage for events that are almost certain to occur.
Further, the discussion of Figures 2.3 and 2.4 indicated that the additional amount
the individual is willing to pay increases as the probability of the event occurring
falls and the magnitude of the potential loss rises. These observations suggest
that the individual will tend to purchase insurance if administrative expenses are
not excessive and that the amount of insurance is inversely related to the loading
portion of the premium. Further, other factors remaining constant, it is reasonable
to expect the individual to purchase insurance coverage for events that precipitate
a large loss and are expected to occur with a low probability. Hence, the theoretical model suggests that components of service associated with a low probability of use and a large potential loss are more likely to be covered by insurance
than those associated with a high probability of use and a low potential loss.

Thus far, the role of the consumer's income has been ignored in the discussion.

Most analysts argue that the income of the individual exerts two distinct effects on the demand for insurance. The first involves the relation of utility to wealth and influences the amount in excess of the pure premium the individual is willing to pay. As indicated by the shape of the actual utility function, the marginal utility of those earning a high income is relatively low while the marginal utility of the less wealthy is relatively high. Hence, these observations suggest that the wealthy and the poor are more likely to self-insure than other intermediate income groups.

The second effect of income on the demand for health insurance is employment related and involves the traditional tax treatment of premium payments. When viewed from the perspective of the employer, contributions to health insurance premiums are regarded as a deductible business expense. Traditionally, the employer's contribution has not been regarded as a component of the employee's income and, as a result, these payments have not been subject to taxation. In addition, the individual's payments for health insurance are tax deductible if total spending exceeds a specified percentage of income.

Concerning the exclusion of contributions from the taxable income of the employee, observe that as earnings derived from employment rise, the marginal tax rate also increases and, as a consequence, the tax subsidy is directly related to the income of the worker. Other things remaining constant, the tax subsidy reduces the price of insurance to the employee, thus inducing the purchase of more coverage.

Offsetting the effects of the tax subsidy on the price of insurance are increases in use, costs, and premiums that result from the behavior of the individual that is termed *moral hazard*. As suggested by Pauly (1968), moral hazard occurs when the quantity of health insurance influences the expected loss. In this regard, moral hazard may influence the probability that an insured event will occur or the magnitude of the loss, given that the event has occurred. For example, the purchase of health insurance may induce the individual to engage in less preventive behavior, resulting in losses or costs that are attributable to the treatment of an avoidable illness. Second, since health insurance reduces the user price of health services, an insured individual who has experienced illness is induced to demand additional units of service, an action that generates a marginal benefit that is less than the corresponding marginal cost.

The effects of moral hazard have been long recognized in the insurance industry and are reduced, with varying degrees of success, by the deductible clauses, coinsurance provisions and upper limits of coverage that are specified in many policies. As indicated below, cost-sharing arrangements not only reduce the effects of moral hazard but also transfer a portion of the fiscal risks of illness or injury to the insured, thereby permitting the insurer to reduce the premium.

A deductible is a fixed amount that the consumer must pay prior to the insurer assuming responsibility for all or a portion of all additional costs. The deductible usually applies to a given service or represents the cumulative amount the insured and, in some cases, family members must pay during a specified period of time.

When viewed from the perspective of moral hazard, the effect of deductibles on use is nonlinear. Until the deductible is satisfied, user and market prices are identical. As suggested by Keeler, Newhouse, and Phelps (1977b) and Ellis (1986), the effects of the deductible on the utilization behavior of the insured depend on the extent to which spending is expected to exceed the fixed amount. In particular, these analyses indicate that the deductible depresses use if the level of spending anticipated by the insured is not expected to exceed the deductible amount. To the extent that deductibles lower use, the transaction costs of processing claims is reduced. The savings in administrative cost might lower the loading factor and the premium, thereby inducing demand for coverage.

Coinsurance is a form of cost sharing that is typically in effect after the deductible is satisfied. The coinsurance rate is usually expressed as a percentage, indicating the fraction of medical expenses in excess of the deductible that is the responsibility of the insured. In general, coinsurance provisions reduce the amount devoted to loading and transfer a portion of the fiscal risks for additional costs to the insured, thus restraining use of health services.

In addition to deductibles and coinsurance provisions, insurers limit benefits to a maximum dollar amount or to the use of a maximum quantity of care. Costs or use that exceed the maximum limit represent the fiscal responsibility of the insured. In the absence of compensating coverage, these provisions transfer the fiscal risks of catastrophic illness from the third party to the insured and might be regarded as an instrument that addresses the effects of extreme moral hazard.

Empirical Findings

Perhaps the most difficult problem encountered in empirical investigations of the demand for health insurance is the development of theoretically appropriate measures of price and quantity (Arnett and Trapnell 1984). The presence of multiple insurers offering multiple plans, each with a given set of benefits and cost-sharing arrangements, clearly complicates the problem of measuring the quantity of coverage. Similarly, as suggested by Pauly (1986), expected benefit levels affect the loading portion of the premium, which is the proper measure of price. Faced with these measurement difficulties, previous research has been forced to adopt crude surrogates for its theoretical counterparts.

The price of insurance has been measured by loading relative to benefits or other surrogates for the loading portion of the premium. On the assumption that administrative costs decline as the number of enrollees increases, the size of the employment group has been used as a surrogate for the loading fee. For example, Phelps (1973), Goldstein and Pauly (1976), Ginsburg (1981), and Taylor and Wilensky (1983) report that the level of coverage increased with growth in the size of the employee group. To the extent that administrative loading costs decline as the number of enrollees increases, these findings are consistent with the predictions derived from the expected utility model.

In general, reported price elasticities are also consistent with the view that higher loading costs depress the demand for health insurance. However, as described below, estimates exhibit considerable variation, ranging from approximately − .2 (Farley and Monheit 1985); to values (e.g., < − 1.0) that suggest the demand for coverage is price elastic (Phelps 1976).

Of perhaps greater interest to policy deliberations are studies that assess the responsiveness of demand for coverage to prices, adjusted for employer contributions and the marginal tax rate of the employee. These studies are of considerable importance to evaluations of the potential effectiveness of eliminating the tax exclusions described previously.

In the first major studies of the demand for health insurance, Phelps (1973, 1976) employed survey data, depicting the health insurance coverage of families in 1963, to estimate price and income elasticities in the context of a hypothetical choice situation that involved a continuum of plans characterized by the same price. Since the marginal tax rates of the families were not available, Phelps employed the size of the employee group as a surrogate for the price of health insurance.

Based on the strength of the relation between the premiums and the size of the group, the price elasticities reported by Phelps were between − .04 to − .07, while the income elasticities were in the range of .12 to .19. As indicated earlier, however, the price surrogate was not adjusted for differences in employer contributions or the marginal tax rate. In a subsequent study, Phelps (1982) employed these findings to estimate the change in employment-related premiums that would result from a reduction in the tax exclusion. The results indicated that an increase of approximately 13 percent in the average price of insurance would reduce premiums from $62 billion to $28 billion, resulting in an arc elasticity of − 2.843.

As suggested by Holmer (1984), conditions prevailing in the insurance market during 1963 may have resulted in an overestimate of the price elasticity suggested by the results reported by Phelps. In particular, insurers were introducing major medical plans, with higher premiums and coverage, and these policies were limited to larger groups. Recognizing that coverage is traditionally more comprehensive in larger than in smaller groups, the introduction of major medical policies may have contributed to the strength of the relation between group size and premiums, resulting in an overestimate of the price elasticity of demand for health insurance.

The response of employees to multiple options has also been examined by Farley and Taylor (1985). Using data derived from the National Medical Care Expenditure Survey (NMCES), the study examined separately the choices of 339 employees who were offered a traditional plan and an HMO, and those of 251 employees who were offered two traditional plans. Concerning the latter aspect of the study, the two plans were regarded as the high and low option with the low option defined as the next less expensive plan available to the employee. The high option plans typically offered lower coinsurance rates and deductible provisions. Serving as a surrogate for price was the difference in the premiums of the high and low options offered the employee.

After controlling for personal attributes such as age, sex, marital status, education, family income, insured benefits and health status, the results suggested that the price surrogate was negative, highly significant ($p \leq .01$) and indicated a demand elasticity of $-.14$. Further, differences in the insured benefits of the traditional plans also exerted significant effects on choice probabilities. Relative to the low option, more generous benefit provisions and lower cost-sharing requirements increased the likelihood of selecting the high option.

Although significant ($p \leq .01$), premium differences exerted a smaller influence on choices between the traditional plan and the HMO. Compared with the low option plan, each $100 in the relative price of a high option reduced the choice probability by 5 percent. For each $100 in the relative price of an HMO, the likelihood of enrollment declined by only 2 percent. Hence, even though the price surrogate behaved as expected, the effects were lower when employees were offered an option of selecting HMO coverage or a traditional plan. These results also indicate that employees value traditional high option benefits and that, if an HMO or a low option alternative is offered, many employees will select comprehensive plans. On the other hand, the results also support the contention that a substantial number of employees prefer a low option to more comprehensive plans.

Employing plausible assumptions concerning risk aversion, the price elasticity of demand for medical care and marginal tax rates, Feldstein and Friedman (1977) calculated an elasticity based on predictions derived from a choice simulation model. Families were offered a choice among several plans that were financed in full by the employer. In the first two simulations, a moderate degree of risk aversion was combined with assumed price elasticities of demand for medical care of approximately $-.23$ and $-.46$. In the third simulation, a high degree of risk aversion was combined with a price elasticity of demand for medical care of approximately $-.46$. The model generated estimates of the aggregate demand for health insurance for a tax policy of full exclusion and a policy that eliminates the subsidy. The calculations indicate that the subsidy exerts a "substantial effect" in insurance coverage. Holmer (1984) employed the results of the simulation model to estimate price elasticities of demand for health insurance in a range extending from $-.6$ to approximately $-.9$.

Based on individual data assembled in the NMCES, Taylor and Wilensky (1983) used variations in the marginal tax rate, t, to calculate price, which was measured by $1-t$. The focus of the analysis was on the influence exerted by the tax-adjusted price and disposable income on the demand for health insurance, as measured by the health insurance premium. Further, since nontaxable sources of income and the tax subsidy were relatively uncorrelated, Taylor and Wilensky were able to calculate price and income elasticities of demand. The results suggested that the price and income elasticity of demand for health insurance were $-.21$ and $.02$, respectively. Recognizing that most of the employees were offered little, if any, choice among plans, Taylor and Wilensky regarded the estimate of $-.21$ as a short-run elasticity and, with multiple options, it was suggested that the demand for insurance might become more price sensitive.

A potential source of error in the Taylor and Wilensky study involved the assumption that the full premium was financed by the contribution of the employer. In a subsequent study, Farley and Wilensky (1983) employed data assembled in the NMCES and adjusted the price variable for variations in employer contributions. Employing many of the independent variables incorporated earlier, a price elasticity of $-.41$ ($p \le .05$) and an income elasticity of .04 ($p \le .05$) were reported in this study.

Farley and Monheit (1985) employed data assembled in the NMCES and the Health Insurance Employer Survey (HIES) to estimate the parameters of a two-stage, least-squares model of demand for health insurance. Information contained in the HIES provided a distribution of benefit provisions, premiums, employee contributions, and employer contributions. Hence, the data enabled Farley and Monheit to examine the demand for health insurance, which was defined as expected out-of-pocket expenditures of the employee. Given the individual's coverage and identical assumptions concerning the actuarial loss for all employees, the insurance variable represented out-of-pocket expenditures and ranged from zero, which corresponded to comprehensive coverage, to an expected value of \$291, an amount that indicated virtually no coverage. The reduction in net price was measured by the product of the employer's contribution and the employee's marginal tax rate. Further, since a given set of benefits is less expensive for a larger than smaller group, the loading portion of the premium was measured by the size of the employer group.

The results indicated that the surrogate for net price behaved as expected. In particular, the elasticity coefficient of .04 indicated that larger groups, and hence lower loading fees, were associated with more comprehensive coverage than smaller groups. Similarly, the elasticity of .22 is consistent with the proposition that the tax subsidy encouraged the purchase of more insurance by those offered multiple options. In addition, among employees who were offered a single policy option, the income elasticity of .06 suggests that an increase in earnings stimulates more comprehensive coverage. As measured by the interaction between the availability of multiple options and the employer's contribution to premiums, the coefficient of .788 suggested that offering employees several plans exacerbated the effects of employer subsidization; hence, the results of the study suggest that the employer's contribution and offering multiple plans are complementary instruments, the effectiveness of which depends on appropriate financial incentives.

Focusing on federal employees, the influence of variation in the employer's contribution on price was given explicit recognition by Holmer (1984). Letting h represent the premium, e the employer contribution, and t the marginal tax rate, Holmer defined the price of insurance by $p = 1\text{-}te/h$. Estimates of a discrete choice model of the demand for health insurance were based on a 1982 survey of plan choices implemented by federal employees who were offered 23 insurance plans that were aggregated into low, medium, and high fee-for-service coverage and an HMO option. Maximum likelihood estimates indicated an average price elasticity for health insurance of $-.16$ and an average price elasticity for sup-plementary insurance of $-.51$. In addition, estimates of the choice model re-vealed an income elasticity of approximately $.01$.

Unfortunately, Holmer was forced to estimate family income and the marginal tax rate, which introduces measurement error in the results. In addition, Pauly (1986) suggests that bias may result from the interaction between plan choice and the self-selection of workers among alternate employment sources. For example, assume that labor compensation is determined by marginal productivity and that less generous coverage or lower contributions by the employer might be exchanged for higher wages. A worker who prefers low coverage should not choose employment in a situation in which a comprehensive option is subsidized by a high employer's contribution. Most workers who select these sources of employment are likely to have a strong preference for insurance, an attribute that might dominate the effects of the tax subsidy.

Marquis and Phelps (1985) focused on the demand for supplemental insurance by families who participated in the Rand Health Insurance Experiment (HIE). Excluded from the experiment were (1) families in which the head was 62 years of age or older, (2) the disabled who were eligible for Medicare, (3) persons eligible for care sponsored by the military, (4) persons who received supplemental security income, and (5) families earning an income in the upper 7 percent of the national distribution. The other salient aspects of the HIE are described in Chapter 3.

At the end of the participation in the experiment, 1,326 families were offered a set of hypothetical plans that were characterized by different prices and re-ductions in the annual maximum dollar expenditure for which the consumer assumed responsibility. The major provisions of the hypothetical plans reduced the family's maximum expenditures during a given year by 33, 67 and 100 percent.

The price of insurance was measured by one plus a loading fee that was derived by comparing the expected monetary value of the benefits of each sup-plemental plan with the corresponding offer price. The effective fees ranged from $-.3$ to $.3$, which includes the effective loading that results from the tax subsidy and the elimination of the exclusions of employer contributions from taxable income. In addition to effective loading, the model also examined the effects of family attributes, location, and the insurance coverage prevailing during the HIE on choice probabilities.

The results of the probit analysis indicated that increases in the loading fee decreased the probability that the family would express interest in the hypothetical offer. Based on predictions derived from the probit analysis, Marquis and Phelps (1985) examined the willingness of respondents to assume greater risk in response to variation in the effective loading fee. The results confirmed, in part, the prediction that when price is positive, full supplementation is less attractive than the risk-sharing arrangements. These results also indicated that respondents were willing to assume financial risks even when the effective loading assumed negative values, an outcome that appears to contradict the expectations derived from the utility maximizing model described earlier.

In addition to those studies that focus on estimates of the price elasticity of demand for health insurance, several other studies have examined the utility maximizing model in terms of individual preferences for different cost-sharing options. As indicated previously, theoretical considerations indicate that risk averse individuals are likely to prefer higher deductibles and coinsurance rates if loading fees are higher for small claims and the actuarial portion of the premium reflects the individual's risk. Further, the model also suggested that, among the risk averse, catastrophic coverage is preferred to policies that finance a larger portion of less expensive illnesses. Accordingly, it is usually expected that individuals prefer catastrophic coverage to policies that offer lower deductibles or coinsurance rates.

Several studies employed cross-sectional data to examine these expectations. For example, results reported by Feldstein and Friedman (1977), Keeler, Morrow, and Newhouse (1977a), and Keeler, Newhouse, and Phelps (1977b) report findings that are consistent with the utility maximizing model. The results of the conjoint analysis reported by Hershey, Kunreuther, Schwartz, and Williams (1984) suggest that respondents prefer policies that cover low-probability, high-cost occurrences relative to plans of equal actuarial value that finance less expensive but more frequent events. These findings suggested, however, that respondents were as likely to choose plans that contain cost-sharing arrangements as they were to select policies without these options.

Medigap: Choices by the Elderly

Perhaps the most frequently cited evidence that contradicts the theoretical model are findings that suggest that two-thirds of Medicare beneficiaries purchase supplemental coverage and that more than half purchase coverage that finances the initial deductible and copayments (Reed and Myers 1967; Cafferata 1984, 1985; Rice and McCall 1985; Pauly 1986). Although total premiums for "Medigap" coverage amounted to $3.94 billion in 1977, private insurance paid approximately 6 percent of the elderly's medical expenses during the year. These policies are more likely to offer coverage for hospital care than outpatient services and for short- rather than long-term care. Further, Rice and McCall (1985) conclude that the supplemental policies purchased by beneficiaries fail to cover the most significant gaps in the Medicare provisions (e.g., nursing home care, prescription drugs and physician fees in excess of allowable reasonable charges) and that those who are least capable of financing the costs of a catastrophic illness are least likely to purchase supplemental coverage. Cafferata (1984) employed data derived from the NMCES to examine the distribution of benefits for nursing home care, the characteristics of the insured, and the total coverage of those with more than one source of coverage. The results indicated that in 1977,

40 percent of Medicare beneficiaries were covered for nursing home care and that among those covered, 85 percent were insured for the copayment provisions that are imposed on days 21 to 100; however, only 16 percent were covered for 365 days or more. Similarly, only 14.4 percent had full coverage for Part *A* copayments and a generous maximum defined as 365 more days of care or a major medical maximum of $100,000 or more.

Among the factors that may have contributed to the purchase of these policies is an asymmetry in the knowledge of the insured and the insurer. As summarized by Cafferata (1984), the literature suggests that (1) the knowledge of the population regarding insurance concepts is quite poor, (2) the elderly mistakenly believe their coverage is inadequate, and (3) the accuracy of knowledge improves with the length of coverage, the extent of coverage, and medical complexity of the plan's provisions. Results reported by Cafferata also indicated that the level of knowledge was lower among the elderly than the general population and poorest among groups exposed to the greatest risks of illness. The relatively poor knowledge of the elderly concerning the insured benefits of the Medicare program may be one of the factors that has contributed to the inadequate coverage of some services and the excessive coverage of others.

Long, Settle, and Link (1982) and Cafferata (1985) present findings that document a positive relation between the probability of purchasing supplemental coverage and income. Long et al. however, concluded that the likelihood that a beneficiary will receive coverage under Medicaid declines precipitously with rising income. Hence, the rate of supplemental coverage among the elderly was relatively uniform throughout the observed income distribution. The analysis also indicates a negative association between the likelihood of purchasing supplemental insurance and age. The inverse relation may be attributable to rising premiums that accompany increases in actuarial risk, an outcome that may reduce the access of the elderly to supplemental coverage.

Focusing on the poor elderly, Berk and Wilensky (1984) concluded that approximately two-thirds of the elderly supplemented their Medicare coverage with private insurance; however, analysis of data assembled in the NMCES suggested that, in comparison to 78 percent of the higher income elderly, only 47 percent of the poor or near-poor had private coverage. The study also suggested that the elderly with Medicare and Medicaid coverage experienced relatively low out-of-pocket expenditures, followed by those with only Medicare coverage and beneficiaries with private insurance.

The Uninsured

In addition to the potential inequities that may result from inadequate supplemental coverage of the elderly, the number of uninsured is also of importance to policy analysts and an evaluation of the health system. Estimates based on sample surveys suggest that 12 to 13 percent of the population are uninsured (Carroll 1978; Cordor 1979; Kasper, Walden, and Wilensky 1980). However, as suggested by Sunshine (1984), previous estimates overstate the number of uninsured. After adjusting for the underreporting of coverage present in survey data, Sunshine concluded that approximately 7 percent or 15 million Americans are uninsured. More recent studies, however, suggest that during the recession of 1983, the number of uninsured ranged from 29 to 35 million (Munnell 1986; Sulvetta and Swartz 1986).

Concerning the composition of those with no coverage, Mulstein (1984) focused on data assembled in the NMCES and the Current Population Survey to examine the distribution of the uninsured with respect to age, employment, income, family status, and geographic location. The results indicated that, among the 25 million uninsured, most tend to be young adults, the poor, and those employed in part-time jobs. Similar results were reported by Wilensky, Walden, and Kasper (1981), who focused on the characteristics of those who were uninsured throughout 1977. Employing data assembled in the NMCES, the results of the logistic regression analysis indicated that the likelihood of being uninsured was greater among (1) those who were 19–24 years of age, (2) females, and (3) nonwhites. Conversely, the probability of being uninsured for the entire year was lower among (1) white-collar employees, relative to their blue-collar counterparts, (2) those who reside in SMSAs, and (3) those who report other than an excellent health status.

The dependence of coverage on employment status has also been documented by Monheit, Hagan, Berk, and Wilensky (1983); Gold, McEachern, and Santoni (1984); and Berki, Wyszewianski, Lichtenstein, Gimothy et al. (1985). Employing data assembled in the NMCES, Monheit et al. (1983) examined the likelihood of health insurance loss among unemployed workers who were covered by private insurance in 1977. Included in the logit model were economic, demographic, and behavioral factors that were thought to influence the loss of coverage. The results indicated that higher levels of household income and the presence of an employed spouse significantly reduced the probability of losing coverage. Similar to results reported by Berki et al. (1985), Monheit et al. found that a longer duration of unemployment and the loss of a job precipitating the receipt of unemployment compensation increase the probability of health insurance loss. Consistent with results reported by Wilensky, Walden, and Kasper (1981), the logit analysis also indicated that the probability of insurance loss rose until 32 years of age and declined thereafter.

Focusing on data assembled on a sample of the unemployed in Detroit, Berki et al. reported that 40 percent of those who received unemployment compensation between 1980 and 1982 also lost their insurance coverage. The study also indicated that the lack of insurance is directly related to the length of time the individual was unemployed. Gold et al. examined a sample of those who benefited from unemployment compensation in Maryland during the week of December 6, 1983, and found that 33 percent lost coverage that was related to their employment status or participation in labor unions. Employing data assembled in the Current Population Survey, Monheit et al. concluded that 13 percent or 1.4

million unemployed persons lost their insurance coverage in 1982. That an increase in the unemployment rate and the proportion of the population under the poverty level contributes to a growing number of Americans who experience difficulty in financing health services has also been demonstrated by Kinzer (1984) and by Davis and Rowland (1983).

Although closely related, participation in the active labor force does not automatically provide workers and their dependents with coverage. Focusing on data assembled in the NMCES and National Medical Care Expenditure and Utilization Survey (NMCEUS), Monheit, Hagan, Berk, and Farley (1985) found that approximately 50 percent of those who were uninsured throughout the year were employed part or all of the year. The findings also indicated that 89 percent of the uninsured workers were not offered coverage and that only 11 percent of the insured work force rejected the offer of employment-related coverage. In particular, those engaged in part-time employment or positions requiring less training or skill were more likely to be uninsured than their skilled and full-time counterparts. Black (1986) contends that the less skilled, part-time employees and their dependents are likely to represent an increasing proportion of the uninsured as changes in the U.S. economy shift employment from manufacturing to service sectors, an outcome that may precipitate a decline in unionization and an increase in part-time employment.

Several options have been suggested as approaches to the problem of financing uncompensated care and providing coverage to the uninsured. Recognizing the recent publication of a book devoted to these issues (Sloan, Blumstein, and Perrin 1986), we provide only a brief discussion of the problem of financing uncompensated care. As described by Bovbjerg and Koller (1986) and Mulstein (1984), insurance pools, implemented in six states, are financed by all insurers who are required to offer coverage and share in the losses of covering the uninsured. Most states impose eligibility requirements on participants, and the pool is available to all residents in only one state, Connecticut. Since most pools are limited to those who are otherwise uninsurable, the adverse health status of participants results in higher use and costs. As indicated by Bovbjerg and Koller, low enrollment, adverse selection, and a failure to pool risks have resulted in large deficits that are financed by increased assessments on insurers and, indirectly, by a drain on the resources of the state treasury.

An alternative to the state pool is the proposal to employ rate regulation and provisions that require all payers to finance a share of the costs of providing uncompensated care. For example, in Maryland, Massachusetts, New York, and New Jersey, payers contribute a share of the costs of uncompensated care to providers or to a regional pool from which these expenses are financed (Thorpe 1987). Unfortunately, the practice of subsidizing uncollectable accounts reduces incentives to engage in collection efforts, which, in turn, diminishes the need to secure coverage, an outcome that may exacerbate the problem of uncompensated care.

As described by Bovbjerg and Koller (1986), a number of local or private initiatives might be considered as potential solutions to the problem of providing coverage to the uninsured. The first strategy involves a realignment of pool risks. For example, it might be possible to expand the scope of existing groups and thereby extend coverage to (1) dependents of workers, (2) those related to workers, and (3) those who become unemployed. Alternatively, it may be possible to create new pools comprised of those who do not participate in employment-related plans and offer coverage through groups of employers, unions, banks, or insurance brokers. Among the more promising possibilities are multiple employer trusts or multiple employer welfare arrangements that have grown in number, particularly those that are self-insured. The Federal Employee Retirement Income Security Act (FERISA) defines Multiple Employer Welfare arrangements more broadly than multiple employee trusts and enables insurers to group small employment categories for actuarial purposes and market coverages to an industry, association, or other collectivity.

The second major private initiative involves the creation of economies through improved administrative and underwriting techniques. For example, administrative costs and, hence, loading, might be reduced by creating larger risk pools while avoiding adverse selection. Such an approach might result in reduced prices and encourage more coverage among the uninsured. Although the options are many, the dual problems of uncompensated care and the uninsured are issues that are unresolved. As suggested by Etheredge (1986 p. 314), the increased competitive pressures in the health insurance market may exert an increasingly adverse effect on the uninsured, an outcome that "poses a strong challenge for American society in meeting its collective responsibilities."

SUMMARY AND CONCLUSIONS

This chapter reviewed the traditional model of demand for health insurance, which suggests that the decision to purchase coverage is inversely related to the effective loading. Consistent with the views expressed by Pauly (1986), available evidence confirms the view that the price or tax subsidy elasticity is negative and that tax treatment influences the choice of insurance. The precise impact, however, has been obscured by the crude proxies that have been employed for net loading.

In addition to the development of more refined measures of the price of insurance, an empirical assessment of a set of related issues might enhance our understanding of the selection process. For example, it is usually assumed that choices reflect an assessment of expected benefits or costs. Hence, a rational evaluation of alternate policy options requires an understanding of the various benefit packages that are available to the individual. Results reported by Marquis (1983) indicate that the perception of benefits are more congruent with the provisions of the policy when payment structures are simplified. These observations suggest that the complexity of the benefit or payment structure may influence not only the perception of the individual but also the choices that are implemented. Similarly, the expected costs, to include those resulting from coinsurance and deductible provisions, may depend on not only the individual's current health status but also the needs, use and costs that are likely to occur during the life of the policy. For example, Ellis (1985) presents findings that indicate that employees explicitly incorporate expectations concerning future expenditures when selecting among alternate fee-for-service plans and that significant weight is placed on previous expenditures as an indicator of future spending. These findings are of importance to the development of theoretical and empirical assessments of the individual's evaluation of multiple options. Further, since consumers employ previous spending to estimate future expenditures and base health plan choices on these predictions, the findings are also of importance to the problem of examining the influence of coinsurance and deductible provisions on annual utilization behavior. These observations suggest that the decision process and the demand for health insurance are not completely understood and that future research is required to disentangle the effects of previous expenditures from expected ones on the demand for health insurance.

REFERENCES

Arnett, R. H., and G. R. Trapnell. 1984. Private health insurance: New measures of a complex and changing industry. *Health Care Financing Review* 6(2):31–42.

Berk, M. L., and G. R. Wilensky. 1984. Health care of the poor elderly: Supplementing Medicare. Unpublished mimeograph, March.

Berki, S. E., L. Wyszewianski, R. Lichtenstein, P. A. Gimothy et al. 1985. Health insurance coverage of the unemployed. *Medical Care* 23(7):847–54.

Black, J. T. 1986. Comment on 'The employed uninsured and the role of public policy.' *Inquiry* 23(2):209–12.

Blue Cross and Blue Shield Association. 1981. *Blue Cross/Blue Shield Fact Book*, 1980 ed. Chicago, IL:BCBS Association.

Bovbjerg, R. R., and C. F. Koller. 1986. State health insurance pools: Current performance, future prospects. *Inquiry* 23(2):111–21.

Buchanan, J. L., and S. Cretin. 1986. Risk selection of families electing HMO membership. *Medical Care* 24(1):39–51.

Cafferata, G. L. 1984. Knowledge of their health insurance coverage by the elderly. *Medical Care* 22(9):835–47.

Cafferata, G. L. 1985. The elderly's private insurance coverage of nursing home care. *American Journal of Public Health* 75(6):655–56.

Carroll, M. 1978. Private health insurance plans in 1976. *Social Security Bulletin* 41(9):3–16.

Chernick, H. A., M. R. Holmer, and D. H. Weinberg. 1987. Tax policy toward health insurance and the demand for medical services. *Journal of Health Economics* 6(1):1–25.

Chollet, D. J., and Staff. 1984. *Employer-Provided Health Benefits*. Washington, DC: Employee Benefits Research Institute.

Cordor, J. 1979. Health care coverage: United States, 1976. Advance data report no. 44,

National Center for Health Statistics. Washington, DC: Government Printing Office.

Davis, K., and D. Rowland. 1983. Uninsured and underserved: Inequities in health care in the United States. *Milbank Memorial Fund Quarterly* 61(2):149–76.

Ellis, R. P. 1985. The effect of prior-year health expenditures on health coverage plan choice. In R. M. Scheffler and L. F. Rossiter, eds., *Advances in Health Economics and Health Services Research* 6. Greenwich, CT: JAI Press, 149–70.

Ellis, R. P. 1986. Rational behavior in the presence of coverage ceilings and deductibles. *Rand Journal of Economics* 17(2):158–75.

Enthoven, A. C. 1978. Consumer-choice health plan. *New England Journal of Medicine* 298(12,13):650–58, 709–20.

Etheredge, L. 1986. Ethics and the new insurance market. *Inquiry* 23(3):308–15.

Farley, P. J., and A. C. Monheit. 1985. Selectivity in the demand for health insurance and health care. In R. M. Scheffler and L. F. Rossiter, eds., *Advances in Health Economics and Health Services Research* 6. Greenwich, CT: JAI Press, 231–48.

Farley, P. J., and A. K. Taylor. 1985. Premiums, benefits and employee choice of health insurance options. Paper presented to the Eastern Economic Association, March.

Farley, P., and G. R. Wilensky, 1983. Options, incentives and employment-related health insurance coverage. In R. M. Scheffler and L. F. Rossiter, eds., *Advances in Health Economics and Health Services Research* 4. Greenwich, CT: JAI Press, 57–82.

Feldman, R. D., and B. E. Dowd. 1982. Simulation of a health insurance market with adverse selection. *Operations Research* 39(6):1027–42.

Feldstein, M. S., and B. Friedman. 1977. Tax subsidies, the rational demand for insurance, and the health care crisis. *Journal of Public Economy* 7(2):155–78.

Freeman, R. B. 1981. The effect of unionism on fringe benefits. *Industrial and Labor Relations Review* 34(4):489–509.

Gibson, R. M., and D. R. Waldo. 1982. National health expenditures, 1981. *Health Care Financing Review* 4(1):1–35.

Ginsburg, P. G. 1981. Altering the tax treatment of employment-based health plans. *Milbank Memorial Fund Quarterly* 59(2):224–55.

Gold, M., Y. McEachern, and T. Santoni. 1984. Health insurance loss among the unemployed: Extent of the problem and policy options. Paper presented at the Annual Meeting of the American Public Health Association, November.

Goldstein, G. S., and M. Pauly. 1976. Group health insurance as a local public good. In R. N. Rosett, ed., *The Role of Health Insurance in the Health Services Sector.* New York: National Bureau of Economic Research.

Hershey, J. C., H. Kunreuther, J. S. Schwartz, and S. V. Williams. 1984. Health insurance under competition: Would people choose what is expected? *Inquiry* 24(4):349–60.

Holmer, M. 1984. Tax policy and the demand for health insurance. *Journal of Health Economics* 3(3):203–21.

Jensen, G., R. Feldman, and B. Dowd. 1984. Corporate benefit policies and health insurance costs. *Journal of Health Economics* 3(3):275–96.

Kasper, J. A., D. C. Walden, and G. R. Wilensky. 1980. Who are the uninsured? Data review, National Center for Health Services Research. Washington, DC: Government Printing Office.

Keeler, E. B., D. T. Morrow, and J. P. Newhouse. 1977a. The demand for supplementary health insurance, or, do deductibles matter? *Journal of Political Economy* 85(4):789–801.

Keeler, E. B., J. P. Newhouse, and C. E. Phelps. 1977b. Deductibles and the demand for medical care services. *Econometrica* 45(3):641–55.

Kinzer, D. M. 1984. Care of the poor revisited. *Inquiry* 21(1):5–16.

Long, S. H., R. F. Settle, and C. R. Link. 1982. Who bears the burden of Medicare cost sharing? *Inquiry* 19(3):222–34.

Marquis, M. S. 1983. Consumers' knowledge about their health insurance coverage. *Health Care Financing Review* 5(1):65–80.

Marquis, S., and C. E. Phelps. 1985. Demand for supplementary health insurance. Report no. R–3285HHS. Santa Monica, CA: Rand Corporation.

Monheit, A. C., M. M. Hagan, M. C. Berk, and G. R. Wilensky. 1983. Unemployment health insurance and medical care utilization. National Center for Health Services Research, November.

Monheit, A. C., M. M. Hagan, M. L. Berk, and P. J. Farley. 1985. The employed uninsured and the role of public policy. *Inquiry* 22(4):348–64.

Mulstein, S. 1984. The uninsured and the financing of uncompensated care: Scope, costs, and policy options. *Inquiry* 21(3):214–29.

Munnell, A. 1986. Ensuring entitlement to health care services. *Bulletin of the New York Academy of Medicine* 62(1):61–74.

Neipp, J., and R. Zeckhauser. 1985. Persistence in the choice of health plans. In R. M. Scheffler, and L. F. Rossiter, eds., *Advances in Health Economics and Health Services Research* 6. Greenwich, CT: JAI Press, 47–74.

Palmetto-Lowcountry Health Systems Agency, Inc. 1984. Trident Industrial Health Co-alition: Model health insurance benefits design study.

Pauly, M. V. 1968. The economics of moral hazard: Comment. *American Economic Review* 58(3):531–57.

Pauly, M. V. 1980. Overinsurance: The conceptual issues. In M. V. Pauly, ed., *What Now, What Later, What Never?* Washington, DC: American Enterprise Institute, pp. 201–19.

Pauly, M. V. 1986. Taxation, health insurance, and market failure in the medical economy. *Journal of Economic Literature* 24(2):629–75.

Phelps, C. E. 1973. *The Demand for Health Insurance: A Theoretical and Empirical Investigation.* Santa Monica, CA: Rand Corporation.

Phelps, C. E. 1976. Demand for reimbursement insurance. In R. N. Rosett, ed., *The Role of Health Insurance in the Health Services Sector.* New York: National Bureau of Economic Research.

Phelps, C. E. 1982. *Health Care Costs: The Consequences of Increased Cost Sharing.* Rand Corp. Report R–2970-RC. Santa Monica, CA: Rand Corporation, November.

Price, J. R., and J. W. Mays. 1985. Biased selection in the Federal Employees Health Benefits Programs. *Inquiry* 22(1):67–77.

Price, J. R., J. W. Mays, and G. R. Trapnell. 1983. Stability in the Federal Employees Health Benefits Program. *Journal of Health Economics* 2(3):207–23.

Reed, L., and R. Myers. 1967. Health insurance coverage complementary to Medicare. *Social Security Bulletin* 30:3.

Rice, R. G. 1966. Skill, earnings, and the growth of wage supplements. *American Economics Review* 56(2):583–93.

Rice, T., and N. McCall. 1985. The extent of ownership and the characteristics of medicare supplemental policies. *Inquiry* 22(2):188–200.

Rossiter, L. F., and A. K. Taylor. 1982. Union effects on the provision of health insurance. *Industrial Relations* 21(2):167–77.

Rothschild, M., and J. E. Stiglitz. 1976. Equilibrium in competitive insurance markets: An essay on the economics of imperfect information. *Quarterly Journal of Economics* 90(4):629–49.

Sloan, F. A., J. F. Blumstein, and J. M. Perrin, eds. 1986. *Uncompensated Hospital Care: Rights and Responsibilities*. Baltimore, MD: Johns Hopkins University Press.

Sulvetta, M. B., and K. Swartz. 1986. *The Uninsured and Uncompensated Care: A Chartbook*. Washington, DC: National Health Policy Forum, George Washington University.

Sunshine, J. H. 1984. How many Americans lack outside sources of payment for major health care costs? *Journal of Health and Human Resources Administration* 6(3):341–60.

Taylor, A. K., and G. R. Wilensky. 1983. Tax expenditures and the demand for private health insurance. In J. Meyer, *Market Oriented Reforms in Federal Health Policy*. American Enterprise Institute for Public Policy Research.

Thorpe, K. 1987. Does all-payer rate setting work? The case of the New York prospective hospital reimbursement methodology. *Journal of Health Politics, Policy and Law* 12(3):391–408.

Wilensky, G. R., D. C. Walden, and J. A. Kasper. 1981. The uninsured and their use of health services. Paper presented at 141st Annual Meeting of the American Statistical Association, August.

Wilensky, G. R., P. J. Farley, and A. K. Taylor. 1984. Variations in health insurance coverage: Benefits vs. premiums. *Milbank Memorial Fund Quarterly* 62(1):53–81.

Wilensky, G. R., and L. F. Rossiter. 1986. Patient self-selection in HMOs. *Health Affairs* 5(1):66–80.

Woodbury, S. A. 1980. Estimating preferences for wage and non-wage benefits. Paper prepared for a National Bureau of Economic Research sponsored conference on the Economics of Compensation, Cambridge, MA, November.

3

THE DEMAND FOR HEALTH SERVICES

As indicated in Chapter 1, persistent inflationary pressures in the health industry are attributable, in part, to increases in the demand for medical care. Since the use and costs of medical care are inextricably related, the formation of policy designed to control expenditures requires an understanding of the factors that affect the demand for health services. The primary objectives of demand analysis are to identify the factors that determine the quantity of health care consumed and to measure the extent to which each affects utilization behavior. An understanding of these interrelated issues enables the analyst to isolate instrumental variables and incorporate these factors in policies designed to reduce use and, hence, control aggregate expenditures on health care. Further, a knowledge of factors that affect demand constitutes the basis for formulating policy designed to redistribute health services. For example, it might be desirable to reduce or eliminate inequities in the distribution of care by altering the utilization experience of certain groups in society. An understanding of factors influencing demand constitutes the basis for implementing policies that enhance the use of service by members of the group.

In addition to the formation of public policy instruments, an understanding of those factors that affect demand enables the analyst to explain the variation in the utilization experience of individuals, population groups and different geographic areas. Further, an explanation of the variation in the use of health care is a prerequisite to developing not only more accurate forecasts of future use but also plans concerning the distribution of health resources. For these and other reasons, demand analysis is of vital importance to policy analysts, administrators, planners, and academics.

The purpose of this chapter is twofold. The first is to review theoretical models that have been proposed for examining the determinants of consumer behavior and the demand for health care. The second objective is to assess previous empirical research in terms of the theoretical models of demand.

Concerning the organization of this chapter, the traditional economic theory of demand constitutes the basis for much of the research and empirical evidence regarding the determinants of consumer behavior. Accordingly, the discussion is devoted initially to a consideration of the conventional model of a sovereign consumer as the basis for explaining the decision to seek care and the volume of service consumed. Following this discussion, the focus is on (1) the behavioral model proposed by Andersen (1968) and by Andersen and Newman (1973), (2) the investment model of demand developed by Grossman (1972), as modified by Muurinen (1982), among others, and (3) the model of physician-induced demand suggested by Fuchs and Kramer (1972), Evans (1974) and Fuchs (1978). Recognizing the potential role of the physician in determining utilization patterns, the chapter concludes with a consideration of the theoretical model proposed by Mechanic (1978) and explores the social-psychological determinants of care-seeking behavior or patient-initiated demand.

TRADITIONAL THEORY OF DEMAND

The Basic Framework

Demand is a term that refers to the quantity of a good or service a consumer will purchase at different prices during a given period of time. The conventional microeconomic model assumes that the objective of consumers is to maximize utility and that choices are determined by the tastes or preferences of the individual, the constraints imposed by income limitations and the prices of goods and services. To illustrate the role of these factors, this section considers the case of a consumer with a given amount of income that might be used to purchase two goods, X and Y.

The role of tastes or preferences in the traditional theory of consumer behavior is specified by the utility function:

$$TU = f(X, Y) \tag{3.1}$$

where TU represents the total utility or satisfaction derived from consuming different amounts of good X and good Y; X represents the quantity of good X consumed per time period; and Y represents the quantity of good Y consumed per time period.

Consider next the role played by income and relative prices in determining the consumer's budget set, and let M represent the income of the consumer; P_x and P_Y correspond to the price per unit of X and Y respectively; and X and Y denote the amounts of X and Y consumed. Employing this notation and assuming that the fixed income is spent on X and Y, the limitation imposed by the budget constraint is given by:

$$M = P_x X + P_y Y \tag{3.2}$$

Consider next the combination of X and Y that maximizes total utility, specified by equation 3.1, subject to the budget constraint, specified by equation 3.2. The following employs LaGrange's method of solution and an artificial multiplier, λ, which ensures that the number of unknowns is equal to the number of equations. The objective function may be expressed in the form

$$Z = f(X, Y) - \lambda [M - (P_x X) - (P_y Y)] \tag{3.3}$$

The first order conditions for utility maximization require the partial derivatives of Z with respect to each variable. Forcing each to equal zero yields:

$$\partial Z / \partial X = \partial TU / \partial X - \lambda P_x = 0 \tag{3.4}$$

$$\partial Z / \partial Y = \partial TU / \partial Y - \lambda P_y = 0 \tag{3.5}$$

$$\partial Z / \partial \lambda = M - P_x X - P_y Y = 0 \tag{3.6}$$

Solving these equations simultaneously, it can be shown that the condition

$$(\partial TU / \partial x)/P_x = (\partial TU / \partial Y)/P_y \tag{3.7}$$

maximizes utility. Since $\partial TU / \partial Y$ and $\partial TU / \partial x$ are the marginal utilities of Y and X respectively, equation 3.7 is equivalent to

$$MU_x / P_x = MU_y / P_y \tag{3.8}$$

which is the more familiar form for the condition that yields maximum utility.

Other things remaining constant, equation 3.8 implies that a decline in P_x will result in the inequality

$$MU_x / P_x > MU_y / P_y$$

which induces the consumer to purchase more units of product X. Hence, normative theory posits an inverse relation between price and quantity demanded.

Further inspection of the objective function (equation 3.3) indicates that the ability to purchase additional units of X and Y is constrained by the consumer's money income. Thus a rational individual who seeks to maximize utility would increase consumption of normal goods, such as X and Y, if money income is increased. In Figure 3.1, the response to an increase in income is reflected by a shift of the demand curve for product X from D_1 to D_2.

In summary, traditional economic theory posits that consumers act to maximize utility or satisfaction and that choices are consistent with preferences as depicted by the utility function. If the product market is competitive and the commodities

Figure 3.1
The Effect of a Change in Income on Demand

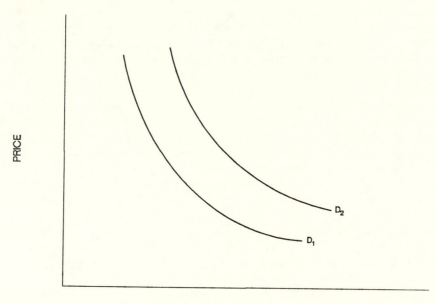

are normal goods, the analysis presented in this section suggests testable hypotheses concerning consumer demand. Among the most important are the following. Holding other factors constant, an increase in the price of a given commodity reduces the quantity demanded by the consumer. Consistent with the discussion of a shift in the demand curve, the analysis indicates that, *ceteris paribus*, an increase in the income available to the individual results in an increase in consumption.

The Empirical Evidence: The Demand for Health Care

Based on the conventional microeconomic model of a sovereign consumer, the focus of most empirical analyses is on a demand function of the general form:

$$D = f(M, P, Z)$$

where D represents the demand for health services; M corresponds to income; P corresponds to the price of service; and Z is a vector of factors that influence the preference for health care (i.e., education, health status, etc.).

The volume of service (e.g., days of care, number of visits, number of admissions) or expenditures on various components of health care are frequently employed as dependent variables in estimated demand equations. In addition to the economic variables, sociodemographic factors and measures of health status are included as independent variables that are assumed to affect the preference for care.

Several comments concerning the surrogates that are commonly used in empirical studies are worthy of note. First, although physical units, such as the number of visits or patient days, appear to reflect resource consumption, these surrogates fail to capture the intensity of service use. For example, the day of care and length of stay do not measure the mix of ancillary or general support services consumed. Similarly, the physician visit fails to capture the mix of services or diagnostic procedures consumed, suggesting that the number of visits does not measure variation in the intensity of care.

As is well known, expenditures on medical care are measured in monetary units and represent the value of the mix of care consumed. However, the use of expenditures as a surrogate for the traditional concept of demand suffers from several important weaknesses. First, if contrary to the assumptions of perfect competition, prices fail to correspond to marginal costs, Newhouse (1981), among others, suggests that variation in expenditures creates ambiguous welfare implications. Further, it is important to note that the price, quantity and quality of care combine to determine the level of expenditure on health services. Thus, in the absence of differential prices, elasticities derived from expenditure data reflect both the quality and the quantity of care consumed. It is also possible that prices are income dependent and that wealthy members of society are charged higher fees than their less affluent counterparts. As a result, elasticity coefficients based on expenditure data measure not only the relation between the quantity of care consumed and income but also the relation between price and income.

Among the most striking aspects of previous research are differences in studies of the same general phenomenon. For example, the unit of analysis might be the individual, residents of a geographic area, the family or family members, with a separate analysis for children or adults. The numeric information selected for analysis has been derived from micro sources, insurance claims, state averages and national surveys. Also found in the literature are studies that examine overall utilization patterns, explain variations in consumer demand or purport to identify the determinants of the use of specific components of service, such as illness/ injury and preventive care. In addition, several econometric techniques have been employed previously. For example, a number of studies estimate a single demand function while others employ a simultaneous equation model. Dependent variables reflect not only the volume of service consumed, including or excluding nonusers of care, but also categorical variables, resulting in an estimate of the influence exerted by factors on the likelihood of using service.

The Influence of Income

Recognizing the differences extant in the various studies of the same general phenomenon, this section focuses on those analyses that are based on the conventional microeconomic model. A number of studies have attempted to estimate the relationship between economic factors and expenditures on medical care, expenditures on physician and hospital care, and the volume of service, as measured by admissions, patient days, or physician visits. As the following indicates, results are typically expressed as elasticities with respect to price or income, and are, in general, consistent with expectations derived from the model of consumer demand.

In general, previous findings concerning the elasticity of demand with respect to income are consistent with expectations derived from the traditional theory of consumer behavior. Employing expenditure data as the dependent variable, the estimates of 1.0 and 1.2 reported by Feldstein and Carr (1964) and Silver (1970) suggest that the demand for health care is responsive to differences in income. Coefficients in the range of .02 to .85, however, suggest that demand is inelastic with respect to income (Feldstein and Carr 1964; Andersen and Benham 1970; Silver 1970; Wilensky and Holahan 1972; Rosett and Huang 1973; Phelps 1975; Chiswick 1976; Newhouse and Phelps 1976; Coffey 1983; Scheffler 1984; Stano 1985; Cromwell and Mitchell 1986).

Rather than rely on expenditure data, a number of studies have focused on physical measures to estimate income elasticities. The demand for physician services has been measured by the use or nonuse of service, the number of visits per user and the number of visits, resulting in estimates of income elasticity ranging from .01 to .72 (Fuchs and Kramer 1972; Acton 1976; Newhouse and Phelps 1976; Stano 1985). Similarly, measuring the demand for hospital care by the length of stay, admissions and days of care per period, income elasticities in the range .04 to .54 have been reported previously (Feldstein 1971; Phelps 1975; Newhouse and Phelps 1976). Hence, the weight of the evidence indicates that demand is increased by rising income, but most of the elasticity estimates are less than one, suggesting that the percentage change in demand is less than the rate of increase in income.

Although previous findings suggest that demand is income inelastic, it is possible to identify several factors that have reduced the responsiveness of utilization behavior to changes in income. First, the growth in insurance coverage is income related and, as is well known, reduces the financial liability of the consumer. It is common to argue that reductions in out-of-pocket expenditures precipitated by the growth in insurance coverage have reduced the historical dependence of demand for health care on income.

Further, elasticity coefficients derived from survey data probably understate the responsiveness of demand to changes in income. The permanent income hypothesis suggests that consumers adjust consumption not only to current income but to previous earnings and, in particular, to previous peak income. Further, the actual or reported income of a given period consists of the sum of permanent and transitory components. Available evidence indicates that permanent consumption is determined by permanent income and that consumption is neither increased nor decreased in response to transitory changes (Andersen and Benham 1970). Further, it is possible that illness or injury reduces the ability of the individual to perform normal economic roles, resulting in a negative transitory component of reported income. As a consequence, it is likely that the earnings reported by users of health care are less than their permanent income. These observations suggest that the relationship between the demand for medical care and income is understated by studies in which survey data are used to estimate elasticity coefficients.

The Influence of Price

As indicated previously, the rationing function performed by the pricing mechanism is of fundamental importance to the conventional model of consumer behavior. In addition, the elasticity of demand with respect to price is of importance when viewed from a policy perspective. For example, the evaluation of alternate financing mechanisms requires an estimate of the monetary costs for which the funding agency is responsible, a process for which demand elasticities are a necessary ingredient. Normative models of alternate insurance mechanisms developed by Zeckhauser (1970), M. S. Feldstein (1973), and Arrow (1973) depend on the elasticity of demand.

Perhaps the most difficult problem in empirical analysis of demand is the specification and measurement of relevant prices. Ideally, price data employed in these investigations should measure variation in the out-of-pocket expenditures of consumers. Since estimates of these expenditures are seldom available from state or national surveys, stated prices or an average price for the mix of care consumed have been used as surrogates for the charges that are the financial responsibility of the patient. As is well recognized, however, health insurance reduces the effective price of service and, as a result, stated or average charges not only overstate out-of-pocket expenditures but also yield distorted estimates of the price elasticity of demand for health care.

Appearing in Table 3.1 are representative findings concerning the relation between the demand for health care and the price of services. In general, previous results are consistent with expectations derived from the conventional model of consumer behavior and support the contention that the quantity demanded is inversely related to price. These data also indicate that the demand for health services is price inelastic (i.e., the percentage change in demand is less than the percentage change in price).

Recently, a number of analysts have employed the insurance mechanism as a vehicle for estimating net price and the effects of cost sharing on the demand for health care. Among the most prominent of these are studies based on insurance claims, comparisons of individuals with different insurance policies, and the results of natural or controlled experiments. Since the literature that focuses on the insurance mechanism as a vehicle for estimating the elasticity of demand with respect to price is vast, the following is devoted to a brief review of the methods, findings and the strengths and weaknesses of these approaches.

Insurance Claims. Consider first, the use of insurance claims as a source of

Table 3.1
Representative Findings Concerning the Elasticity of Demand with Respect to Price

Source (Year)	Dependent Variable	Coefficient
Cromwell and Mitchell (1986)	Surgical procedures	-.14
McCarthy (1985)	Physician visits	-3.07 to -3.32
Stano (1985)	Physician visits	-.06
Lee and Hadley (1981)	Physician visits	-2.8 to -5.1
Newhouse and Phelps (1976)	Physician visits	-.27
	User/nonuser	-.11
	Physician visits/user	-.16
Phelps (1975)	Physician visits	-.2
Fuchs and Kramer (1972)	Physician visits	-.14
Davis and Russell (1972)	Outpatient visits	-.10
Phelps and Newhouse (1972)	Physician home visits	-.35
	Physician visits	-.14
Feldman and Dowd (1986)	Patients days	-.74 to -.80
	Admissions	-1.1

Study	Measure	Value
Newhouse and Phelps (1976)	Patient days	-.2
Phelps (1975)	Admissions	.033
Davis and Russell (1972)	Patient days	-.32 to -.46
M. Feldstein (1971)	Admissions	-.43
	Patient days	-.67
Rosenthal (1970)	Patient days	-.0 to -.67 (by diagnosis)
Manning et al. (1987)	Admissions	-.14 to -.17
Manning et al. (1987a)	Total expenditures	-.18
Rosett and Huang (1973)	Hospital and physician expenditures	-.35 (20% coinsurance)
		-1.5 (80% coinsurance)
Fuchs and Kramer (1972)	Physician expenditures	-.15 to -.35
Lamberton, Ellington and Spear (1986)	Nursing home utilization	-.76
Henry (1970)	Nursing home utilization	-.51
Chiswick (1976)	Nursing home utilization	-.73 to -2.35

data for estimating the elasticity of demand. Typically, these studies employ coinsurance and deductible rates as a surrogate for net price. Focusing on expenditures for hospital and physician services, expenditures for hospital care and expenditures for dental services, previous analyses have examined the responsiveness of demand to differences in coinsurance rates and deductible provisions. Results reported by Phelps and Newhouse (1974) suggest that a reduction in the coinsurance rate from 25 to 10 percent increased the demand for physician and hospital care by 6 percent. Similar results are reported by Freiberg and Scutchfield (1976) who concluded that a reduction in the out-of-pocket expenditures per day of hospital care, resulting from a decline in the coinsurance rate from 50 percent to approximately zero, increased admissions by 50 percent. Consistent with these results are the conclusions advanced by Phelps and Newhouse (1974) who found that an increase of 30 percent in the demand for dental care was associated with a 20 percent decline in the coinsurance rate. Accordingly, these results are consistent with traditional expectations and indicate that, as out-of-pocket expenditures decrease, the demand for health services increases.

Perhaps the major advantage of using insurance claims to develop a surrogate for out-of-pocket expenditures is the precision with which changes in the coinsurance rate are measured. In addition, Newhouse (1981) argues that, since the data pertain to individuals associated with a single employer, the nature of the benefit package and the coinsurance rate are exogenous, implying that the problem of adverse selection is minimal.

Unfortunately, the use of insurance claims as a source of data is accompanied by several disadvantages. First, information derived from insurance claims rarely depicts the individual's actual or perceived health status, previous medical history and other factors, such as educational attainment, access to care or the usual source of care, each of which is believed to influence the preference for health services. Second, these data fail to measure the use of those services that are not insured benefits, thus preventing an assessment of cross-price elasticities.

Natural Experiments. In addition to insurance claims, a number of studies employed natural experiments to compare the use of service before and after a change in the extent of cost sharing. For example, Scheffler (1984) examined changes in the use of hospital and physician care that were attributed, in part, to the introduction of a cost-sharing program for active and retired coal miners. Implemented on July 1, 1977, the program involved a $250 inpatient deductible, a maximum annual financial liability of $500 per family, and a 40 percent coinsurance rate that applied to physician and other sources of outpatient care. Prior to the introduction of these cost-sharing arrangements, the United Mine Workers of America (UMW) Health and Retirement Fund offered first-dollar coverage with no limit imposed on family expenditures.

The study compared the utilization experience of 2,600 families during the baseline period, which was defined as the five months prior to the introduction of cost sharing, with use during a five-month period following the imposition of the coinsurance and deductible provisions. Scheffler employed a two-stage approach in which the first assessed the influence of cost sharing on the likelihood of experiencing an episode of hospitalization or a physician visit. The second focused on users of service and investigated the influence of cost sharing on hospital expenditures, the length of stay, expenditures on physician care, and the number of visits.

The results were consistent with expectations and suggested that the imposition of cost sharing reduced the likelihood of experiencing an episode of hospitalization by 38 percent and the probability of a physician visit by 28 percent. Even though the cost-sharing program increased the length of stay, the results suggested that those who used physician care consumed 28.4 percent fewer visits and lowered their expenditures by 38 percent. Based on these findings, Scheffler (1984, p. 247) concluded that "behavioral adjustments to cost sharing are fairly rapid and long lasting."

Three factors that might confound the results were identified by Scheffler. First, beneficiaries of the program may have believed that the imposition of cost sharing was temporary, a factor that may have depressed use relative to the period in which comprehensive coverage was provided. Also reducing use were the unusually inclement conditions that prevailed during the period of cost sharing. Finally, results may have been confounded by methods of compensating providers before and after the imposition of cost sharing. Prior to the imposition of cost sharing, 30 percent of the providers were compensated on a retainer basis. Concurrent with the imposition of the cost-sharing program, the fee-for-service mechanism was used to compensate all physicians, an outcome that may increase use.

Roddy, Wallen, and Meyers (1986) extended the initial analysis of the UMW experience and compared the utilization of retired beneficiaries of the fund during the first and second year of copayment with the baseline period of complete coverage (January 1977 to July 1977). Contrary to the expectations expressed by Scheffler, the response to the imposition of cost sharing was temporary. Roddy et al. found that the initial decline in use was reversed as the visit rate and hospitalizations returned to baseline levels during the second year of co-payment.

Employing a similar methodological approach, Scitovsky and McCall (1977) examined the demand for physician care by Stanford University employees before and after the coinsurance rate increased from zero to 25 percent. The results indicated that the increase in the coinsurance rate reduced the number of visits by 25 percent, a decline that persisted four years after the adjustment. In an earlier study, Roemer, Hopkins, Carr, and Gartside (1975) found that a $1 copayment for the use of physician care by recipients of the California Medicaid program reduced the number of visits but increased the use of hospital care and total expenditures. That a change in the coinsurance rate evokes a response in demand that is consistent with the normative economic model has also been documented by Heaney and Riedel (1970), who focused on hospital use, and by Morehead, Donaldson, and Zanes (1971) who examined the demand for medical care.

Experimental Studies. Closely related to studies that rely on natural experiments are those that are based on controlled experiments. Perhaps the most ambitious of these is the Rand Health Insurance Experiment, which was designed to avoid the bias that results from the treatment of insurance as an exogenous variable in cross-sectional studies of the demand elasticity with respect to price. Biased selection occurs when those who anticipate higher medical expenditures select more comprehensive coverage, while more comprehensive coverage induces the individual to increase spending on medical care, an outcome that results from moral hazard.

In addition to deriving a more precise estimate of the responsiveness of demand to insurance coverage, the study was designed to examine not only differences in the demand response among the poor and nonpoor but also the variation in coinsurance elasticities among various types of medical care. A third major objective was to assess the effects of changes in the consumption of medical services on the health status of participants in the experiment. Discussed in Chapter 11, the Rand Health Insurance Experiment also sought to disaggregate the effects of favorable selection from those of efficiency on the relatively low costs in HMOs.

As described by Newhouse, Manning, Morris et al. (1981) and Manning, Newhouse, Duan, Keeler et al. (1987a), families participating in the experiment were assigned to one of 14 different fee-for-service insurance plans or to a prepaid group practice. The fee-for-service plans differed in terms of the coinsurance rate (0, 25, 50 and 95 percent) and the maximum expenditure the family might incur during a given year. One of the plans financed all inpatient services but featured a 95 percent coinsurance rate for outpatient services, subject to an annual limit on out-of-pocket expenditures of $150 per person or $450 per family. Hence, the cost sharing was limited to an individual deductible for outpatient services.

Based on 20 characteristics, the Finite Selection Model was used to assign families to one of the plans. The approach was employed so as to ensure that the distribution of participants among the plans was as similar as possible and that families were assigned randomly. Excluded from the experiment were (1) those who were 62 years of age or older, (2) the disabled who were eligible for Medicare benefits, (3) those earning an income in excess of $58,000, measured in 1984 dollars, (4) those who were in military service and their dependents, (5) those who were institutionalized, and (6) veterans with service-connected disabilities. Accordingly, the extent to which the results of the experiment are generalizable to the entire population is reduced by the exclusion of these groups, particularly the elderly.

Based on the initial 40 percent of the data, which represented the experience of 2,756 families, interim results supported several conclusions that are consistent with the traditional economic model. As reported by Newhouse et al. (1981), findings indicated that per capita expenditures by participants who were subject to a coinsurance rate of 95 percent were 50 percent lower than those of families assigned to the plan with no cost sharing. These differences were attributed to variations in the quantity of care consumed rather than to a systematic dependence of the price per visit on the attributes of the various options. These findings indicate that increases in the coinsurance rate reduce the quantity of care consumed and that higher coinsurance rates induced a decline in not only the probability of experiencing at least one episode of hospitalization and one physician visit but also the number of visits consumed by the individual.

Although participants in the deductible plan used less inpatient care than their counterparts on the free plan, the costs per hospitalized participant were found, in general, to be independent of differences in the various policies. Hence, the interim results were consistent, in large part, with expectations derived from traditional theory.

Recently, Manning et al. (1987a) and Lohr, Brook, Kamberg, Goldberg et al. (1986) reported a more complete set of findings concerning the response of demand to various cost sharing arrangements. Manning et al. focused primarily on estimates of the main effects exerted by insurance coverage on the probability of using medical services, the probability of at least one admission and the annual medical expenditures of those who consumed service. Employing the individual as the unit of analysis, the first equation employed probit analysis to estimate the likelihood that the participant will receive care from either an inpatient or outpatient source. Focusing on areas of medical care, the second was also a probit equation depicting the probability that the individual will experience at least one episode of hospitalization. The third equation focused on the logarithmic transformation of annual medical expenses among the users of care.

Lohr et al. (1986) performed a disaggregated analysis of the effects exerted by cost sharing on the use of outpatient care. This analysis examined the influence of cost sharing on (1) the probability of an episode of care, by diagnosis; (2) the use of specific components of care, grouped by relative effectiveness; and (3) the use of selected drugs and procedures. The major objective was to assess the effects of cost sharing on these dimensions of demand by subgroups defined primarily in terms of age and income. With the exception of the findings pertaining to the use of drugs and procedures, the investigation focused on an episode of care that was constructed from treatment history codes and specific time spans between consecutive visits for a given diagnosis. The episodes of use were defined in terms of well care, acute conditions, chronic conditions, and those that could be either chronic or acute. The following focuses on the aggregate results reported by Manning et al. (1987a), and is supplemented with a discussion of the more detailed findings described by Lohr et al. (1986).

The findings reported by Manning et al. indicated that the probabilities of medical service use by those subjected to a coinsurance rate of 0, 25, 50 and 95 percent were .87, .79, .74, and .68 respectively. When contrasted with the likelihood associated with the free plan, the differences were statistically significant, with t-values ranging from -6.33 to -11.57. Accordingly, these results are consistent with the view that, as the coinsurance rate increases, the propensity to use medical service declines.

Focusing on the effects of cost sharing on demand by subgroups, the analysis revealed that higher coinsurance rates were accompanied by a significant decline in the likelihood of children and adults demanding service from inpatient or outpatient sources. As expected, holding the attributes of plan coverage constant, the likelihood of demanding service increased with rising income; however, as Manning et al. note, these differences were influenced by the dependence of the family's maximum expenditures on income. An assessment of the difference indicated that the partial effects of income on the propensity to use service were small, significant, and dominated by other factors correlated with family earnings (Manning et al. 1987b).

The likelihood of experiencing at least one hospital admission also exhibited an inverse relation to the coinsurance rate. The probability of at least one episode of hospitalization declined from .10, which was associated with participants in the free plan, to approximately .08, a likelihood that pertained to those enrolled in the plan that featured a coinsurance rate of 95 percent. When contrasted with the free plan, coinsurance rates of 25, 50 and 95 percent significantly reduced the likelihood of use, as evidenced by t-ratios that ranged from -4.8 to -2.7.

The data also suggested that, among those participants in plans characterized by coinsurance rates of 25, 50 and 95 percent, the likelihood of at least one hospital episode declined with rising income. Family income however, failed to exert a significant effect on the likelihood of using inpatient care by those who were assigned to the free or deductible options.

Results reported by Manning et al. (1987a) indicated that cost sharing exerted an insignificant effect on the probability of using inpatient services. In an analysis of a subset of the data, however, the admission rate and the probability of at least one hospital episode appeared to be plan-sensitive. Similarly, when compared to the free plan, the admissions rate and the probability of using inpatient services among adults declined with rising coinsurance rates (Newhouse et al. 1981; Leibowitz et al. 1985; Manning et al. 1987a).

Consistent with expectations, annual medical expenditures, measured in 1984 dollars, ranged from $777 among those enrolled in the free plan, to $534 for participants in the plan characterized by 95 percent coinsurance rate. When contrasted with the free plan, increases in the coinsurance rate were found to exert a significant reduction in spending. A similar pattern of spending among children and adults was observed, while annual medical expenditures exhibited a *U-shaped* relation with income.

For purposes of comparison, Manning et al. (1987a) computed arc elasticities, using average and "pure" coinsurance rates. The latter approach focuses on the episode of care and assumes that, among those who have not exceeded the maximum expenditure, marginal spending on medical care is influenced by the nominal price, discounted by the probability of exceeding the deductible (Keeler, Newhouse, and Phelps 1977; Ellis 1986). The pure coinsurance elasticities were based on episodes of care among those whose spending was $400 or more below their maximum and were assumed to assign a value of near zero to the probability of exceeding the upper limit.

Elasticities based on pure coinsurance rates were calculated for acute, chronic, and well care episodes of use. The results indicated that arc elasticities were slightly higher in the 0 to 25 percent range than in the 25 to 95 percent range of cost sharing. For all components of care, elasticities were $-.17$ for coinsurance rates in the 0 to 25 percent range and $-.22$ for the 25 to 95 percent range. Arc elasticities, based on average coinsurance rates, ranged from $-.2$, a value calculated for 0–16 percent and all components of care, to $-.21$ which pertains to coinsurance rates of 16 to 31 percent and the use of outpatient services.

Consider next the results of the detailed analysis reported by Lohr et al. (1986) and Manning et al. (1984, 1986a, 1986b). As indicated previously, Lohr et al. focused on the use of outpatient services and, with the exception of drugs and procedures, used the episode of treatment as the unit of analysis. Similar to the results reported by Manning et al., Lohr et al. found that, when compared to the free plan, cost sharing reduced the probability that participants would seek care for acute conditions (i.e., those that are unforeseen and treatment is not deferrable), well care, and chronic conditions. The decline appeared to be greater for chronic conditions than other categories analyzed. The percentage reductions that were attributed to cost sharing were larger among poor adults for 11 of 13 diagnostic categories and among poor children for 10 of the 11 groups. Although cost sharing reduced the likelihood of an episode of treatment, the deterrent effect was found to be greatest among the children of the poor.

Lohr et al. also examined the effects of cost sharing on an episode of care, grouped in terms of relative effectiveness. Diagnoses were assigned to seven groups that were defined in terms of varying degrees of the predicted effectiveness of medical care. An iterative ranking process that involved the participation of physicians at Rand was used to form the groups.

Relative to the free plan, cost sharing was found to reduce the likelihood of seeking treatment but failed to discriminate among the various degrees of effectiveness. The findings suggested that the reduction in the probability of using outpatient care was larger among the poor than their wealthier counterparts. Of potential concern is the conclusion that the effects of cost sharing were greatest among the poor children, and, in particular, in their use of effective treatment for acute conditions.

Focusing on seven categories of procedures provided by outpatient sources and 24 categories of prescribed medications, the analysis suggested that the probability of using prescribed medications and most of the procedures was lower among adults who participated in cost-sharing arrangements than their counterparts enrolled in the free plan. Similar to previous findings, poor adults who participated in the free and cost-sharing plans were less likely to use these components of care than their wealthier counterparts. These results were particularly dramatic for standard tests employed in response to acute or chronic conditions. Although children rarely used many of the prescribed medications, cost sharing reduced their consumption, and the effect was, once again, pronounced among the poor. Similar results pertaining to the use of outpatient procedures by all children and children of the poor were reported by Lohr et al.

Manning, Wells, Duan, Newhouse, and Ware (1984); Ware, Manning, Duan, Wells, and Newhouse (1984); and Wells, Manning, Duan, Newhouse, and Ware (1987) also used data derived from the Rand Health Insurance Experiment to examine the influence of cost sharing on the demand for mental health service. Focusing on expenditures on mental health services provided in an ambulatory setting, Manning et al. found that lower coinsurance rates significantly increased expenditures. Most of the response in spending to variation in cost sharing was traceable to the probability of using service. For example, participants in the free plan were twice as likely to use mental health care as those who were enrolled in the plan featuring a 95 percent coinsurance rate.

Similar results are reported by Manning, Bailit, Benjamin, and Newhouse (1985), who examined the effects of cost sharing on the demand for dental care. The study separated "transitory" from steady state demand and found that, after the initial effects of cost sharing were dissipated, expenditures and the use of dental care were increased significantly by lower coinsurance rates. In addition, it was estimated that approximately two-thirds of the response to cost sharing was in the probability of any use. Concerning the assessment of the transitory changes in demand, the study indicated that the increase in spending per enrollee between the free and 95 percent plans was approximately twice as large in the first as in the second year. Temporary changes were also observed in the plans featuring intermediate coinsurance rates.

Given the findings concerning the effects of cost sharing on the likelihood of use, it is conceivable that higher coinsurance rates might indirectly exert an adverse effect on health status. Using data collected prior to the Health Insurance Experiment and after its conclusion, the Rand researchers compared the health status of experimental subjects who were assigned to the free-care plans against that of the subjects who were assigned to plans that contained cost-sharing provisions (Brook, Ware, Rogers 1983). Their analysis of the entire sample suggested that free care had no effect for the average enrollee on any of five general self-assessed measures of health. In the analysis of the subgroup of individuals who entered the experiment with a below average health status, however, the researchers found that the health status of individuals with myopia and hypertension was positively associated with assignment to the free-care plan.

In a related paper, Keeler, Sloss, Brook, Operskalski, Goldberg, and Newhouse (1987) extended the earlier study and focused on an additional 20 measures of health status and 9 measures of health practice. The results indicated that those subject to cost sharing scored better on 12 measures and worse on one. Further, the analysis supported the conclusion that, with the exception of hypertension or vision problems, "the effects of cost sharing on health were minor" (Keeler et al. 1987, p. 279). It is important to note that the path of causality leading from free care to increased utilization to improved health status was not examined. As a consequence, it was not possible to determine "whether higher use by persons with free care reflects overuse or whether lower use by those with income-related catastrophic coverage reflects under-use" (Newhouse et al. 1981, p. 1501).

Insurance Coverage. The influence of variation in the coinsurance rate on the demand for health care has also been examined by comparing the use of service by individuals or households with different insurance policies. Based on surveys or area averages, these studies combine price and demand data with other factors that influence the preference for health care and estimate elasticities with respect to the coinsurance rate. As shown in Table 3.1, these studies report estimates that exhibit considerable variation. Among the highest estimates are those found by Rosett and Huang (1973), who estimated elasticities of approximately $-.35$ associated with a coinsurance rate of .2 and -1.5 at a rate of 80 percent. The estimates of approximately $-.1$ found by Newhouse, Phelps, and Marquis (1980) are consistent with elasticities of demand reported in studies that employ alternate methods.

The comparability of results reported in studies that examine the effects of differences in insurance coverage on demand is reduced by several factors. Perhaps the most important of these is the wide variation in insured benefits and other dimensions, a factor that prevents a complete classification of differences in coverage. As suggested by Newhouse (1970, 1981), however, average coinsurance rates, which are commonly used to estimate elasticities, frequently result in biased and inconsistent coefficients. Similarly, imprecise information concerning out-of-pocket expenditures has forced analysts to estimate price by the ratio of expenditures to the quantity demanded. As is well known, however, errors in measuring the amount consumed frequently result in biased and inconsistent estimates of the elasticity of demand with respect to price.

In addition to the effects of variation in the price of a given service and the demand for that component of care, the traditional model of consumer behavior implies that a change in relative prices induces the individual to substitute less expensive services for more costly ones. Evidence reported by Davis and Russell (1972) suggests that a percentage change in the price of inpatient care induces an approximately equal percentage increase in the demand for outpatient visits. Similarly, the regression estimates developed by Davis and Russell indicate that a one percent increase in the price of outpatient care results in a .25 percent increase in hospital admissions. In addition to confirming the results of Davis and Russell, Gold (1984) concluded that the demand for outpatient services is related to the availability and the price of other sources of care (e.g., primary-care physician, specialty physicians, or inpatient services), insurance coverage, per capita income, and a set of demographic variables. Thus, in addition to supporting the expectation that price exerts a negative impact on demand, the results are consistent with the expectation that an increase in the relative price of hospitalization results in a substitution of outpatient for inpatient care.

BEHAVIORAL MODEL OF DEMAND

The behavioral model developed by Andersen (1968) is an extension of the traditional theory of consumer behavior and provides a framework for assessing the influence of economic variables and other factors that influence the preference for health care. The conceptual approach relates the decision to use health care to predisposing, enabling, and need components. Concerning the first, a predisposition to consult a physician is assumed to exist prior to the perception of illness or the recognition of one or more symptoms. As such, the predisposition to such care is influenced by demographic and social-structural variables such as age, sex, marital status, family or household composition, and residence, as well as by beliefs or attitudes concerning illness and the efficacy of medical care. The model further assumes that the enabling component either facilitates or impedes the use of service by those who are predisposed to such care. The enabling factors represent not only financial resources of the individual, such as income, personal assets, and insurance coverage, but also the availability and accessibility of health services.

As posited by Andersen and Newman (1973), the final component consists of two types of health need. The first refers to the individual's perception of differences between actual and desired health status. Commonly used measures of perceived or self-reported need are the number of days of restricted or limited activity resulting from disease or injury, the number of reported symptoms, and the individual's evaluation of his or her general health status. The second type of need, defined by professional medical opinion, refers to the extent that self-reported symptoms should precipitate care-seeking behavior.

The conceptual approach developed by Andersen has been used extensively in studies of health behavior. Among the predisposing factors, age is probably the most important determinant of health services use. Although several studies suggest that age is not an important predictor of physician use (Hershey, Luft, and Gianaris 1975; Kennedy 1979; Leavitt 1979), the weight of evidence supports the contention that the relation between use and age is curvilinear (see, for example, Broyles, Manga, Binder, Angus, and Charette 1983; Manga, Broyles, and Angus 1987; Aday and Andersen 1975; Andersen, Lion, and Anderson 1976; Colle and Grossman 1978; Aday, Andersen, and Fleming 1980). In particular, relative to other population groups, the prevalence of chronic and acute disease among the elderly and young respectively results in a greater use of health services. For example, the young and elderly not only are more likely to visit a physician but also consume a greater volume of care than other members of society. Similarly, rates of admission and the length of stay also increase with advancing age. It is important to note, however, that the observed relation between age and utilization behavior is probably attributable to the differential prevalence of morbidity among the elderly and young. In fact, when measures of health status are included in multivariate analyses of use, the effect of age is diminished. That the observed relation between use and age is attributable to morbidity was also indicated by results reported by Andersen and Aday (1978), who used ordinary least squares regression to develop a path model. Although no significant direct influence was found, the analysis revealed that age exerted an indirect effect on use through illness and need surrogates.

Concerning the other predisposing variables, previous findings suggest that females use more service than their male counterparts (Aday and Andersen 1975; Andersen et al. 1976; Chamberlain and Drui 1975; Kennedy 1979). Although differences are attributable, in part, to obstetrical needs, women use more service relative to health status. Specifically, previous findings suggest that females are more likely to visit a physician and consume more ambulatory care than males. Although males tend to experience longer episodes of hospitalization, admission and discharge rates are higher among females (Andersen et al. 1976; Ferguson, Lee, and Wallace 1976; Aday et al. 1980; Haupt 1980).

Closely related to the effects of age, sex, and morbidity are those exerted by marital status, family composition, and social structural factors on utilization behavior. For example, those who have never married consume the lowest number of physician visits and are least likely to experience an episode of hospitalization, while the consumption of ambulatory care and the likelihood of experiencing an episode of hospitalization are highest among those who were formerly married. Although findings concerning family size are mixed, previous studies suggest that those living alone consume more physician services, are more likely to report multiple episodes of hospitalization, and experience longer lengths of stay than other members of society.

Attitudes concerning illness and beliefs regarding the efficacy of medical care have been found to exert inconsistent effects on utilization behavior. For example, positive beliefs concerning the efficacy of medical care, higher levels of family concern regarding health matters, and a positive attitude toward physicians seem to increase the use of ambulatory care, particularly preventive services (Kravits 1975; Becker, Nathanson, Drachman, and Kirscht 1977; Berki and Ashcraft 1979). Conversely, other studies report findings that suggest that these factors exert little, if any, influence on the use of health services (Anderson and Eggers 1976; Kirscht, Becker, and Eveland 1976; Colle and Grossman 1978).

Consider next the effects of the enabling component on utilization behavior. Socioeconomic status—a combination of income, education, and occupation—clearly exerts an effect on the use of physician care. In general, socioeconomic status is positively associated with the use of physician care and, in particular, preventive services. Consistent with results summarized in the previous section, wealthier members of society are more likely to visit a physician than are the poor. Although differences in the volume of physician care used by the poor and nonpoor have been reduced, the less wealthy use fewer services relative to their medical needs than their wealthier counterparts. With respect to the use of hospital care, previous studies suggest that the admission rate and length of stay are higher among the poor than the nonpoor, an outcome that is probably attributable to the moderating effects of publicly funded programs that reduce the net price of these services.

As posited by the behavioral model, the availability and accessibility of health care represent enabling variables that influence utilization. On the assumption that health resources are more plentiful in urban than in rural areas, place of residence is frequently used as a surrogate for the availability of care. Previous studies (Aday and Andersen 1975; Andersen et al. 1976; Aday et al. 1980) suggest that the likelihood of visiting a physician and the volume of ambulatory care consumed are greater among residents of SMSAs and other urban centers than among those living in rural areas. Conversely, Long (1981) assessed the effects of residential location on the use of inpatient hospital care. These results suggest that consumer location is a better proxy for sociodemographic, economic, and need variables than for the availability of health resources. The availability of health resources, as measured by the physician–bed population ratio and bed population ratio, have been shown to increase the likelihood of contacting a provider and the volume of care consumed. In addition, those reporting a regular source of service are not only more likely to contact a physician and experience an episode of hospitalization but also consume more physician care and preventive services than individuals lacking a regular source of care.

Perhaps the most consistent and important correlate of utilization behavior is health status or medical need. Commonly used surrogates for medical need are reported symptoms, chronic conditions, acute conditions, chronic limitations, disability days, severity of condition, and episodes of illness. In general, the measures of health status and medical need are the most important determinants of the propensity to use service and the volume of care consumed. More specifically, results reported by Stoller (1982) suggest that need factors are more important determinants of the volume of care consumed by the elderly than the likelihood of an initial physician contact. Focusing on five narrowly defined diagnoses, Goldfarb, Hornbrook, and Higgins (1983) found that measures of case severity were among the most important and consistent determinants of the length of stay and the use of ancillary services. Similarly, Becker and Sloan (1983) report findings that confirm the expectation that the use of inpatient care is significantly influenced by case mix while Becker and Steinwald (1981) documented the importance of diagnostic mix in explaining differences in the use and costs of care provided by teaching and nonteaching hospitals.

As suggested by Newhouse (1981), however, the observed relationship between health status and utilization behavior may represent reverse causation. Previous research frequently relies on data derived from a household survey that contains information depicting health status at the time of the interview, measures of medical need during the past year, and the use of service over the past 12 months. Obviously, relating use during the past 12 months to health status at the time of the interview violates the conditions that must be satisfied in order to demonstrate causality. Further, it is possible that previous contact may modify reported perceptions of health status, resulting in inconsistent and biased regression estimates of the relation between medical need and use.

In addition to the concerns expressed by Newhouse, the results reported by Wolinsky (1981) suggest that the predisposing and enabling components were unrelated to the use of physician care. These data also seem to imply that the conceptual support for these variables has changed over time and that these components are unstable predictors of use. Apart from source of payment, Shortell (1975) also found that provider characteristics and pattern of care variables are more important determinants of utilization behavior than the predisposing and the other enabling variables. Also documenting the importance of provider characteristics in explaining the variation in the use of ambulatory care are the results reported by Kronenfield (1980). Consistent with these findings, the behavioral model might be revised so as to emphasize the role of characteristics and incentives that are specific to the provider in determining use, an issue that is discussed later in this chapter.

INVESTMENT MODEL OF DEMAND

Initially developed by Grossman (1972), the investment model of demand regards health as a capital good that is inherited and depreciates or deteriorates over time. The theory suggests further that investment in health is a process in which medical care is combined with other factors to produce new health, thus offsetting, in part, the deterioration in the stock of health. When viewed from the perspective of the investment model, the demand for medical care is derived from a demand for new health that in turn is related to two benefits. The first is a consumption benefit and corresponds to the effects of improved health on utility (e.g., relief of pain or discomfort). Hence, the consumption benefits of improved health are represented by increases in utility derived from a decline in sick time. The second desirable aspect of improved health is an investment benefit and is derived from an increased amount of healthy time that enables the individual to engage in activities such as work, leisure, or consumption, to include the use of medical care, and to improve the capacity to perform necessary tasks.

The major implications of the investment model are threefold. The first involves the specification of the effects exerted by age on the demand for health and medical care. As suggested by Muurinen (1982), a change in the stock of health occurs if the gross investment in health differs from the deterioration in the stock. Further, the rate of depreciation in health is a function of age and a set of exogenous variables, such as environmental, occupational, or life-style factors, that might adversely affect health status. Thus, age is posited to exert an effect on the demand for health and medical care through the age-specific component of depreciation. In particular, it is assumed that advancing age is accompanied by increases in the rate of depreciation in the stock of health. Further, the model posits that gross increases in investment are dependent on not only the use of medical care but also the productivity of these services in producing health. For example, Grossman found that the elasticity of health with respect to medical care varies between .1 and .3. In general, it is plausible to argue that the productivity of medical care in producing health probably declines during later stages of the life cycle, thus requiring an increased use of service in order to produce a given increment in new health. Hence, the model suggests that, in order to compensate for increases in the rate of depreciation and declines in the productivity of medical care, consumers increase their expenditures on, and their use of, medical care during their life cycles.

The second implication involves the effects of education and other exogenous factors on the demand for health and medical care. As suggested previously, the model initially proposed by Grossman posits that medical services are combined with other inputs, which the individual supplies, to produce health. Grossman argues that education increases health productivity, implying that the better educated are more skillful in combining inputs to produce health. Thus, if the price elasticity with respect to health is less than one, education diminishes the demand for medical care. Results reported by Acton (1975) suggest that the net change in the use of ambulatory services produced by increasing education is negative, thus supporting expectations derived from Grossman's model.

As modified by Muurinen, the investment model suggests that educational attainment, among other factors, influences the rate of deterioration in health. Rather than increasing the nonmarket productivity of the individual, Muurinen argues that education operates on a more aggregate level and redirects the choice of production processes, resulting in a life style that is less use-intensive in terms of health. Among the major advantages of the approach is the increased potential for assessing the influence of environmental and occupational factors on the deterioration in health and, hence, on the demand for medical care. For example, Cropper (1977) developed a model in which investment in health during the life cycle is assessed in terms of occupational choice and exposure to hazards in the workplace. Similarly, Ippolito (1981) examined the optimal age profiles of consuming goods that are hazardous to health.

The third implication of the investment model involves a more precise specification of influence exerted by wage and nonwage income on the demand for medical care. In general, the theory suggests that, as wages increase, the value of time devoted to the consumption of medical services and the value of additional healthy time or reductions in sick time rise. It is possible that a consumer earning a high-wage rate will substitute the use of medical services for his or her own time when producing health. As a consequence, the model posits a positive relation between wage rates and expenditures on medical care.

The importance of the exogenous factors and income on the demand for health and medical services has been explored empirically. For example, Auster, Leveson, and Saracheck (1969) investigated the relationship between health, as measured by mortality, medical care expenditures, and a set of "environmental factors" including income and education. The results indicated that the elasticity of health with respect to the consumption of medical services was approximately − .1 (i.e., a 1 percent increase in the consumption of medical care reduced mortality by .1 percent). Although educational attainment was twice as effective as medical care in producing health, income exhibited a positive relationship with mortality. Employing mortality and sick time as indicators of health, Grossman (1972) also reported negative income elasticities with regard to health even though the elasticity of income with respect to medical care was positive.

The findings regarding the influence of income on health are probably attributable to life style or occupational factors. For example, rising income may be associated with consuming adverse diets, purchasing faster cars, and engaging in less exercise. Conversely, in order to obtain a higher income, it may be necessary to engage in occupations characterized by more strain, higher stress, and greater exposure to risks that result in illness or injury. Thus, it is possible that, after some level, the detrimental effects of income on health production exceed the beneficial effects, resulting in an inverted- U relation between health and income.

A related issue involves the effects of opportunity costs on the use of medical services. As suggested by Grossman, health investment is produced by the use of medical care and own-time as measured by the wage rate. Further, the initial specification implicitly assumed that time and medical care are equally effective in producing health, a feature that ignores the amount of time required per unit of service. In this regard it is possible to define the total price of medical care as the sum of the time-and-money price of securing services. As suggested by Acton (1975), and by Phelps and Newhouse (1974), a reduction in out-of-pocket expenditure, holding the monetary value of travel and waiting time constant, is expected to increase the sensitivity of demand to changes in time prices. Similarly, it is expected that as time prices decline, observed elasticities of demand with respect to money prices should rise.

Empirical results reported by Acton (1975), Phelps and Newhouse (1974), Salkever (1976), Inman (1976), Luft, Hershey, and Morrell (1976) and Taylor, Wilensky, and Rossiter (1981) are consistent with these expectations. Similarly, Coffey (1983) reports findings that support the contention that the time price of using medical care reduces the probability of seeking service but exerts virtually no effect on the number of visits consumed during the year. That time prices exert a significant influence on the demand for medical care is also documented by findings reported by Dor, Gertler, and van der Gaag (1987), Cauley (1987), Colle and Grossman (1978) and Van de Ven and van der Gaag (1982). As a consequence, it is possible to encounter a situation in which the quantity of health demanded is reduced while the quantity of health services demanded is increased. The first of these outcomes might be attributable to a rising cost of an incremental unit of health as income and the importance of the accompanying detrimental effects are increased while the second is traceable to declines in the money cost of medical care relative to travel or waiting time as wage rates rise.

In perhaps the most complete empirical treatment to date, Wagstaff (1986) employed data assembled in the Danish Welfare Survey of 1976 to estimate the parameters of the consumption and investment components of the model proposed by Grossman. For both submodels, the study derived estimates of a reduced form and a recursive equation system in which health capital was regarded as a latent variable. Since results derived for the two submodels were similar, the following focuses, in general, on estimates derived for the investment component of Grossman's model.

Employed as measures of utilization were the number of physician visits, the number of days respondents remained in a general hospital, and the number of complaints for which the respondent used medication. Indicators that were used to derive a surrogate for health reflected the degree of mobility, mental disorders, respiratory problems, and pain, while sex, the age composition of the respondent's family, marital status, and location of residence served to reflect use-related depreciation. In addition, the work environment, including exposure to hazardous substances, physical stress, temperature and mental stress, was also used to measure use-related depreciation. Further, recognizing that user charges are nonexistent in the Danish health system, the hourly wage rate and foregone earnings resulting from utilization were used to measure time cost while availability was indicated by the physician and bed per 1000 rates.

Concerning the results derived for the investment model, reduced form estimates of the demand for medical care were generally consistent with expectations. However, only a few significant coefficients were reported. For example, education, measured by the number of years of schooling, was significant and negative in the examination of physician visits, suggesting that education improves nonmarket productivity. Further, none of the time cost variables differed significantly from zero. Concerning the measures of use-related depreciation, all coefficients relating age to use were positive, and two were significant, an outcome that was consistent with results reported by Grossman. Similarly, the coefficients on measures of the work environment were positive and two were significant. However, coefficients on the other use-related depreciation variables were less consistent with expectations.

Employing maximum likelihood procedures, the structural model focused on the demand for health and medical care. Linking health capital to the set of health indicators, the variable HEALTH indicated an increasingly good health status. Although the results pertaining to the demand for health were consistent with the reduced form specification of the demand for medical care, several estimates of the parameters of the recursive system were inconsistent with the investment model. Of importance in this regard are estimates that implied that the elasticity of the marginal efficiency of capital schedule is negative. In addition, the results of the recursive systems were also inconsistent with the hypothesis concerning use-related depreciation and the expectation that demand is derived from differences between the actual and desired health stock. Assuming the elasticity of demand for health capital is positive, the hypothesis concerning use-related depreciation suggests that the coefficients on health damaging variables should be positive and those for factors that promote health ought to be negative. However, 10 of the 14 coefficients on the variables depicting use-related depreciation were of the "wrong" sign. As suggested by Wagstaff, these unexpected results may be attributable to the gestation period between exposure to risk and the resultant influence on the depreciation rate. Consistent with the derived demand hypothesis, individuals are expected to increase consumption when the actual stock of health is less than the desired stock, suggesting that coefficients on the HEALTH variable should be positive. These estimates were negative and significant, however, in the structural model of demand for all components of care.

Results that were inconsistent with expectations regarding the effects of education were also reported. The model proposed by Grossman suggests that the efficiency of producing health improves with education; estimates of the structural model of the demand for care indicated that, in general, the better educated consumed more care than the poorly educated, a result that was attributed to the possibility that the better educated assign a lower marginal benefit to medical care consumption or enjoy a more favorable relationship with their physicians than the poorly educated. The results also documented the difficulty of disentangling the effects of education from those of lifetime wealth on the demand for care.

Perhaps the most striking aspect of the estimates of the consumption component of the model were findings that suggested that the optimal stock of health is dependent on initial assets, stage of the life cycle, and lifetime wages. These results appear to contradict Grossman's model that predicts that health investment decisions are independent of initial wealth. In a related paper Dardanoni and Wagstaff (1987) demonstrate that, when uncertainty is introduced in the model, consumption and investment decisions are determined simultaneously and that the wealthy invest more in health capital than those endowed with a relatively low initial stock of financial capital.

Although contradictory evidence has been reported, the model of demand proposed by Grossman is of importance when viewed from a policy perspective. By focusing on health rather than health services, the model emphasizes the role of environmental, occupational, and life-style factors in determining morbidity and, hence, the use of service. Given the importance of the positive relationship between education and the efficiency of producing health, the model also suggests that the primary focus of public policy should be on the provision of health information rather than health services. Further, the investment theory of demand implies that public policy should be designed to reduce the effects of factors that are detrimental and enhance the influence of those that are beneficial to health status.

SUPPLIER-INDUCED DEMAND

As implied earlier, the neoclassical theory of demand focuses on a sovereign consumer who selects the mix of goods and services that maximizes utility. As such, the conventional model ignores the role of the physician in determining the volume of service consumed. In 1985, spending on physician services comprised less than 20 percent of all expenditures on health care (Waldo, Levit, and Lazenby 1986); however, since physicians dominate decisions concerning admissions, discharges, the use of surgical procedures, and the consumption of ancillary services, Blumberg (1979) estimated that physicians control 70 percent of the total spending on health care. Accordingly, the physician must be regarded as playing an important role in determining the quantity and composition of care provided.

Although most recognize the importance of the provider in the process of determining the mix of care consumed, it is common to assume that the physician acts as a perfect agent for the patient. As suggested previously, empirical studies that are based on the conventional model focus on the characteristics of the patient as determinants of demand and rarely evaluate the effects of the physician's objectives or constraints on utilization behavior.

Among the most compelling reasons for examining the role of the physician in determining the use of care is the difference in the amount of information possessed by providers and patients. Due to the complexity of medical knowledge and technology, it is common to argue that the physician possesses more information concerning alternative modes of treatment and the potential efficacy of each than the patient. Commenting on these disparities, Arrow (1963) notes that the need for medical care is "irregular and unpredictable," that uncertainties concerning quality are more pervasive in the health industry than in other markets, and that recovery from disease or injury is as unpredictable as its incidence. Each of these considerations impairs the ability of the consumer to evaluate alternate sources of care or modes of treatment. Consequently, consumers reach decisions that are based on an inadequate knowledge of the utility of consumption.

Although most markets are characterized by self-corrective mechanisms, the problem of inadequate information is acute in the health industry. As suggested by Richardson (1981), the course of illness or injury, without treatment, is uncertain. Further, homeostasis may occur, which, in turn, prevents patients from comparing their welfare prior to treatment with their welfare without treatment. Since the potential efficacy of alternate modes of treatment is at best uncertain, the informational problem is an impediment to the process of evaluation and the elimination of errors.

The inability of consumers to assess uncertainties concerning the need for care, alternate sources of service, different modes of treatment and the efficacy of each tends to distinguish medical care from other goods and services. With the exception of trivial illnesses, episodes of morbidity are frequently unique to the patient, suggesting that the individual is unable to rely on previous experience as the basis for evaluating alternate courses of action. Although the individual might consult with others concerning the diagnosis and treatment of illness, the experiences of lay patients are also limited and they possess different homeostatic properties. Alternatively, an individual might obtain several medical opinions

Figure 3.2
The Inducement Hypothesis

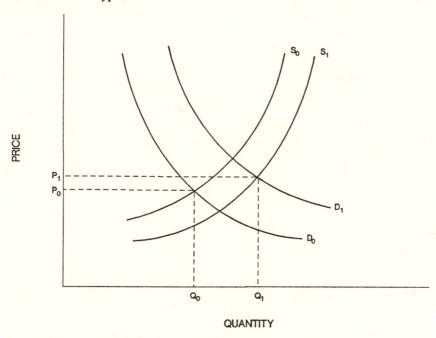

concerning the diagnosis and treatment of illness; however, recognizing that medicine is an inexact science, considerable latitude exists for legitimate differences in professional judgement. In addition to the time and costs of obtaining multiple professional opinions, the individual not only must be aware of the potential advantages of investigation but also must possess the ability to conduct the inquiry and evaluate its results. Since it seems unreasonable to ascribe these idealized attributes to patients, the informational impediment described above suggests that the physician rather than the patient dominates decisions concerning the mix of care consumed.

The conceptual basis for interpreting empirical assessments of the inducement hypothesis may be examined by referring to Figure 3.2. In this figure, it is assumed that the initial supply, demand, price and quantity conditions are represented by S_o, D_o, P_o and Q_o, respectively. Observe that an increase in the number of providers in the market area shifts the supply curve from S_o to S_1, resulting in a reduction in price and an increase in the quantity of care. Assuming that demand is inelastic with respect to price, professional incomes are expected to decline, which induces physicians to exploit consumer ignorance by prescribing additional units of service, resulting in a shift in the demand curve from D_o to D_1. In this case, both price and quantity increase in response to the physician-induced demand. In contrast to the expectation that an increase in supply increases quantity and reduces price, findings that suggest an increase in the supply of physicians is accompanied by an increase in quantity and a constant or rising price are consistent with the demand shift hypothesis.

Perhaps the most contentious issue concerning the inducement hypothesis involves the set of factors that limit the extent to which providers exploit their dominant role in the process of determining the mix of care required by a given patient. As summarized by Phelps (1986), the conceptual approach developed by Dranove (1985) suggests that the severity of the illness limits the aggressiveness of the physician and represents a threshold below which treatment will not be recommended. When viewed from the patient's perspective, the probability of seeking care is dependent on the physician's reputation and is expected to vary inversely with the aggressiveness of the recommended course of treatment. Hence, the model developed by Dranove implies that the demand curve confronting the physician shifts downward and to the left as attempts to induce demand increase.

The expected response to aggressive recommendations and attempts to induce demand is predicated on the assumption that patients are able to detect attempts to induce demand. Mitigating against this assumption is the disparity between the knowledge of the patient and physician; however, second opinions, recommendations of friends, and the joint production of treatment and knowledge may precipitate behavior that is consistent with Dranove's model.

The conceptual framework developed by Farley (1986) not only reconciles the neoclassical model and the target income hypothesis advanced by Evans (1974) but also imposes constraints on physician behavior. The synthesis offered by Farley suggests that the difference between the neoclassical model and the target income hypothesis involves the distribution of income. Concerning the target income hypothesis, an ethical constraint is typically entered in the utility function of the physician as a negative argument, implying that the provider balances the increment in utility resulting from additional income with the disutility of exploiting patients (Evans 1974; Wilensky and Rossiter 1981). Specifications of the hypothesis usually involve the assumption that one value is assigned to the target income, irrespective of the effects on the patient, or that behavior is influenced by a flexible target and a continuous evaluation of the interests of the patient and the physician. Conversely, the market-oriented approach assumes that patients are able to evaluate recommended courses of treatment and that the decision to consume care is determined by the advice offered by the physician.

Farley assumed that the utility function of the physician contains arguments defined by the profits earned from medical practice and the patient's utility function. The model also suggests that profits are maximized for a given level of patient welfare by selecting the quantity of care that equates marginal benefits and marginal costs. Farley also demonstrates that both theories of provider behavior are consistent with the proposition that pricing and prescribing decisions are influenced by the physician's welfare and the welfare of patients. Hence, the distribution of gains between patients and physicians is determined by professional ethics and the constraints imposed by competitive forces.

Although the constraints suggested by Dranove and Farley have not been examined empirically, a number of studies have explored the extent to which physicians exploit their superordinate position in the provider-patient relationship and prescribe excessive service so as to increase personal income. Fuchs and Kramer (1972) used cross-sectional data among states to assess the extent of supplier-induced demand. Holding income, the average price of physician care, insurance coverage, and the number of beds per capita constant, the results indicated that an increase in the supply of physicians resulted in a decrease in the number of visits per physician. The elasticities of supply with respect to the number of physicians per person ranged from $-.49$ to $-.67$ suggesting that the decline in the number of visits per physician precipitated a reduction in the professional income of the average provider. Consistent with the demand shift hypothesis, the results also revealed a positive association between the number of visits per person and the physician-population ratio. Holding the price of physician care constant, elasticities relating the number of visits per person to the physician population ratio were significant ($p \leq .01$) and ranged from .34 to .51. Although of smaller absolute value, elasticities reported by Evans (1974) are also consistent with the demand shift hypothesis and indicate that physicians are able to partially offset decreases in their workloads, which result from an increase in the supply of physicians.

Among the criticisms of the conclusions advanced by Fuchs and Kramer is a failure to explore the effects exerted by an increase in the supply of physicians on the time costs of using care and the possibility that changes in quality might explain the positive association between per capita use and the physician–population ratio. Concerning the first of these, it is likely that an increase in the supply of physicians reduces travel and waiting time, thus diminishing the total price of care (Mueller 1985). Similarly, it is conceivable that an increase in the supply of physicians results in longer visits and an improvement in the quality of care, both of which might increase the use per person. Thus, the total price, to include money and time costs, for a quality adjusted visit might be lower than the observed unadjusted prices that remained constant or increased.

In response to these criticisms, Fuchs (1978) assessed the relation between hospital surgical rates and the supply of surgeons to examine the demand shift hypothesis. The focus on the use of surgical procedures by inpatients addresses the criticisms of the initial study in two ways. First, as Fuchs observes, time costs are less relevant for inpatient operative procedures, since the psychic and time costs of surgery are large relative to the time costs of search, travel, and waiting. Second, a number of studies (Luft, Bunker, and Enthoven 1979; Shortell and LoGerfo 1981; Farber, Kaiser, and Wenzel 1981; Hughes, Hunt, and Luft 1987) found that results improve as the frequency of performing operative procedures increases, which, of course, addresses criticisms regarding the previously ignored effects of changes in quality on utilization behavior. Controlling for demographic factors such as age, sex, education, and ethnicity, the results reported by Fuchs suggest that a 10 percent increase in the surgeon population ratio results in a 3 percent increase in the surgical rate. Further, these results indicate that an increase in supply exerts a perverse effect on price, as evidenced by a positive association between surgical fees and the surgeon population ratio. Newhouse (1970), Reinhardt (1975), Blumberg (1979), and Yang (1986) also found a positive relation between fees and the supply of physicians.

In perhaps the most recent investigation of the inducement hypothesis to date, Cromwell and Mitchell (1986) developed a simultaneous equation model of physician demand and fees for surgery. Endogenous variables included in the analysis were surgical rates for total, elective and nonelective procedures, surgeon-physician ratios, workloads, and average fees. Exogenous factors were represented by a vector of demand characteristics, a vector of variables that influence cost or productivity, and a vector of variables that reflected professional and community amenities.

Employing data assembled in the Health Interview Surveys (HIS) of 1969 through 1976, two-stage least-squares methods were used to examine the inducement hypothesis. In the first stage, the endogenous variables were related to the set of exogenous factors. Their computed values were then used to estimate structural coefficients in the second stage of the analysis. Further, the data derived from the HIS were used to derive regional (defined in terms of SMSAs) and national estimates of parameters depicting physician inducement of demand.

Concerning the national focus of the study, the results indicated that, holding fees and other factors constant, surgeon density exerted a positive and significant effect on both the total and elective surgical rates. Further, surgeon density exhibited a significant and positive association with equilibrium fees. The analysis suggested that a 10 percent increase in physician density resulted in a 1.3 percent increase in elective surgery, a .9 percent increase in the total surgical rate, and a 9 percent increase in the fee per procedure.

In the regional analysis, the model was estimated for three subsamples that were defined as Nonmetropolitan Primary Sampling Units, small SMSAs, and large SMSAs (i.e., those characterized by populations in excess of 500,000). Concerning the nonmetropolitan areas, the analysis indicated that increases in the surgeon density were accompanied by decreases in fees and no discernible inducement of demand. The analysis of large metropolitan areas, however, suggested that surgeon density exhibited a significant and positive association with equilibrium fees. The coefficients relating surgeon density to the total and elective surgical rates were positive but not significant individually; however, when the samples were comingled, the coefficients combined to form a significant effect on use.

Finally, the study examined the approach suggested by Green (1978) who contended that direct estimates of the shift effect might be derived by separating observations into excess demand and supply regions. Segmenting the sample in terms of the mean work load, the results indicated that in "shortage" areas, rates of use were almost exclusively related to the density of surgeons and unrelated to fees or socioeconomic characteristics. In "surplus" areas, however, demand characteristics significantly influenced use, while the density of physicians continued to exert a significant and positive influence on surgical rates.

Although strongly supporting the inducement hypothesis, the results of the study were flawed by essentially three considerations identified by Phelps (1986). Perhaps the most important of these is the failure to incorporate a direct measure of insurance coverage for surgical fees. Although Cromwell and Mitchell (1986) included a measure of the coinsurance rate for hospital costs, Phelps contended that the approach represented a cross-price for services that complement surgery and may introduce bias in reported results. In addition, Phelps argued that the likely presence of serial correlation among observations may overstate the precision of estimates and that corrections for the correlation among observations might reduce the significance of reported coefficients. The final concern expressed by Phelps involved the use of files maintained by the AMA to measure the physician supply in the regional analysis. In this regard, a failure to adjust for the full- or part-time status of physicians to construct the measure of surgeon density may also bias reported results.

Rather than focus on use rates, Wilensky and Rossiter (1981) explored the hypothesis of demand shift by relying on data derived from the NMCES, which contains direct measures of follow-up visits initiated by physicians. Essentially four sets of independent variables were used to examine the probability that a visit was initiated by the physician. The first set represents the patient's demand for service, measured by the proportion of the bill paid by the family, as well as market conditions represented by waiting time and physician density. The second set depicts characteristics of the patient that reflect arguments of the utility function. The third set of variables included the provider's age and outside income, which, of course, reflect the physician's utility function. The final set represented characteristics of the physician's practice and the cost function of the provider.

The findings of the study suggested that physicians initiated 38 percent of all visits; patients initiated 54 percent of all visits, and the balance, 8 percent, were initiated by unknown means. After controlling for patient, physician, and practice characteristics, results of the multivariate analysis indicated that economic and market conditions were important determinants of the proportion of physician-initiated visits. Decreases in the proportion of the bill paid by the family significantly increased the proportion of physician-generated visits, while waiting time was found to be negatively associated with demand inducement. Consistent with the inducement hypothesis, the proportion of visits initiated by the provider was found to increase as the physician population ratio increased. The results also suggested that inducement is greater among specialty than among primary or secondary physicians.

In a companion paper, Rossiter and Wilensky (1984) extended their analysis and examined the extent to which the initiation of visits reflects the self interest of the physician or the behavior of an agent representing the interests of the patient. Employed as dependent variables were physician initiated expenditures for all medical services, including inpatient physician services, inpatient hospital services, and prescribed medication as well as ambulatory care expenditures that were physician initiated. Controlling for physician and patient characteristics, the findings indicated that measures of health status exerted a significant ($p \leq$ .05) and positive effect on both measures of physician-initiated expenditures. These results are consistent with the traditional view of the role of the physician, acting as an agent for the patient. Holding insurance coverage, health status, and other demographic characteristics constant, the results also indicated that physician density exerted a significant ($p \leq$ .05) and positive effect on expenditures on provider-initiated ambulatory care. In this case, elasticity coefficients at the mean ranged from .11 to .13. Since the density ratio exerted no significant effect on all medical services, the findings indicate that inducement is limited to discretionary services and that the overall effect is small ($.07 to $.08).

In addition to those that evaluated the outcomes that are derived from the inducement hypothesis, several studies have assessed the effects of disparities in the information possessed by physicians and patients on utilization behavior. For example, Pauly and Satterthwaite (1981) examined the inducement hypothesis within the context of a model that suggests that consumer information concerning the quality of local physicians declines as physician density increases. If, as suggested by this study, consumer information decreases as the supply of physicians increases, disparities in knowledge might be regarded as a permissive factor that supports the inducement hypothesis; however, the approach addressed only one dimension of consumer information, and the empirical results suffer from limitations imposed by the aggregate data employed in the empirical investigation.

Bunker and Brown (1974) assessed the effects of differential information on utilization behavior by comparing surgical rates in a sample of physicians and their spouses with those of other professional groups. The study examined the hypothesis that physicians and their spouses use less surgery than their professional counterparts who exhibited similar sociodemographic attributes but lacked medical knowledge. Among the seven surgical procedures examined were appendectomies and hysterectomies, both of which are subject to abuse and are characterized by indications that are regarded as imprecise. The results indicated that the standardized use rate by physicians and their spouses was 20 to 30 percent higher than the professional groups studied. Further, the rates of operative procedures for physicians and their spouses were significantly higher or did not differ from the utilization experience of the comparison group, an outcome that is inconsistent with the inducement hypothesis.

Several limitations of the Bunker and Brown results are worthy of note, however. First, the study was based on the utilization experience of those appearing on membership lists of professional and alumni associations in Northern

California, suggesting that the results are not representative of the general population. Further, the study failed to control for differences in the full price of service. In this regard, it is possible that physicians and their spouses are better insured, receive medical care under the auspices of professional courtesy, and experience shorter travel and waiting times, each of which reduces the total cost of service. In addition, the study failed to control for factors such as education, income, family size, and health status.

The major defects in the Bunker and Brown study were rectified by Hay and Leahy (1982), who examined the use of physician office and hospital visits by individuals grouped into one of four occupational groups. In addition to blue- and white-collar designations, individuals were classified into two medical occupations. The first contained individuals related to a family in which at least one member was employed as a physician, dentist, nurse, dietician, or therapist. Individuals were assigned to the second health-related group if at least one family member was employed as a health technologist or technician. As before, the study examined the hypothesis that those associated with health professionals use less service than other occupational groups. In addition to the surrogate for medical information, the study examined independent variables that represented biographical attributes, insurance coverage, time costs, and perceived health status.

Similar to the results reported by Bunker and Brown, the findings failed to support the demand-inducement hypothesis. In particular, Hay and Leahy found that medical professionals and their families are as likely or more likely to visit a physician than others; however, neither of the variables depicting employment in a health-related occupation exerted a significant influence on the volume of physician service consumed, an outcome that also fails to support the inducement hypothesis.

It is also important to note that the significant results found by Hay and Leahy pertain to the propensity to initiate care, and the insignificant findings occurred when examining the physician-generated phase of the utilization process. Unfortunately previous assessments of the effects of imbalances in information on physician use failed to control for the diagnosis or the medical condition that precipitated the utilization process. When defined in clinical terms, diagnosis dictates, in varying degrees of precision, the appropriate course of treatment, which influences the latitude for discretion and the extent of demand inducement. Further, for a given medical condition, those with more medical knowledge may expect and receive more service than their less well-informed counterparts, thus reducing differences in use that otherwise might be attributable to demand inducement.

Several studies report evidence that challenges the demand-inducement hypothesis. Wennberg (1984) reviewed a number of studies that correct for border-crossing and focused on surgical problems for which there is little professional consensus regarding appropriate treatment. A substantial variation in operations per capita exists, which is not explained by physician-population or hospital bed–population ratios. Further, these variations have been observed in different countries (United States, Canada, United Kingdom, and Norway) that use different schemes to compensate physicians. It is possible that disparities in medical practice are due to differences in "physician beliefs" as to the efficacy of surgical intervention. This contention is supported by the relatively small variation in medical practice for procedures characterized by a high degree of professional consensus. Additional support for Wennberg's hypothesis is provided by Brook, Lohr, Chassin, Kosecoff, Fink, and Solomon (1984), Stano, Cromwell, Velky, and Saad (1985), and Stano (1986).

McCarthy (1985) empirically tested a structural model of the physician services market, which included functions for demand, waiting time, production, supply of physician hours, and demand for labor inputs. Results from the two-stage least-squares regression analysis suggest that consumers are sensitive to physician pricing and scheduling choices and, to a less certain extent, physician quality. Collaborative evidence is provided by Newhouse, Williams, Bennett, and Schwartz (1982) and Sweeney (1982).

Mixed results for supplier-induced demand are provided by Stano (1985). The hypothesis was supported by the results of a multivariate analysis that employed aggregated physician data in Michigan. The findings indicate a positive relationship between physician visits per 1,000 population and the ratio of physicians-to-population. The analysis of data from individual physician practices, however, does not indicate that physicians treat their patients more intensively as the availability of physicians increases, as is hypothesized to occur under supplier-induced demand.

Stano reconciles the disparity in the results obtained in the analysis of aggregated and disaggregated data by arguing that the aggregated analysis suffers from three methodological problems found in other studies of supplier-induced demand. First, per capita use rates could be seriously distorted by patient border-crossing, which may not be adequately controlled in the analysis of aggregated market area data. Second, many aggregated studies failed to treat the physician-population ratio as endogenous; hence, their estimated coefficient may be biased. Third, as demonstrated by Auster and Oaxaca (1981), the demand equation in usual formulations of supplier-induced demand is not identified.

Similar to the investment theory of demand, the inducement hypothesis is of importance when viewed from a public policy perspective. Consider first the implications of supplier-induced demand on policy instruments designed to control spending on health care. As is well known, decisions to expand the capacity of American medical schools and to encourage the immigration of foreign medical graduates were predicated on the assumption that an increase in supply of physicians reduces fees and, *ceteris paribus*, spending on health services. The inducement hypothesis, however, suggests that increases in physician density exert a perverse effect on fees, use, and costs.

As suggested by Evans (1974), the inducement hypothesis challenges the wisdom and potential effectiveness of increased cost sharing as a vehicle for controlling utilization and moderating the costs of health care. Rather, an increased dependence on cost sharing and the accompanying decline in consumer-initiated demand not only reduces the professional income of physicians but also induces providers to expand demand, thereby reducing the effects of higher prices on total spending.

Further, the inducement hypothesis suggests that limitations imposed on the fees charged by physicians are unlikely to control spending on health services. Rather, price controls are likely to expand utilization and induce the substitution of more expensive services for less costly ones. As Evans (1974) suggests, such limitations are also likely to induce physicians to increase billings to compensate for their impaired ability to adjust fees. Findings reported by Dyckman (1978) are clearly consistent with these expectations and suggest that the largest two-year increase in physician use occurred during fiscal years 1973 and 1974, a period in which price controls were in effect. More normal patterns of utilization increases were resumed during the two years following the removal of price controls. These observations suggest that policies designed to control physician fees are unlikely to contain costs and may exert perverse effects on total spending.

THE DECISION TO SEEK CARE: A SOCIAL-PSYCHOLOGICAL APPROACH

As suggested by Mechanic (1978), the decision to consult a physician is dependent on a set of social and psychological factors that influence the individual's response to illness or symptoms. Accordingly, the model is predicated on the assumption that illness behavior and the decision to seek care are culturally and socially conditioned responses to the onset of symptoms.

As developed by Mechanic, the decision to seek care is determined by (1) the visibility and recognition of symptoms; (2) the extent to which the symptoms are perceived as serious; (3) the extent to which the symptoms disrupt the performance of normal social and economic roles; (4) the frequency and persistence of symptoms; (5) tolerance to the symptoms; (6) needs that lead to denial or compete with illness responses; (7) information or knowledge; (8) competing interpretations of recognized symptoms; (9) the availability and physical proximity of health resources; and (10) the financial and psychological costs of care-seeking behavior.

The model posits that the set of factors and the individual's definitions of the situation combine to determine whether or not health care is sought. As described by Mechanic, the determinants of illness behavior operate at two levels. The first involves the individual's perception and definition of the situation. As such, Mechanic argues that perceptions are formed by the individual's cultural background, past experiences, and the socialization process. The second level involves a social component and refers to the attempts of others to define symptoms, alert the individual to their presence, and identify appropriate or alternate courses of action.

Compared to other models of demand, the social-psychological approach to explaining health behavior has not been the subject of extensive empirical research. Although the structure of the model is intuitively appealing, the failure of the theory to specify the interrelationships between the various determinants and the levels of definition is an impediment that has probably prevented empirical investigation and validation.

According to several recent reviews, available evidence indicates that, after controlling for medical need, social structure, organizational attributes, social networks, and social-psychological variables have exerted an inconsistent effect on the use of health services. Viewed from the perspective of social structure, Andersen, Kravits, and Anderson (1975), among others, demonstrated that commonly reported effects of age on use are attributable, in large part, to health status. Similarly, ethnicity, which was identified as a determinant of utilization behavior by Andersen et al., was unrelated to use in the National Interview Surveys examined by Wolinsky (1978). Further, publicly funded programs have apparently reduced differences in utilization that are attributable to income, and, although sex usually exerts an effect on physician use, Andersen et al. found no significant relationship.

Inconsistent findings regarding the influence of social network on physician demand have also been reported. For example, Reeder and Berkanovic (1973) conclude that those with networks dominated by friends were less likely to use physician services than their counterparts who reported networks comprised of relatives. Conversely, McKinlay (1972) and Salloway and Dillon (1973) concluded that individuals with networks dominated by friends tended to use physician care more frequently than those with relative networks. Among the variables depicting social network characteristics and health orientation, Berkanovic, Telesky, and Reeder (1981) report that only the index measuring the frequency of contact and the physical proximity of network members exerted a significant effect on use. In particular, the results indicate that those with more contact were less likely to seek care during the study period. When viewed from the perspective of specific symptoms, the study indicated that the size of the network and the frequency of contact increased the likelihood that the respondent consulted a physician.

Concerning the social-psychological level, fragmentary evidence suggests that health orientation and beliefs concerning the efficacy of care influence utilization behavior. Among the variables depicting health beliefs and orientation examined by Berkanovic et al. (1981), the perceived efficacy of care, the perceived seriousness of the symptom, and the perceived likelihood of recurrence were the strongest predictors of utilization behavior. Suchman (1964) reported that the health beliefs of the individual influence the decision to seek care; however, results reported by Geersten, Klauber, Rindflesh, Kane, and Gray (1975) and by Reeder and Berkanovic (1973) indicate that the same indicators failed to produce an influence on care-seeking behavior. Similarly, Andersen (1975) reports findings that fail to establish a relation between utilization and variables depicting health beliefs and orientation.

Perhaps the most important, but least extensively examined component of Mechanic's model is the role played by the individual's experiences in forming perceptions concerning symptoms and deciding to consult a physician. As suggested by Jones, Wiese, Moore, and Haley (1981), perceived seriousness is a more powerful determinant of symptom definition than familiarity, embarrassment caused by the symptom, or personal responsibility for its onset. Focusing on 11 indicators of illness, Tanner, Cockerman, and Spaeth (1983) assessed the influence of the perceived seriousness of those symptoms that were experienced by respondents during the past twelve months. The results of the study indicated that, when combined with standard multivariate and social-psychological variables, respondent-evaluated symptoms provide an efficient prediction of utilization.

In addition to those mentioned previously, Mechanic posits that psychological and financial costs influence the decision to seek care. Although financial barriers have been assessed extensively, as documented earlier, the effects of psychological costs on use have received limited attention. Previous findings reported by Dutton (1978) indicate that the indigent who seek care from hospital outpatient departments, emergency rooms, and public health clinics experience a poor patient-physician relationship and a long waiting time resulting from a queue of patients seeking service. These results suggest that the low use of service by some of the poor is attributable, in part, to unpleasant experiences and related psychological costs that, when combined with the perceived high financial costs of items that are not financed by publicly funded programs, are impediments to care-seeking behavior. These observations are also supported by findings reported by Tanner et al. (1983), who concluded that greater access to private sources of health care might increase the use of service by minorities and other disadvantaged members of society.

In addition to the poor who underutilize health services, Medicaid officials are concerned about the unnecessary costs generated by beneficiaries who not only practice indiscriminate "doctor shopping," which results in excessive tests, prescriptions, and office visits, but also use inappropriate and costly facilities (i.e., emergency rooms) for primary care (Freund 1984). Although costly, the Medicaid beneficiary, whose care is not structured in a way that assures appropriately coordinated care and an on-going doctor-patient relationship, may not be receiving good care (Freund and Neuschler 1986). Accordingly, managed care programs, which are part of the "competitive approach" discussed in Chapter 11, have been proposed as a solution to the cost, access, and quality problems facing the Medicaid program.

FUTURE RESEARCH AND POLICY IMPLICATIONS

The review presented in this chapter suggests several implications concerning directions for future research. Among the most important deficiencies in previous analyses of demand, as defined by traditional economic theory, is the specification of the dependent variable. As indicated, many studies have examined surrogates that fail to distinguish between patient-initiated use, which is conceptually consistent with traditional definitions of demand, and consumption that is dominated by the physician.

A potentially fruitful approach to resolving the problem of misspecifying the dependent variable is to employ the episode of illness as the unit of analysis. As indicated in Chapters 5 and 12, a focus on the episode of illness is also germane to the formulation of public policy designed to control costs and ensure an equitable distribution of health services.

As suggested by Stoddart and Barer (1981), the episode of illness may be defined as a process that consists of a patient-initiated phase and a physician-generated or dominated phase. As such, the two components of the consumption process enable the analyst to distinguish consumption behavior that is initiated by the patient and is congruent with the traditional theory of demand from utilization that is generated or dominated by the physician. As is well known, empirical analyses are frequently designed to assess the effectiveness of public policy to control cost or ensure an equitable distribution of service, objectives for which the episode of illness is well suited. For example, analyses designed to assess the extent to which policy controls cost or utilization behavior and ensures an equitable distribution of services might focus on both components of the consumption process. Similarly, investigations designed to examine the effects of incentives that are specific to the provider on costs and use should focus on the physician-dominated phase. Finally, analyses of impediments to access and the demand for care, as defined by traditional concepts, should be limited to the patient initiated phase.

The use of the episode of illness as the unit of analysis is also consistent with differential applications of one or more of the models proposed previously. For example, the social psychological model, the traditional theory of demand and the behavioral model, where need is defined symptomatically, might be combined in an analysis of the use or nonuse of service among members of the study group. Similarly, the Grossman model, the behavioral model, where need is defined clinically, and the supply-inducement theory might be employed in examinations of consumption that occurs during the physician-dominated phase of use. In particular, the effects of life style, environmental, and occupational factors in relation to health risks, medical need, and the use of health services might be productively examined within the context of the Grossman framework.

In addition to those described previously, the episode of illness is also germane to the formulation of public policy concerning the problem of financing the use of care, controlling costs, and ensuring an equitable distribution of service. For example, this review suggests that cost-sharing arrangements are perhaps most effective when applied to the patient-initiated phase; hence, deductible provisions or coinsurance payments should apply to initial visits, where, in accordance with findings reported by Newhouse et al. (1981), the magnitude of cost sharing is adjusted for differential abilities to pay. Conversely, consumption and the costs of care provided during the provider-dominated phase might be controlled by a system of rewards and penalties that induce physicians to prescribe medically required services and to avoid providing those units of care that are medically unnecessary, as defined clinically, and are prescribed solely for the purpose of augmenting personal income. Although the episode of illness, to include the related use of hospital care, might be difficult to define operationally, explicit recognition of the patient- and physician-dominated phases of the consumption process may result in the formation of policies that are more likely to control costs and ensure an equitable distribution of service than those that currently dominate the fiscal environment of the American health industry.

REFERENCES

Acton, J. 1975. Nonmonetary factors in the demand for medical services: Some empirical evidence. *Journal of Political Economy* 83(3):595–614.

Acton, J. 1976. Demand for health care among the urban poor with special emphasis on the role of time. In R. Rosett, ed., *The Role of Health Insurance in the Health Services Sector*. New York: National Bureau of Economic Research.

Aday, L., and R. Andersen. 1975. *Development of Indices of Access to Medical Care*. Ann Arbor, MI: Health Administration Press.

Aday, L., R. Andersen, and G. Fleming. 1980. *Health Care in the U.S.: Equitable for Whom?* Beverly Hills, CA: Sage Publications.

Andersen, R. 1968. A behavior model of families' use of health services, research series 25. Chicago, IL: Center for Health Administration Studies, University of Chicago.

Andersen, R., 1975. Health service distribution and equity. In R. Andersen, J. Kravits, and O. Anderson, eds., *Equity in Health Services*. Cambridge, MA: Ballinger.

Andersen, R., and L. Benham. 1970. Factors affecting the relationship between family income and medical care consumption. In H. Klarman, ed., *Empirical Studies in Health Economics*. Baltimore, MD: Johns Hopkins University Press.

Andersen, R., and J. Newman. 1973. Societal and individual determinants of medical care utilization in the United States. *Milbank Memorial Fund Quarterly* 51(1):95–124.

Andersen, R., and L. A. Aday. 1978. Access to medical care in the U.S.: Realized and potential. *Medical Care* 16(7):533–46.

Andersen R., J. Kravits, and O. Anderson, eds. 1975. *Equity in Health Services*. Cambridge, MA: Ballinger.

Andersen R., J. Lion, and O. Anderson. 1976. *Two Decades of Health Services: Social Survey Trends in Use and Expenditures*. Cambridge, MA: Ballinger.

Anderson, J. G., and P. W. Eggers. 1976. Patterns of utilization among members of a prepaid group practice. *Inquiry* 13(4):382–94.

Anderson, O. W. 1963. The utilization of health services. In H. A. Freeman, S. Levin, L. G. Reeder et al., eds., *Handbook of Medical Sociology*. Englewood Cliffs, NJ: Prentice-Hall.

Arrow, K. 1963. Uncertainty and the welfare economics of medical care. *American Economic Review* 53(5):941–73.

Arrow, K. 1973. Welfare analysis of changes in health care insurance rates. Santa Monica, CA: Rand Corporation.

Auster, R. D., and R. L. Oaxaca. 1981. Identification of supplier induced demand in the health care sector. *Journal of Human Resources* 16(3):327–42.

Auster, R., I. Leveson, and D. Saracheck. 1969. The production of health: An explanatory study. *Journal of Human Resources* 4(4):411–36.

Beck, R. 1974. The effects of copayment on the poor. *Journal of Human Resources* 9(1):129–42.

Becker, E., and A. Steinwald. 1981. Determinants of hospitals case-mix complexity. *Health Services Research* 16(4):439–58.

Becker, E., and F. Sloan. 1983. Utilization of hospital services: The roles of teaching, case-mix, and reimbursement. *Inquiry* 20(3):248–57.

Becker, M., R. Nathanson, R. Drachman, and J. Kirscht. 1977. Mothers' health beliefs and children's clinic visits: A prospective study. *Journal of Community Health* 3(2):125–35.

Berkanovic, E., C. Telesky, and S. Reeder. 1981. Structural and social psychological factors in the decision to seek medical care for symptoms. *Medical Care* 19(7):693–709.

Berki, S., and M. Ashcraft. 1979. On the analysis of ambulatory utilization: An investigation of the roles of need, access and price as predictions of illness and preventive visits. *Medical Care* 17(12):1163–81.

Blumberg, M. 1979. Rational provider prices: Provider price changes for improved health care use. In G. Chacho, ed., *Health Handbook*. Amsterdam: North-Holland.

Brook, R., J. E. Ware, and W. Rogers et al. 1983. Does free care improve adults' health: Results from a randomized controlled trial. *New England Journal of Medicine* 309(23):1426–34.

Brook, R. H., K. N. Lohr, M. Chassin, J. Kosecoff, A. Fink, and D. Solomon. 1984. Geographic variations in the use of services: Do they have any clinical significance? *Health Affairs* 3(2):63–73.

Broyles, R. W., P. Manga, D. A. Binder, D. E. Angus, and A. Charette. 1983. The use of physician services under a national health insurance scheme: An examination of the Canada health survey. *Medical Care* 21(11):1037–54.

Bunker, J., and B. Brown. 1974. The physician-patient as an informed consumer of surgical services. *New England Journal of Medicine* 290:1051–55.

Cauley, S. 1987. The time price of medical care. *Review of Economics and Statistics* 7:59–66.

Chamberlain, H., and A. Drui. 1975. Content of care in rural primary health care practices. *Medical Care* 13(3):230–40.

Chiswick, B. R. 1976. The demand for nursing home care: An analysis of the substitution between institutional and noninstitutional care. *Journal of Human Resources* 11(3):245–316.

Coffey, R. M. 1983. The effect of time price on the demand for medical care services. *Journal of Human Resources* 18(3):407–24.

Cohen, D. 1980. The use of prenatal cytogenetic diagnosis: A comparison of rates in prepaid group practices and the general population. *Medical Care* 18(5):513–19.

Colle, A., and M. Grossman. 1978. Determinants of pediatric care utilization. *Journal of Human Resources* 13 (Supp.):115–53.

Cromwell, J., and J. B. Mitchell. 1986. Physician-induced demand for surgery. *Journal of Health Economics* 5(4):293–313.

Cropper, M. 1977. Health, investment in health and occupational choice. *Journal of Political Economy* 85(6):1273–94.

Custer, W. S. 1986. Hospital attributes and physician prices. *Southern Economic Journal* 52(4):1010–27.

Dardanoni, V., and A. Wagstaff. 1987. Uncertainty, inequalities in health and the demand for health. *Journal of Health Economics* 6(4):283–290.

Davis, K., and L. Russell. 1972. The substitution of hospital outpatient care for inpatient care: *Review of Economics and Statistics* 54(2):109–20.

Dor, A., P. Gertler and J. van der Gaag (1987). Non-price rationing and the choice of medical care providers in rural Côte d'Ivoire. *Journal of Health Economics* 6(4):291–304.

Dranove, D. 1985. Demand inducement of the physician-patient relationship. Working paper, Chicago, IL: University of Chicago.

Dutton, D. 1978. Explaining the low use of health services by the poor: Costs, attitudes or delivery system? *American Sociological Review* 43(3):348–68.

Dyckman, Z. 1978. A study of physicians' fees. Washington, DC: Council on Wage and Price Stability, Executive Office of the President.

Ellis, R. P. 1986. Rational behavior in the presence of coverage ceilings and deductibles. *Rand Journal of Economics* 17(2):158–75.

Evans, R. G. 1974. Supplier-induced demand: Some empirical evidence and implications. In M. Perlman, ed., *The Economics of Health and Medical Care*. New York: John Wiley.

Ezzati, T. M. 1980. The national ambulatory medical care survey 1977 summary, National Center for Health Statistics, Vital and Health Statistics, Series 13, No. 44.

Farber, B., D. Kaiser, and R. Wenzel. 1981. Relation between surgical volume and incidence of postoperative wound infection. *New England Journal of Medicine* 305(4):200–204.

Farley, P. J. 1986. Theories of the price and quantity of physician services: A synthesis and critique. *Journal of Health Economics* 5(4):315–33.

Feldman, R., and B. Dowd. 1986. Is there a competitive market for hospital services? *Journal of Health Economics* 5(3):277–92.

Feldstein, M. S. 1971. Hospital cost inflation: A study of nonprofit price dynamics. *American Economic Review* 61(5):853–71.

Feldstein, M. S. 1973. The welfare loss of excess health insurance. *Journal of Political Economy* 81(5):853–72.

Feldstein, P. J., and J. Carr. 1964. The effect of income on medical care spending. Proceedings of the Social Statistics Section of the American Statistical Association.

Feldstein, P. J., and R. Severson. 1964. The demand for medical care, report of the commission on the costs of medical care. Chicago, IL: American Medical Association.

Ferguson, C., M. Lee, and R. Wallace. 1976. Effects of medicare on hospital use: A disease specific study. *Medical Care* 14(7):574–89.

Freiberg, L., and F. Scutchfield. 1976. Insurance and the demand for hospital care: An examination of moral hazard. *Inquiry* 13 (1):54–60.

Freund, D. A. 1984. *Medicaid Reform: Four Studies of Case Management*. Washington, DC: American Enterprise Institute.

Freund, D. A., and E. Neuschler. 1986. Overview of Medicaid capitation and case-management initiatives. *Health Care Financing Review* (Annual Supplement):21–30.

Fuchs, V. 1978. The supply of physicians and the demand for operations. *Journal of Human Resources* 13(Supp.):35–56.

Fuchs, V., and M. Kramer. 1972. Determinants of expenditures for physician services in the United States 1948–1968. New York: National Bureau of Economic Research.

Geersten R., M. R. Klauber, M. Rindflesh, R. L. Kane, and R. Gray. 1975. A reexamination of Suchman's views on social factors in health care utilization. *Journal of Health and Social Behavior* 16(2):226–37.

Givens, J. D. 1978. Current estimates from the health interview survey. *Vital and Health Statistics* Series 10, No. 130: 17, 25, 34.

Gold, M. 1984. The demand for hospital outpatient services. *Health Services Research* 19(3):383–412.

Goldfarb, M., M. Hornbrook, and C. Higgins. 1983. Determinants of hospital use: A cross diagnostic analysis. *Medical Care* 21(1):48–66.

Green, J. 1978. Physician-induced demand for medical care. *Journal of Human Resources* 13 (Supplement):21–34.

Grossman, M. 1972. On the concept of health capital and the demand for health. *Journal of Political Economy* 80(2):223–55.

Haupt, B. 1980. Utilization of short stay hospitals: Annual summary for the United States, 1978, Vital and Health Statistics, National Center for Health Statistics, Series 13, No. 46.

Hay, J., and M. Leahy. 1982. Physician induced demand: An empirical analysis of the consumer information gap. *Journal of Health Economics* 1(3):231–44.

Heaney, C., and D. Riedel. 1970. From indemnity to full coverage: Changes in hospital utilization research series. Chicago, IL: Blue Cross Association.

Henry, L. H. 1970. The impact of medicare and medicaid on the supply and demand conditions of nursing homes. Unpublished doctoral dissertation, University of Notre Dame.

Hershey, J. C., H. Luft, and J. Gianaris. 1975. Making sense out of utilization data. *Medical Care* 13(10):838–54.

Hughes, R., S. Hunt, and H. Luft. 1987. Effects of surgeon volume and hospital volume on quality of care in hospitals. *Medical Care* 25(6):489–503.

Hulka, B. S., and J. R. Wheat. 1985. Patterns of utilization: The patient perspective. *Medical Care* 23(5):438–60.

Inman, R. P. 1976. The family provision of children's health: An economic analysis. In R. N. Rosett, ed., *The Role of Health Insurance in the Health Services Sector*. New York: National Bureau of Economic Research, 215–59.

Ippolito, P. 1981. Information and the life cycle consumption of hazardous goals. *Economic Inquiry* 19(4):529–58.

Jones, R. A., H. J. Wiese, R. W. Moore, and J. V. Haley. 1981. On the perceived meaning of symptoms. *Medical Care* 19(7):710–17.

Keeler, E. B., and J. E. Rolph. 1982. The demand for episodes of medical treatment: Interim results from the Health Insurance Experiment. Report to the Department of Health and Human Services R–2829-HHS, Santa Monica, CA:Rand Corporation.

Keeler, E. B., J. P. Newhouse, and C. E. Phelps. 1977. Deductibles and the demand for medical care services: The theory of a consumer facing a variable price schedule under uncertainty. *Econometrica* 45(3):641–56.

Keeler, E. B., E. M. Sloss, R. H. Brook, B. H. Operskalski, G. A. Goldberg, and J. P. Newhouse. 1987. Effects of cost sharing on physiological health, health practices and worry. *Health Services Research* 22(3):279–306.

Kennedy, V. 1979. Rural access to a regular source of medical care. *Journal of Community Health* 4(3):199–203.

Kirscht, J., M. Becker, and J. Eveland. 1976. Psychological and social factors as predictions of medical behavior. *Medical Care* 14(5):422–31.

Kravits, J. 1975. The relationship of attitudes to discretionary physician and dentist use by race and income. In R. Andersen et al., eds., *Equity in Health Services: Empirical Analysis in Social Policy*. Cambridge, MA: Ballinger.

Kronenfield, J. 1980. Sources of ambulatory care and utilization models. *Health Services Research* 15(1):3–20.

Lamberton, C. E., W. D. Ellington, and K. R. Spear. 1986. Factors determining the demand for nursing home services. *Quarterly Review of Economics and Business* 26(4):74–90.

Leavitt, F. 1979. The health belief model and utilization of ambulatory care services. *Social Science and Medicine* 13A:105–12.

Lee, R., and J. Hadley. 1981. Physicians' fees and public medical care programs. *Health Services Research* 16(2):185–203.

Leibowitz, A., W. G. Manning, E. B. Keeler et al. 1985. Effect of cost sharing on the use of medical services by children: Interim results from a randomized controlled trial. *Pediatrics* 75(5):942–51.

Lohr, K. N., R. H. Brook, C. J. Kamberg, G. A. Goldberg et al. 1986. Use of medical care in the Rand Insurance Experiment: Diagnosis- and service-specific analyses in a randomized controlled trial. *Medical Care* 24(9) Supplement.

Long, M. 1981. The role of consumer locations in the demand for inpatient care. *Inquiry* 18(3):226–73.

Luft, H. S., J. C. Hershey, and J. Morrell. 1976. Factors affecting the use of physician services in a rural community. *American Journal of Public Health* 66(9):865–71.

Luft, H. S., J. Bunker, and A. Enthoven. 1979. Should operations be regionalized? The empirical relation between surgical volume and mortality. *New England Journal of Medicine* 301(25):1364–69.

Manga, P., R. W. Broyles, and D. E. Angus. 1987. The determinants of hospital utilization under a universal public insurance program in Canada. *Medical Care* 25(7):658–70.

Manning, W. G., Jr., K. B. Wells, N. Duan, J. P. Newhouse, and J. E. Ware. 1984. Cost sharing and the use of ambulatory mental health services. *American Psychologist* 39(10):1077–89.

Manning, W. G., Jr., H. L. Bailit, B. Benjamin, and J. P. Newhouse. 1985. The demand for dental care: Evidence from a randomized trial in health insurance. *Journal of the American Dental Association* 110(6):895–902.

Manning, W. G., Jr., K. B. Wells, N. Duan et al. 1986a. How cost sharing affects the use of ambulatory mental health services. *Journal of the American Medical Association* 256(14):1930–34.

Manning, W. G., Jr., et al. 1986b. *Health Insurance and the Demand for Dental Care:*

Evidence from a Randomized Experiment. Pub. No. R–3225-HHS, Santa Monica, CA: Rand Corporation.

Manning, W. G., Jr., J. P. Newhouse, N. Duan, E. B. Keeler, A. Leibowitz, and M. S. Marquis. 1987a. Health insurance and the demand for medical care: Evidence from a randomized experiment. *American Economic Review* 77(3):251–77.

Manning, W. G. et al. 1987b. *Health Insurance and the Demand for Medical Care: Evidence from a Randomized Experiment.* Pub. No. R–3476-HHS, Santa Monica, CA: Rand Corporation.

McCarthy, T. R. 1985. The competitive nature of the primary-care physician services market. *Journal of Health Economics* 4(2):93–117.

McKinlay, J. B. 1972. Some approaches and problems in the study of the use of services: An overview. *Journal of Health and Social Behavior* 13(2):115–52.

Mechanic, D. 1978. *Medical Sociology.* 2nd ed. New York: Free Press.

Morehead, M., R. Donaldson, and A. Zanes. 1971. Dental service at a Teamster comprehensive care program. *Journal of the American Dental Association* 83:607–13.

Mueller, C. D. 1985. Waiting for physicians' services: Model and evidence. *Journal of Business* 58(2):173–190.

Muurinen, J. 1982. Demand for health: A generalized Grossman model. *Journal of Health Economics* 1(1):5–28.

Nathanson, C. A. 1977. Sex, illness and medical care: A review of data, theory, and method. *Social Science and Medicine* 11(1):13–25.

Newhouse, J. 1970. A model of physician pricing. *Southern Economic Journal* 37(2):174–83.

Newhouse, J. P. 1981. The demand for medical care services: A retrospect and prospect. In J. van der Gaag and M. Perlman, eds., *Health, Economics, and Health Economics.* Amsterdam: North-Holland.

Newhouse, J. P., and C. E. Phelps. 1976. New estimates of price and income elasticities for medical services. In R. N. Rosett, ed., *The Role of Health Insurance in the Health Services Sector.* New York: NBER.

Newhouse, J. P., C. E. Phelps, and M. Marquis. 1980. On having your cake and eating it too: Econometric problems in estimating the demand for health services. *Journal of Econometrics* 13:365–90.

Newhouse, J. P., W. Manning, C. Morris et al. 1981. Some interim results from a controlled trial of cost-sharing in health insurance. *New England Journal of Medicine* 303(25):1501–7.

Newhouse, J. P., A. P. Williams, B. W. Bennett, and W. B. Schwartz. 1982. Does the geographical distribution of physicians reflect market failure? *Bell Journal of Economics* 13(2):493–505.

Pauly, M., and M. Satterthwaite. 1981. In pricing of primary care physicians' service: A test of the role of consumer information. *Bell Journal of Economics* 12(2):488–506.

Phelps, C. E. 1975. Effects of insurance on demand for medical care. In R. Anderson, ed., *Equity in Health Services,* Cambridge, MA: Ballinger.

Phelps, C. E. 1982. Health care costs: The consequences of increased cost sharing. Report R–2970-RC, Santa Monica, CA: Rand Corporation.

Phelps, C. E. 1986. Induced demand: Can we ever know its extent? *Journal of Health Economics* 5(4):355–65.

Phelps, C. E., and J. P. Newhouse. 1972. The effect of coinsurance: A multivariate analysis. *Social Security Bulletin* 35(6):20–28.

Phelps, C. E., and J. Newhouse. 1974. Coinsurance, the price of time and the demand for medical services. *Review of Economics and Statistics* 56(3):334–42.

Phelps, C. E. and J. Newhouse. 1979. Coinsurance and the demand for medical services. Santa Monica, CA: Rand Corporation.

Reeder, L. B., and E. Berkanovic. 1973. Sociological concomitants of health orientations: A partial replication of Suchman. *Journal of Health and Social Behavior* 14(2):134–43.

Reinhardt, U. 1975. *Physician Productivity and the Demand for Health Manpower*. Cambridge, MA: Ballinger.

Richardson, J. 1981. The inducement hypothesis: That doctors generate demand for their own services. In J. Van der Gaag and M. Perlman, eds., *Health, Economics and Health Economics*. Amsterdam: North-Holland.

Roddy, P. C., J. Wallen, and S. M. Meyers. 1986. Cost sharing and use of health services: The United Mine Workers of America Health Plan. *Medical Care* 24(9):873–7.

Roemer, M., C. Hopkins, L. Carr, and F. Gartside. 1975. Copayments for ambulatory care: Penny-wise, pound foolish. *Medical Care* 13(6):457–66.

Rosenthal, G. 1970. Price elasticity of demand for short term general hospital services. In H. Klarman, ed., *Empirical Studies in Health Economics*. Baltimore, MD: Johns Hopkins University Press.

Rosett, R., and L. Huang. 1973. The effect of health insurance on the demand for medical care. *Journal of Political Economy* 81(2):281–305.

Rossiter, L., and G. Wilensky. 1984. Identification of physician-induced demand. *Journal of Human Resources* 19(2):231–44.

Salkever, D. S. 1976. Accessibility and the demand for preventive care. *Social Science and Medicine* 10(9/10):469–75.

Salloway, J. C., and D. Dillon. 1973. A comparison of family networks in health care utilization. *Journal of Comparative Studies* 4:137.

Scanlon, W. J. 1980. A theory of the nursing home market. *Inquiry* 17(1):25–41.

Scheffler, R. M. 1984. The United Mine Workers' Health Plan: An analysis of the cost-sharing program. *Medical Care* 22(3):247–54.

Scitovsky, A., and N. McCall. 1977. Coinsurance and the demand for physician services: Four years later. *Social Security Bulletin* 40(5):19–27.

Shortell, S. 1975. The effects of patterns and medical care on utilization and continuity of services. In R. Andersen, J. Kravits and O. Anderson, eds., *Equity in Health Services*. Cambridge, MA: Ballinger, 191–216.

Shortell, S., and J. LoGerfo. 1981. Hospital medical staff organization and quality of care: Results for myocardial infarction and appendectomy. *Medical Care* 19(10):1041–55.

Silver, M. 1970. An economic analysis of variations in medical expenses and work loss rates. In H. Klarman, ed., *Empirical Studies in Health Economics*. Baltimore, MD: Johns Hopkins University Press.

Stano, M. 1985. An analysis of the evidence on competition in the physician services markets. *Journal of Health Economics* 4(3):197–211.

Stano, M. 1986. A further analysis of the "variations in practice style" phenomenon. *Inquiry* 23(2):176–82.

Stano, M., J. Cromwell, J. Velky, and A. Saad. 1985. The effect of physician availability on fees and the demand for doctors' services. *Atlantic Economic Journal* 13(2):51–60.

Stoddart, G., and M. Barer. 1981. Analyses of demand and utilization through episodes of medical service. In J. van der Gaag and M. Perlman, eds., *Health, Economics and Health Economics*. Amsterdam: North-Holland Publishing Company.

Stoller, E. 1982. Patterns of physician utilization by the elderly: A multivariate analysis. *Medical Care* 20(11):1080–9.

Suchman, E. A. 1964. Sociomedical variations among ethnic groups. *American Journal of Sociology* 70(3):319–31.

Sweeney, G. H. 1982. The market for physicians' services: Theoretical implications and an empirical test of the target income hypothesis. *Southern Economic Journal* 48(3):594–614.

Tanner, J. L., W. Cockerman, and J. Spaeth. 1983. Predicting physician utilization. *Medical Care* 21(3):360–69.

Taylor, A. K., G. R. Wilensky, and L. F. Rossiter. 1981. The role of money and time in the demand for medical care. Paper presented at Annual meeting of the American Economic Association, Washington, DC, December.

Van de Ven, W., and J. van der Gaag. 1982. Health as an observable: A MIMIC model of the demand for health care. *Journal of Health Economics* 1(2):157–183.

Wagstaff, A. 1986. The demand for health: Some new empirical evidence. *Journal of Health Economics* 5(3):195–233.

Waldo, D., K. Levit, and H. Lazenby. 1986. National health expenditures, 1985. *Health Care Financing Review* 8(3):1–21.

Ware, J. E., W. G. Manning, N. Duan, K. B. Wells, and J. P. Newhouse. 1984. Health status and the use of outpatient mental health services. *American Psychologist* 39(10):1090–1100.

Wells, K. B., W. G. Manning, N. Duan, J. P. Newhouse, and J. E. Ware. 1987. Cost-sharing and the use of general medical physicians for outpatient mental health care. *Health Services Research* 22(1):1–17.

Wennberg, J. E. 1984. Dealing with medical practice variations: A proposal for action. *Health Affairs* 3(2):6–32.

Wilensky, G., and J. Holahan. 1972. National health insurance: Costs and distributional effects. Washington, DC: The Urban Institute.

Wilensky, G., and L. Rossiter. 1981. The magnitude and determinants of physician-initiated visits in the United States. In J. van der Gaag and M. Perlman, eds., *Health, Economics and Health Economics*. Amsterdam: North-Holland.

Wolinsky, F. D. 1978. Assessing the effects of predisposing, enabling and illness-morbidity characteristics on health service utilization. *Journal of Health and Social Behavior* 19(4):384–96.

Wolinsky, F. 1981. The problems for academic and entrepreneurial research in the use of health services: The case of unstable structural relationships. *Social Science Quarterly* 22:207–23.

Yang, B. M. 1986. Do physicians induce patient demand for medical care: An empirical analysis. *Journal of Economic Development* 11(2):83–102.

Zeckhauser, R. 1970. Medical insurance: A case study of the trade-off between risk spreading and appropriate incentives. *Journal of Economic Theory* 2(1):10–26.

Part III
Supply-Side Analysis

4

BEHAVIORAL MODELS OF
HOSPITALS AND OTHER HEALTH
CARE ORGANIZATIONS

In this chapter, our focus turns toward a review of the major conceptual models of the behavior of hospitals and other health care organizations. Rather than examine empirical validation of these models, we will emphasize the concepts and issues that will facilitate an understanding of the empirical work reviewed in the succeeding chapters, including development of output measures, production-function analysis, cost function analysis, and an assessment of prospective payment programs. Economic models have been used commonly for two purposes: to explain past behavior, or to predict future behavior. There is no consensus as to a theory of behavior for health care organizations. Instead a number of different theories have emerged. Associated with each theory is a different model of organizational behavior. As our analysis will reveal, each model was developed to represent a particular phenomenon that occurred in the health care industry. Accordingly, it may not be appropriate to evaluate models comparatively. For example, a model developed to explain the restriction of staff privileges (Pauly and Redisch 1973) may not predict responses to prospective payment well, even though it performs satisfactorily for its intended purpose.

Most of the development and testing of models in the health care industry have focused on hospital behavior. Accordingly, we begin this chapter by examining the hypothesized objectives of hospitals. This examination will be followed by a review of major models of hospital behavior. Finally, the available literature concerning economic models of other organizational participants in the health care industry will be reviewed.

An economic model typically has two components: an objective function and a set of constraints. For example, a hospital can be hypothesized as maximizing output subject to a minimum profit constraint. Both components are important. The objective function indicates the goals that the organization will attempt to pursue. The constraints limit the courses of action available to the institution.

A hospital can increase output by reducing its price because it faces a downward-sloping demand curve; however, the hospital is limited in doing so by the profit constraint. This brief example illustrates the necessity for appropriate goals and constraints in economic models.

HOSPITAL OBJECTIVES

Unfortunately, the goals of hospitals are not well understood. At the end of an extensive literature review, Berki concluded, "If the literature on the objectives of hospitals agrees on a central point, it is that the objectives are vague, ill-defined, contradictory, and sometimes non-existent" (Berki 1972, p. 28).

Some of the hypothesized objective functions of hospitals include:

1. profit maximization or satisficing and its variants: cash-flow maximization, utility maximization, net revenue maximization (Davis 1971);
2. social welfare maximization subject to the constraint of solvency (P. Feldstein 1961);
3. maximization of the number of patients treated, (Klarman 1965) or maximizing the weighted number of patients treated, the weights being the professional prestige of the doctors attending them (Reder 1965);
4. maximization of the hospital's scope of services, prestige, reputation, and excellence (Lee 1971);
5. maximization of amenities subject to profit maximization (Rice 1966);
6. maximization of quality and quantity of service (Newhouse 1970; M. Feldstein 1971);
7. maximization of physician income (Penshansky and Rosenthal 1965; Pauly and Redisch 1973; Shalit 1977; Pauly 1980; Morrisey, Conrad, Shortell, and Cook 1984; Frank, Weiner, Steinwachs, and Salkever 1987).

PROFIT-MAXIMIZING MODELS

P. J. Feldstein (1979) developed one of the simplest models of hospital behavior. For expository purposes, he assumed that the hospital acts as a profit-maximizing firm with monopoly power (i.e., it has a downward-sloping demand curve). To maximize profits, hospitals will produce the quantity of output indicated by the intersection of the marginal revenue, MR, and marginal cost, MC, curves. This is given as Q_1 in Figure 4.1. The demand curve, D, indicates that to sell Q_1 output, the hospital must charge price P_1.

Feldstein extends this model to a situation where the hospital is a multiproduct firm with different payers. Under these conditions, his model predicts that the hospital will practice price-discrimination by charging different prices for its different services and classes of patients according to the price elasticity of demand for each class of patient and type of service. Assuming there are n classes of patients and k types of services, the following criteria will be observed when setting prices:

Figure 4.1
Short-Run Equilibrium Under Monopoly

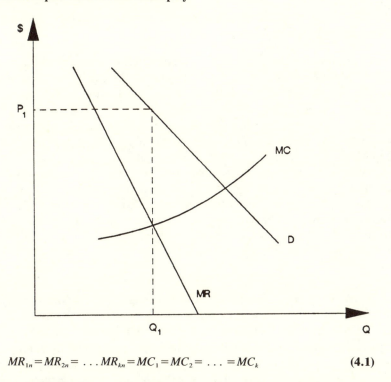

$$MR_{1n} = MR_{2n} = \ldots MR_{kn} = MC_1 = MC_2 = \ldots = MC_k \qquad (4.1)$$

Although Feldstein's model is based on the standard microeconomic model of the profit-maximizing monopolist, it does predict some forms of hospital behavior quite well. For example, the Feldstein model predicts that if there is an increase in demand, hospitals will increase price and quantity. Hospitals responded to the introduction of Medicare and Medicaid, public insurance programs that increased demand for hospital services, in accordance with predictions of the Feldstein model. This model also predicts that price-discriminating hospitals will charge higher mark-ups for those services, and that class of patients, whose demands are price inelastic. Feldstein verifies the accuracy of this prediction by observing that hospitals usually have higher markups for inpatient ancillary services, for which demand tends to be inelastic, than for outpatient services, for which demand is likely to be more price sensitive due to the availability of more substitutes.

Despite these correct predictions, Feldstein's expository model has many flaws that are due to its simplicity. For example, in contrast to common observations, his model predicts that hospitals will attempt to minimize the cost of providing service. Further, the model predicts that hospitals will invest in projects solely on the basis of criteria pertaining to profitability. Perhaps the most serious flaw in the model is that it does not recognize that hospital decision makers have objectives other than the maximization of profits.

QUANTITY-MAXIMIZING MODELS

Since the theory of the for-profit firm is not very relevant to the American hospital industry, which is dominated by nonprofit organizations, a number of alternative theories of behavior have been developed. Among these are models that posit the hospital as a quantity maximizer (Long 1964; Klarman 1965; Reder 1965; Rice 1966; Brown 1970). The incentives for hospital decision makers to pursue strategies designed to promote institutional growth are well documented. For example, Lawrence and Lorsch (1969) argue that healthy institutions are always under pressure to grow. Saltman and Young (1983) contend that administrators and physicians provide most of the impetus for hospitals to grow. Hospital growth is a multidimensional concept that can be measured along several continua, including (1) size, complexity, and comprehensiveness of the hospital's programs and facilities; (2) the number, background, and reputation of the physicians on the institution's medical staff; (3) the extent and image of the institution's research efforts; (4) total patient volume; and (5) total revenue (Saltman and Young 1983).

First, we will discuss the incentives that induce administrators to pursue an institutional growth strategy. The results of a survey conducted by Schulz and Rose (1973) suggest that administrators believe that trustees evaluate their performance on the basis of institutional growth. More specifically, the survey found that trustees place emphasis (in descending order) on institutional solvency, quality of services, intraorganizational harmony, and organizational growth. Although institutional growth was ranked fourth by trustees, it is possible that expansion enables the administrator to achieve the three higher-order objectives of the trustees (Rosko 1984).

McClure (1976) and Mechanic (1980) argue that by increasing the size of the hospital the administrator may help ensure the institution's fiscal solvency, because larger hospitals tend to enjoy greater financial flexibility (i.e., access to more sources of capital and a greater ability to obtain quantity discounts) and thus, tend to be more viable. Further, in the short-run, an increase in patient volume, *ceteris paribus*, should result in a reduction in the cost per unit of service because, in the short-run, fixed costs will be spread over more units of output.

Regarding the relationship between growth and quality, changes in technology may require hospitals to add new programs and services in order to maintain or enhance the quality of care. Further, a growing body of evidence indicates that a positive relationship exists between the volume of services provided and the quality of care (Shortell and LoGerfo 1981; Farber, Kaiser, and Wenzel 1981; Flood, Scott, and Ewy 1984; Hughes, Hunt, and Luft 1987). Accordingly, institutional growth may facilitate increases in quality in these areas. Finally, Harris (1977) argues that conflicts among administrators, medical staff, and other interest groups can often be resolved through growth in available programs and other resources.

Besides institutional obligations, a desire for professional advancement may also motivate hospital administrators to pursue a strategy of institutional growth. For example, it is well known that the reputation of a chief executive officer is closely linked to the reputation of his/her hospital; and the image of the hospital is related to the five dimensions of growth listed by Saltman and Young (1983). Consequently, hospital administrators have a number of internal and external incentives to make decisions that favor the growth of hospitals.

Physicians act on a set of professional and financial incentives to behave in a manner that would encourage institutional growth. Regarding professional influences, Schroeder (1980) argues that the social contract between the physician and patient is the most common and important reason for the physician's decisions. This social contract requires the physician to act as the patient's advocate and to order any potentially efficacious procedure, irrespective of cost. Thus, as diagnostic and therapeutic advances occur, it is likely that the volume of services ordered by physicians will increase.

The socialization that occurs in medical school encourages physicians to use the most recent technology in the practice of medicine (Miller and Miller 1981). This orientation is reinforced by the expectations of peers (Freidson 1970) and patients (Mechanic 1974). Consequently, hospitals may add new services or acquire new resources in order to induce physicians to join or remain on their medical staffs (Rosko and Broyles 1987).

Financial incentives also induce physicians to increase the volume of hospital services. Concern about professional liability has resulted in the practice of "defensive medicine," in which the decisions of physicians to order additional tests and procedures are based more on legal considerations than on judgments about the patient's health status (Havighurst 1984). Further, concerns about potential liability may reinforce the technological orientation of physicians.

Monetary considerations may also induce the physician, who operates a fee-for-service medical practice, to order excessive amounts of medical services. This behavior has been examined in a number of studies of supplier-induced demand, which are discussed in Chapter 3 (Newhouse 1970; Evans 1974; Wennberg 1984).

Rice's (1966) model, which is depicted in Figure 4.2, is representative of the early quantity-maximizing models. The graph indicates that total costs are directly related to output. The slope of the total-cost curve increases as output expands, an outcome that reflects the affect of diminishing marginal productivity on marginal costs. The revenue curve is drawn with a slope that decreases as output increases. This reflects decreases in marginal revenue associated with a declining price elasticity of demand, which occurs as quantity produced (and sold) increases. Total surplus, or profit, is equal to total revenue minus total cost. An inspection of Figure 4.2 reveals that the break-even volume is Q_1, surplus is maximized at Q_2 and losses are incurred if the hospital attempts to

Figure 4.2
Model of an Output-Maximizing Firm with No Subsidy

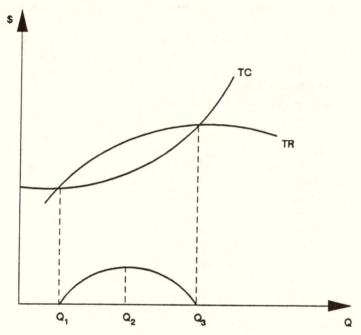

Source: Rice, R. 1966. Analysis of the hospital as an economic
organism. The Modern Hospital 106(4): 89.

Reprint with permission from MODERN HEALTHCARE MAGAZINE. Copyright
Crain Communications, Inc., 740 N. Rush St., Chicago, IL 60611.

produce more than Q_3 units of output. Accordingly, if the hospital's goal is to
maximize output while avoiding a financial loss, the model predicts that output
Q_3 will be produced. If the break-even constraint is altered and profits (losses)
are permitted, output is expected to be larger (smaller) than Q_3.

Rice's model exhibits many of the deficiencies of the early models of hospital
behavior. Most of these models used a vague definition of output. As our summary of hospital objectives suggests, several output-related variables were used.
Among them were patients treated, an actual output measure, and services offered, a variable pertaining to capacity. In addition to these, Feldstein (1971)
used patient days, another direct output measure. All of these measures are vague
and do not indicate a preference for the type of patients treated. Only one of the
early models (Reder 1965) explicitly recognized that the output of the hospital
was not homogeneous. Product heterogeneity was recognized in this model by
weighting patients according to the prestige of the physicians attending them.

A second problem of the quantity-maximizing models pertains to their treatment of quality. Long (1964) enters quality into his model as a constraint: the services provided must be the best possible given the available resources. Feldstein (1961) treats quality as a given. These views of quality are not consistent with goals expressed in many hospital mission statements: to provide the best quality services possible.

The quantity-maximizing models of hospital behavior were an improvement over the general economic model of the for-profit firm, which they were designed to replace. Unfortunately, they were too simple and consequently did not include all of the relevant objectives of the key hospital decision makers.

The neoclassical, microeconomic view of the firm as a profit maximizer has been criticized by many who argue that, in organizations characterized by a separation of ownership (i.e., stockholders) and control (i.e., management), profit maximization is no longer relevant (Miller 1978). Unlike the early industrialists who owned and managed their firms, contemporary managers of publicly held corporations do not gain directly from the profits of their corporations, unless they are also owners (i.e., stockholders). Consequently, theories of discretionary managerial behavior, in which managers are assumed to maximize utility (i.e., salary, prestige, etc.) rather than profits, have gained favor. This type of model is intuitively appealing for the hospital industry, because most of its participants are organized on a not-for-profit basis. The view of the hospital executive as a utility maximizer is also consistent with theories of organizational behavior developed by management scientists (Simon 1965; Barnard 1968).

UTILITY-MAXIMIZING MODELS

In this section our focus turns to a wide variety of utility-maximizing models ranging from the early quality-quantity models to the more sophisticated multioutput models. Among the earliest of the utility maximizing models of hospital behavior were those developed by Newhouse (1970), Lee (1971) and M. Feldstein (1971). Newhouse attempted to depict the impact of retrospective, cost-based reimbursement on hospital behavior. Feldstein focused on price/output dynamics, including retrospective reimbursement, during the 1960s. Lee developed a conspicuous production theory of hospital behavior that reflected the growth of excessive amounts of sophisticated inputs and services (i.e., open-heart units, cardiopulmonary units) that occurred in the hospital industry during the 1960s. According to Lee, the investment behavior of hospitals was distinguished from that of businesses by the acquisition of equipment and facilities without an adequate regard for the contributions of inputs to output.

Lee (1971) postulated that hospital administrators attempt to maximize their utility, which is a function of salary, prestige, security, power, and professional satisfaction. Further, Lee argued that the determinants of utility were directly related to the number and types of sophisticated inputs and services employed by the hospital. It is obvious that the operation of a sophisticated service, such as an open-heart facility, enhances the ego gratification components of Lee's hypothesized utility function (i.e., prestige, power, and professional satisfaction). The acquisition of sophisticated services will enhance the income and security aspects of the administrator's utility function in a more indirect manner. The availability of technical inputs and sophisticated components of care enables the hospital to attract more physicians and patients. Consequently, the hospital administrator will be rewarded by the board of trustees. Since the governing board reinforces the administrator's behavior, conspicuous production will result in unnecessary duplication of facilities and overhiring of staff.

Although Lee's view of the hospital as an organization that competes with others by increasing services reflects a phenomenon that occurred in the hospital industry, his model does not go far enough. Lee (1971, p. 54) argues that it is easy for hospitals to finance service offerings by raising prices because "the price elasticity of demand (over the relevant range) for hospital care is zero or nearly so." This formulation fails to impose a constraint on prices, output, or the range of services. Contrary to Lee's assumptions, revenue is not unlimited and hospital administrators must make trade-offs between the level of quality and the quantity of services their institutions can provide.

The absence of explicit recognition of this trade-off constitutes a serious deficiency in Lee's model. Newhouse (1970) and Feldstein (1971) developed theories of hospital behavior that included a quantity-quality trade-off. Although their models were developed for different purposes, Feldstein and Newhouse each hypothesized the existence of a utility function and a production-possibility curve, each having quality and quantity of hospital services as its arguments. Although the phenomena that Feldstein sought to explain are not entirely relevant today, his model will be emphasized in this section because it has been adapted by others to explain hospital responses to contemporary rate regulation programs.

Feldstein (1971) developed a utility-maximizing model of hospital behavior as part of a twelve equation model (including specifications for demand, price adjustments, costs, and capacity) of nonprofit hospital price dynamics. The portion of the model that pertains to the hospital's quality-quantity trade-off is depicted in Figure 4.3. Feldstein's model is based on the simplifying assumption that, given a fixed budget, hospital decision makers face the opportunity locus (or product transformation curve) AB. This curve depicts a situation in which the hospital faces a trade-off between patient days (PDS) provided and the quality of hospital care (QH). Although this model can be extended to include additional outputs, three or more products cannot be shown graphically. In Feldstein's model, quality is defined as the intensity of services provided (i.e., the number of inputs per patient day). Unfortunately, the intensity of service use is probably a poor measure of quality for an empirical model. Dowling, House, Lehman et al. (1976) reported serious difficulties in acquiring valid and reliable measures of intensity. Therefore, it is assumed that, as used in the Feldstein model, quality pertains to something that can be conceptualized but cannot be measured.

The opportunity locus in Feldstein's model is drawn concave with respect to

Figure 4.3
Feldstein's Utility-Maximizing Model of Hospital Behavior

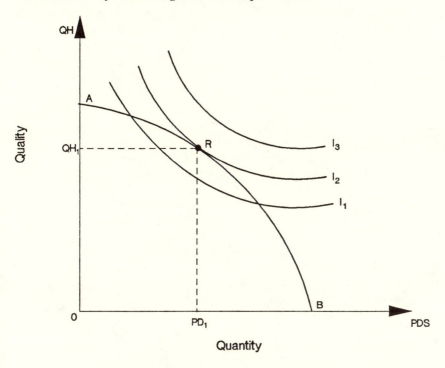

Source: Feldstein, M.S. 1971. Hospital cost inflation : A study of
nonprofit price dynamics. <u>American Economic Review</u> 61(5) : 858.

the origin. This indicates that as the hospital moves from point *B* toward point *A* on the product transformation curve, an increasing amount of *PDS* must be sacrificed to obtain each extra unit of *QH*. This reflects rising marginal costs as *QH* is increased. The model also includes indifference curves I_i, which indicate that the utility of the decision maker is a function of patient days and quality. The indifference curves are drawn convex with respect to the origin, which reflects the assumption that the administrator's marginal evaluation of quality decreases as the level of quality increases. The model predicts that the decision maker will attempt to maximize utility by operating the hospital at point *R* in Figure 4.3, where the level of quality is QH_1, and the number of patient days provided is PD_1. This is consistent with theories of discretionary managerial behavior that are frequently found in the economic literature (Miller 1978). Similar objective functions for hospitals were developed by Newhouse (1970) and Evans (1971).

Feldstein's model must be altered in order to show the effects of prospective

Figure 4.4
Effect of Prospective Payment on Hospital Revenue-Seeking Behavior

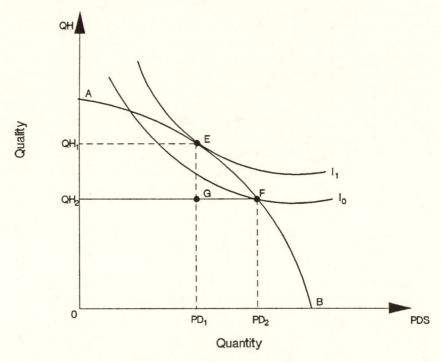

payment on hospital behavior. As shown in Figure 4.4, the revenue constraint imposed by prospective payment can be entered into the model as a price ceiling for each patient day. Cromwell (1976) depicted the ceiling as a kink in the product transformation curve. This is labeled as QH_2 in Figure 4.4. The hospital's opportunity locus becomes QH_2GFB because the revenue ceiling imposed by prospective payment does not allow the hospital to provide care that is more expensive than the value of the inputs needed to provide QH_2 amount of quality per patient day. At the new equilibrium position, point F, the hospital will provide more patient days but at a lower level of quality than prior to the imposition of revenue controls. The hospital can increase the volume of patient days by increasing either the average length of stay or the admission rate. The average length of stay can be increased by extending the patient's period of convalescence in the hospital. Patient days during this period are likely to require a less than average amount of resources, which may result in a cost per day that is below the prospective per diem rate. Hence, hospitals can use profits earned during these days to subsidize losses that occur during the earlier, more service-intensive period of the patient's hospital stay. If excess capacity exists after increasing the length of stay, the hospital may attempt to increase the rate of admissions. Since the per diem rates established by the regulators do not reflect costs associated with case-mix differences, the system induces hospitals to admit patients who present conditions less complex, and, hence, less costly to treat.

The model of hospital responses to prospective payment can be altered to reflect a rate regulation program that relies on cases treated as the unit of payment. Substituting cases treated for patient days on the horizontal axis of Figure 4.4, the kink in the production possibility curve, QH_2F, now pertains to a revenue ceiling per case treated. The reader can verify that the response of hospitals to this form of prospective payment will be to reduce quality and increase the quantity of cases treated. Unlike the per diem system, however, the cases treated payment mechanism creates an incentive to decrease the average length of stay.

Returning to per diem-based prospective payment, let us consider how a hospital can operate at the initial equilibrium position, point E, even with the price ceiling in effect. This can be done if the hospital is willing to suffer a loss per patient day equal to the vertical distance EG in Figure 4.4. PD_1E is equal to the cost per patient day when QH_1 quality and PD_1 patient days are provided; PD_1G is the per diem prospective rate set for this hospital. Alternatively, the hospital can avoid suffering a loss if it is able to subsidize the losses associated with the care provided to regulated patients by raising charges to nonregulated patients or by increasing its level of endowment. Cross-subsidization may be preferred to debt financing as a response to prospective payment because it does not threaten the solvency of hospitals if successfully carried out. Indirect support for this premise is provided by Rosko (1984), whose study is reviewed in Chapter 12.

In contrast to the earlier models of hospital behavior, Goldfarb, Hornbrook, and Rafferty (1980) explicitly recognized the multiproduct nature of the hospital by incorporating trade-offs among various competing goals. Their model is based on the assumption that hospital decision makers attempt to maximize utility, which is a function of the number of admissions, case-mix, quality, and profits. The constraints consisted of reimbursement policies, technology, patient availability, and general resources. They also assume that the hospital decision makers face trade-offs between the components of the objective function and that the criterion for resolving conflicting objectives is to equalize (where possible) the marginal utilities of each of the components of the objective function. This criterion is theoretically appealing because it is consistent with classical microeconomic conditions for utility maximization; however, more pragmatic considerations suggest that the model is of limited use. One weakness of their model development is that Goldfarb et al. fail to discuss how utility is measured by the decision makers. Consequently, it is difficult to determine how trade-offs occur.

Perhaps, a more serious limitation of the model proposed by Goldfarb et al. (1980) lies with the definition and operationalization of the hospital's objectives. The purpose of the model is to provide a realistic depiction of the hospital's objectives; however, the model is so simplistic (perhaps by necessity) that it departs dramatically from reality. For example, case-mix in the objective function could be used to depict the trade-offs made by physicians in specialties that are competing for an increased share of the hospital's resources. Instead, they use the concept of case-mix necessity, which is defined as "the degree to which the unique facilities of a hospital are required for a successful outcome, as compared to the use of alternative ambulatory services" (Goldfarb et al. 1980, p. 186).

Goldfarb et al. use the model to develop a number of hypotheses pertaining to the effects on endogenous variables (i.e., hospital objectives) caused by changes in exogenous constraints, such as the number of patients and the supply of beds in the area. The authors point out, however, that valid testing of the model was precluded by specification and measurement errors in the data set. Accordingly, we will not discuss their empirical results.

Rosko (1982) used the Cromwell model and extended it to consider the case where managerial slack was included in the maximand. The model predicted that as slack increased, quality and quantity of services would decrease and that cost per unit of service would increase. Further, the model predicted that the imposition of revenue constraints in the form of per diem prospective payments would result in a reduction in slack, an outcome that intensifies efforts to secure factor inputs at the lowest possible prices and to enhance the efficiency of resource utilization. Consequently, expenditures per unit of service would be constrained.

Employing more formal mathematical analysis than either Cromwell or Rosko, Sloan and Steinwald (1980) also used a utility maximizing model of hospital behavior based on the work of Newhouse (1970) and Feldstein (1971). Unlike the earlier models, which assumed that the goal of the hospital was to maximize quality and quantity of services, the Sloan-Steinwald objective function was expressed:

$$\text{Maximize } U = U(X, Y, \pi) \tag{4.2}$$

where X is a service composite that incorporates both quality and quantity dimensions of output; Y represents amenities including those provided to patients as well as physician perquisites; and π represents profit.

The objective function is very general. Different types of hospitals may place different weights on the objectives. Proprietary hospitals may emphasize π, while not-for-profit hospitals may place more emphasis on X or Y. This is consistent with Clarkson's (1972) observations regarding the impact of property rights arrangements upon production decisions in proprietary and not-for-profit hospitals. The Sloan-Steinwald model was used to predict the effects of changes in exogenous variables, including regulation, on X, Y, costs, and factor inputs.

It is interesting to note that Sloan and Steinwald used profit as an argument in the objective function of nonprofit hospitals. Some of the early models, which assumed hospitals acted as profit-maximizing firms, were criticized because this maximand was contrary to their nonprofit status; however, changes in the hospital payment mechanism (i.e., prospective payment) and the "corporatization" of hospitals, have created incentives for the not-for-profit hospital to seek profits (i.e., operating surpluses). Although there are no stockholders to whom an operating surplus could be distributed, it is commonly believed that hospitals attempt to earn profits in some areas in order to subsidize services for which adequate compensation is not received (McClure 1981). Consequently, it is more appropriate to view hospitals as profit-seekers now than 10 or 20 years ago.

The most notable feature of Sloan and Steinwald's model is the extensive reliance on formal mathematical proofs; however, in their efforts to create an elegant model, Sloan and Steinwald may have sacrificed too much realism. For example, the researchers (Sloan and Steinwald 1980, p. 19) argue "parsimony in the choice of variables is crucial. Thus, rather than define separate variables for quantity and quality as others have done, for some analytical purposes it is useful to define a single composite measure of patient services X. In this way, one avoids the amorphous term quality." Sloan and Steinwald recognized the deficiencies of this approach but proceeded to develop their model without an explicit quality-quantity trade-off or an explicit recognition of the trade-offs required in a multiproduct firm with limited resources. Similarly, in their review of the literature, Sloan and Steinwald acknowledged the importance of slack in the objective function of many hospital managers, but did not include it in their formal model. These omissions precluded a prediction of the impact of exogenous changes on product-mix, organizational slack, and quality. Since their model was developed for policy analysis, it was unfortunate that they were not able to predict the impact of rate regulation on other dimensions of hospital performance that governmental authorities may find important to influence.

Finally, the absence of an explicit and well-defined role for physicians constitutes a deficiency in the Sloan-Steinwald model and is a common exclusion in most models of hospital behavior. In contrast to those proposed by economists, models of hospital behavior developed by organizational theorists (Perrow 1961; Roemer and Friedman 1971; Allison 1976) stress the diversity of interests between the administration, the medical staff, and the governing board. Sloan and Steinwald (1980, p. 19) summed up the feelings of many economists regarding the apparently inappropriate reliance on a single objective function in hospital models as follows: "Although the ideas of organizational theorists coincide with the reality many of us [i.e., economists] have observed, at the same time they greatly complicate any attempt to develop explicit models of hospital behavior. For this reason, with some reservations, we have devoted most of this analysis to the traditional economic approach."

MEDICAL STAFF INCOME-MAXIMIZING MODELS

Pauly and Redisch (1973) were the first to emphasize an active role of the physician in a model of hospital behavior. They assumed that the medical staff has de facto control of the hospital at any point in time. Their model posits that the goal of nonprofit hospitals is to maximize the net income per member of

Figure 4.5
Physician Equilibrium in the Pauly-Redisch Model

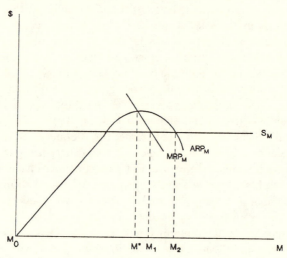

Source: Pauly, M., and M. Redisch. 1973. The not-for-profit hospital
as a physician cooperative. _American Economic Review_ 63 (1) : 92,94.

the medical staff. The objective function is subject to the constraints imposed by the hospital's production function and demand curve. These constraints interact to determine how the maximum output can be produced while maximizing physician income and allowing the hospital to break even.

Pauly and Redisch credit the structure of the model to the work of those who attempted to explain the economic behavior of the Soviet collective farm or the Yugoslav producers' collective (Furubotn and Pejovich 1970; Ward 1958). The model also borrows from the orthodox theory of the firm, which attempts to explain input utilization and pricing decisions made by for-profit firms (Miller 1978).

Pauly and Redisch, whose model is depicted in Figure 4.5, used ARP_M, the average revenue product of the medical staff, as the maximand of the objective function. It is expressed:

$$Y_M = (PQ - cK - wL) /M \qquad\qquad (4.3)$$

where PQ represents total revenue; cK represents expenditures for capital; wL represents expenditures for labor; and M represents the size of the medical staff.

An examination of equation 4.3 implies that the difference between total revenue and hospital operating costs (i.e., $cK + wL$) is distributed to the medical staff. Also appearing in Figure 4.5 is the marginal revenue product, which is equal to the change in the total revenue product associated with a one unit change in the size of the medical staff. The downward-sloping portion of this curve may be attributed to either an elastic demand or a diminishing marginal product of the medical staff. S_M represents the supply curve for physicians.

As indicated in Figure 4.5, the objective function, Y_M, is maximized when M^* physicians are hired. This model suggests that physicians who are members of a "closed staff" that share income equally are willing to add members to the staff as long as the increment increases each member's net income (e.g., increasing staff size from M_o to M^*).

If the assumption of equal sharing is replaced by allowing hospitals to hire physicians at the supply price, OS, the equilibrium staff size will be M_1, where MRP_M equals the supply price. This is the same result found in the standard analysis of the for-profit firm's decision to hire inputs (Miller 1978).

Finally, if an open staff is assumed, the Pauly-Redisch model predicts that the equilibrium size of the medical staff is M_2 where ARP_M equals the supply price OS. There is no incentive to expand the size of the medical staff beyond M_2 because further increases would reduce average income below a level that could be earned in alternative activities.

Although it is obvious that the Pauly-Redisch model was developed to describe discriminatory practices of medical staffs during the 1950s and 1960s, it also can be used to illustrate the impact of reimbursement on the patient management decisions of physicians. The model shown in Figure 4.5 is based on the assumption that the patient pays the full cost of hospitalization. Consequently, the average revenue product curve, ARP_M, is constrained by the rationing effect of price on demand. Pauly and Redisch argue that in the extreme case where every patient is fully insured with cost-based insurance, there would be virtually no constraint on the amount of capital and labor that physicians use to provide service. Therefore, these inputs would be employed up to the point at which the marginal contribution of each physician's revenue was zero. Pauly and Redisch conclude that this would result in hospitals providing "Cadillac quality" medicine to every patient. The amount of resource use is constrained by the restrictions of medical science. Although the extreme case of complete insurance does not exist, this model provides an explanation for the positive relationship between insurance coverage and hospital costs (Feldstein 1971).

The Pauly-Redisch view of the hospital as a physician cooperative, with an objective to maximize physician income, is dramatically different from the previously discussed models of hospital behavior. As we have suggested, the reality of other hospital models suffered from the omission of distinct roles for the medical staff and the administration. Although the inclusion of a specific objective for physicians is appropriate, Pauly and Redisch have made a serious omission by excluding the roles of the administration and the governing board from their model. Their view of the hospital leads to inaccurate predictions such as the minimization of costs and the absence of managerial slack.

Morrisey, Sloan, and Mitchell (1983) adapted the models developed by Pauly and Redisch (1973) and Pauly (1980) to predict hospital responses to a hospital rate regulation program that employs the patient day as the unit of payment. They view the non-profit hospital as an organization that has a single objective: to maximize medical staff net income. They also assume that the proprietary hospital will attempt to maximize the net present value of its operation to its shareholders. Both types of hospitals will pursue their objectives by employing inputs to minimize costs. Moreover, Morrisey et al. also extended their model to consider the more realistic case in which the nonprofit hospital maximizes a utility function subject to a minimum profit constraint rather than maximizing physician income. In this situation, hospital executives are predicted to dissipate their monopoly rents by choosing higher quality and quantity than would the perfectly competitive, profit-maximizing firm. The authors contend that their model is robust over a number of specifications. Although the assumptions regarding the maximand of the hospital influence the optimal levels of the arguments in the objective function, the comparative static predictions of changes caused by shifts in exogenous factors are not affected in most cases. Morrisey et al. do not use formal analysis to support their contention; however, they do refer to a utility maximization model (Hornbrook and Rafferty 1982) that generates predictions, comparable to theirs, for the effects of per diem and case-based rate regulation.

The model developed by Morrisey et al. (1983) is depicted in Figure 4.6. The arguments of the model consist of unit costs ($/X) and output (X). However, unlike earlier models of hospital behavior, which defined the hospital's product in terms of patient days or admissions, the authors viewed output as a bundle of services or characteristics offered by the hospital. Included in this bundle of services are: bed rest, special unit care, specific therapies, tests, lab work-ups, etc. This definition of output is consistent with Lancaster's (1966) product characteristics model. The model proposed by Morrisey et al. predicts that equilibrium will occur at the level of output (X_e) and price (P_e) where marginal costs (MCq_e) equal the marginal valuation of output. This result is similar to the standard microeconomic criterion, marginal cost equals marginal revenue, except that the marginal valuation of output replaces marginal revenue. Another refinement of the standard economic model is the explicit recognition that marginal costs and marginal valuation are dependent on the level of quality. Thus, point A is an equilibrium condition pertaining to a particular level of quality. If quality was changed, MC (q_e) and MV (q_e) would shift, resulting in a new equilibrium at a different price and output level. The curve labeled $A*A*$ represents the locus of equilibrium points. The negatively sloped portion of this curve, which is associated with higher quality levels, reflects rapidly diminishing returns on increases in quality.

Morrisey et al. entered prospective payment into the model as a ceiling, MC (q), that limits average revenues per unit of output. The restriction on revenue is expected to reduce quality; however, the impact on quantity depends on the location of the hospital on the $A*A*$ curve prior to the introduction of rate

Figure 4.6
An Exchange Model of Hospital Responses to Prospective Payment

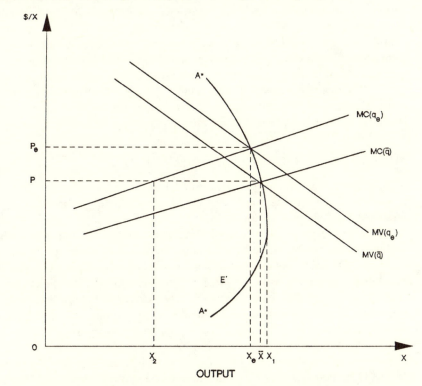

Source: Morrisey, M.A., D.A. Conrad, S.M. Shortell, and K.S. Cook.
1984. Hospital rate review: A theory and an empirical review.
Journal of Health Economics 3(1): 29.

regulation. In the model shown in Figure 4.6, the hospital is on the downward-sloping portion of A^*A^*, a position which the authors argue is likely to occur because of the presence of service-benefit style health insurance. In this situation, the imposition of prospective payment will lead to an increase in output. The authors suggest that under a maximum per diem revenue constraint, hospitals are likely to increase the duration of the hospital stay, thereby reducing the intensity of services per day.

The authors use insights from Barzel (1982) to extend their model and make the following predictions. First, the introduction of prospective payment will result in the unbundling of hospital services. Second, the imposition of revenue constraints will induce hospitals to alter their contractual relationships with physicians. In order to reduce the incentives for physicians to order excessive tests and procedures, Morrisey et al. argue it is likely that hospitals will replace remuneration that is tied to the value of the department's output with straight salary contracts. Since the compensation of pathologists and radiologists is typically determined by the value of departmental output, these professionals are likely candidates for this type of renegotiation.

Although the model developed by Morrisey et al. is based on the Pauly-Redisch (1973) model of physician-income maximization, it is clear that it is also derived from the quality-quantity maximization models developed by Feldstein (1971) and Newhouse (1970). Accordingly, it is not surprising that many of the predictions of hospital responses to prospective payment based on these seemingly different types of models are similar.

MODELS OF NURSING HOME BEHAVIOR

Scanlon (1980) developed a model to explain the existence of excess demand in the market for nursing home care. Separate models for proprietary and nonprofit nursing homes were developed.

The model of proprietary homes, which is illustrated in Figure 4.7, is based on the assumption that these organizations attempt to maximize profit. Accordingly, the standard economic criterion for pricing and output decisions (i.e., equating marginal cost with marginal revenue) is applied. The kinked-demand curve, $D_pABD'_p$, illustrates the existence of two classes of buyers. The horizontal segment, AB, corresponds to the influence of monopsonistic purchasers, such as state Medicaid programs, on demand. Although there are several ways in which nursing home payment rates can be set (see Chapter 12), Scanlon's depiction of nursing homes as price-takers for Medicaid patients is essentially correct. The downward portions of the demand curve represent what Scanlon loosely terms the private market in which he also includes Medicare patients.

D_pA is the portion of the private market that is willing to pay more than the prevailing Medicaid rate and BD'_p represents the demand curve for those who will demand nursing home care only if the price is less than that set by Medicaid. Associated with the two classes of buyers (i.e., private and public) are two marginal revenue curves. The marginal revenue curve for private patients is depicted by MR while the marginal revenue curve for Medicaid patients coincides with segment AB on the demand curve. Since marginal cost equals marginal revenue at point D, proprietary nursing homes will supply Q_s beds. The profit maximizing strategy is to provide Q_p beds at price P_p for private patients and to supply the remaining beds $Q_s - Q_p$ to Medicaid patients at the state-established price of P_m.

Scanlon's model of the nonprofit nursing home market is shown in Figure 4.8. This model reflects the assumption that the objective of nonprofit organizations is to maximize output, subject to a quality constraint and a solvency constraint. To achieve their goal, nonprofit nursing homes must set average revenue equal to average cost, and allocate bed supply, Q_s, between Medicaid and private residents, such that the marginal revenue from each is equal. Ac-

Figure 4.7
Model of the Proprietary Nursing Home Market

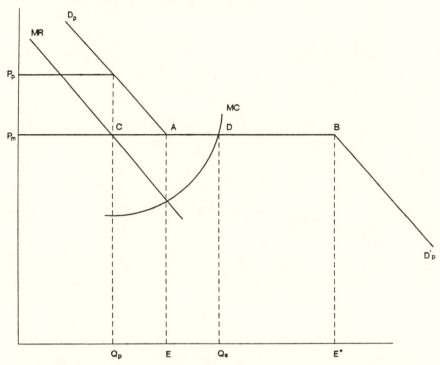

Source: Scanlon, W.J. 1980. A theory of the nursing home
        market. Inquiry 17(1): 29.

cordingly, Q_p beds will be allocated to private patients and the remaining supply, $Q_s - Q_p$, will be allocated to Medicaid patients.

The key point to be drawn from Scanlon's model is that there is no mechanism that guarantees that the quantity of bed days supplied by nonprofit and proprietary homes to Medicaid residents, $Q_s - Q_p$, equals the number of Medicaid eligibles demanding services, $E^* - E$. If the number of beds is not sufficient to satisfy total market demand, the private-pay patients are likely to be given preference because they can be charged a higher price than Medicaid patients. Therefore, the entire shortage of nursing home beds will be borne by Medicaid patients.

Scanlon's analysis suggests that, if the Medicaid reimbursement rate is less than the average total cost for the industry, excess demand will exist even in the long run unless action is taken by the government. Given a limited revenue-base and competing uses for state funds, however, many states are unlikely to increase the rate of compensation for nursing homes.

Figure 4.8
Model of the Nonprofit Nursing Home Market

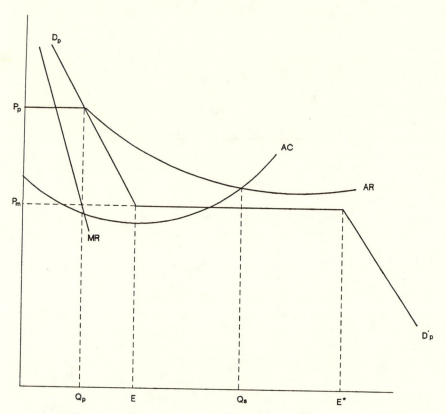

Source: Scanlon, W.J. 1980. A theory of the nursing home
            market. Inquiry 17(1): 31.

Scanlon conducted an indirect test of the excess demand hypothesis. He argued that if the excess demand hypothesis is valid, the unfilled beds variable, defined in terms of the probability of finding a bed, given demand, should affect Medicaid utilization but not private utilization, since the latter is assumed to be satisfied (i.e., extra beds will not lead to more utilization).

Scanlon employed 15 independent variables representing a variety of determinants of demand from a data set compiled from 43 states during the years 1969 and 1973. As expected, significant coefficients ($p \leq .01$) were estimated for the unfilled beds variables in the three equations (i.e., 1969 data, 1973 data, and a combined data set) in which total utilization was used as the dependent variable. In contrast, this variable was insignificant ($p > 0.05$) in the three equations estimated for private demand. This result was also expected.

Scanlon drew several policy implications from this study. First, excess demand for nursing home beds probably exists; however, it is unclear whether the excess demand should be reduced by increasing Medicaid payment rates, by introducing patient cost sharing, or by increasing subsidies for alternatives to nursing homes. Second, given excess demand, nursing homes will be able to implement a more selective admissions policy that discriminates against the more severely ill because these patients are more costly to treat. Consequently, those who have the greatest need for a nursing home bed may not be able to find it. More recent evidence (Nyman, Levey, and Rohrer 1987) suggests that the implementation of severity-adjusted payment rates may not ameliorate this problem in areas where excess demand exists.

SUMMARY

Hospitals and other health care institutions are extremely complex organizations and it is not surprising that models depicting their behavior depart from reality. Our literature review found three common problems in model development. First, the definition of quality is often vague or incomplete. Donabedian (1969) trichotomized quality measurements according to structure (i.e., mix of inputs offered by the institution); process (i.e., the manner in which services were provided); and end results (i.e., the outcome of care). Although the components of Donabedian's quality triad appear to be related (i.e., if competent health professionals adhere to established standards of care and use current medical technology, a positive health outcome should result), there is ample anecdotal evidence about patients recovering despite the type of care provided and vice versa.

Accordingly, it may be more appropriate to use a more comprehensive definition of quality than is usually employed in hospital models. As Donabedian (1969) points out, however, quality is very difficult to measure. Consequently, economic models of hospitals have emphasized structure, which is the easiest aspect of quality to quantify. To the extent that decision makers consider only structural aspects in their evaluations of hospitals, the exclusion of other dimensions of quality is not a serious deficiency. Indeed, given consumer ignorance many hospitals acquire unneeded, sophisticated, and highly visible technical equipment in order to attract patients; however, the image of a hospital within a community is also dependent upon process and outcome results. For example, failure to satisfy standards (process) of medical practice may precipitate malpractice suits in which the plaintiff is successful. Similarly, a hospital with a high mortality rate, irrespective of the hospital's responsibility for it, may have a poor image in the community. These are aspects of quality, not found in many economic models of hospitals, which affect the chief executive officer's job security and level of compensation, as well as the prestige of the hospital. Thus, the absence of these factors, which are likely to determine the decision-maker's level of utility, constitute a serious deficiency in hospital models.

Second, the economic models generally are not clear about to whom the maximand pertains. Vague references to a composite decision maker, consisting of the weighted (but unspecified) preferences of trustees, medical staff, and administrators have been made frequently. However, the trade-offs that are negotiated by these actors are complex and are likely to differ between organizations. Since the purpose of the model is to predict general responses of hospitals to exogenous changes in their environment, it is probably sufficient to develop an appropriate objective function and a set of realistic constraints. Specifying how the organizational participants make their trade-offs is a more appropriate pursuit for organizational theorists.

Third, most of the theories of hospital behavior do not assume that slack or technical inefficiency are desired by the hospital decision makers. Consequently, they predict that hospitals will be cost-minimizers. These assumptions are contradicted by the observations of many health economists (Sloan and Steinwald 1980) that slack exists. Moreover, a survey revealed that institutional harmony is a common criterion that hospital trustees use to evaluate the performance of administrators (Schulz and Rose 1973). Rosko (1984) argued that institutional harmony is related to slack; and, hence, as long as other areas of hospital performance (i.e., financial position, quality of services, and institutional growth) are acceptable, some amount of slack may be desired.

REFERENCES

Allison, R. F. 1976. Administrative responses to prospective reimbursement. *Topics in Health Care Financing* 3(2):97–111.

Barnard, C. I. 1968. *The Function of the Executive*. Cambridge, MA: Harvard University Press.

Barzel, Y. 1982. Measurement cost and the organization of markets. *Journal of Law and Economics* 25(1):24–48.

Berki, S. 1972. *Hospital Economics*. Lexington, MA: Lexington Books, 28.

Brown, M. 1970. Economic analysis of hospital operations. *Hospital Administration* 15:60–74.

Clarkson, K. W. 1972. Some implications of property rights in hospital management. *Journal of Law and Economics* 15(2):363–84.

Cromwell, J. 1976. Hospital productivity trends in short-term general non-teaching hospitals. *Inquiry* 11(2):181–87.

Davis, K. 1971. *Economic Theories of Behavior in Nonprofit, Private Hospitals*. Washington, DC: The Brookings Institute.

Donabedian, A. 1969. *A Guide to Medical Care Administration, Volume II: Medical Care Appraisal—Quality and Utilization*. Washington, DC: American Public Health Association.

Dowling, W. L., P. J. House, J. M. Lehman, G. L. Meade, N. Teague, V. Trivedi, and C. A. Watts. 1976. Impact of the Blue Cross and Medicaid prospective reimbursement systems in downstate New York. Final report on contract HEW-OS-72-2481. Seattle, WA: Dept. of Health Services, University of Washington.

Evans, R. 1971. Behavioral cost functions for hospitals. *Canadian Journal of Economics* 4(2):198–215.

Evans, R. 1974. Supply-induced demand: Some empirical evidence and implications. In M. Perlman, ed., *The Economics of Health and Medical Care*. New York: Wiley, 155–66.

Farber, B., D. Kaiser, and R. Wenzel. 1981. Relation between surgical volume and incidence of postoperative wound infection. *New England Journal of Medicine* 305(4):200–204.

Feldstein, M. 1971. Hospital cost inflation: A study of nonprofit price dynamics. *American Economic Review* 61(5):853–72.

Feldstein, P. 1961. *An Empirical Investigation of the Marginal Cost of Hospital Services*. Chicago: University of Chicago, p. 66.

Feldstein, P. J. 1979. *Health Care Economics*. New York: John Wiley and Sons.

Flood A., W. Scott, and W. Ewy. 1984. Does practice make perfect? The relation between hospital volume and outcomes for selected diagnostic categories. *Medical Care* 22(2):98–114.

Frank, R., J. Weiner, D. Steinwachs, and D. Salkever. 1987. Economic rents derived from hospital privileges in the market for podiatric services. *Journal of Health Economics* 6(4):319–37.

Freidson, E. 1970. *Professional Dominance: The Social Structure of Medical Care*. New York: Atherton.

Furubotn, E., and S. Pejovich. 1970. Tax policy and investment decisions of the Yugoslav firm. *National Tax Journal* 23(3):335–57.

Goldfarb, M., M. Hornbrook, and J. Rafferty. 1980. Behavior of the multiproduct firm: A model of the nonprofit hospital system. *Medical Care* 18(2):185–201.

Harris, J. E. 1977. The internal organization of hospitals: Some economic implications. *Bell Journal of Economics* 8(2):467–82.

Havighurst, C. C. 1984. Reforming malpractice law through consumer choice. *Health Affairs* 3(4):63–70.

Hornbrook, M., and J. Rafferty. 1982. The economics of hospital reimbursement. In R. M. Scheffler, and L. F. Rossiter, eds., *Advances in Health Economics and Health Services Research* 3. Greenwich, CT: JAI Press, pp. 79–115.

Hughes, R., S. Hunt, and H. Luft. 1987. Effects of surgeon volume and hospital volume on quality of care in hospitals. *Medical Care* 25(6):489–503.

Klarman, H. 1965. *The Economics of Health*. New York: Columbia University Press, 121.

Lancaster, K. 1966. A new approach to consumer theory. *Journal of Political Economy* 74(2):132–57.

Lawrence, P. R., and J. W. Lorsch. 1969. *Organization and Environment*. Homewood, IL: Richard D. Irwin.

Lee, M. L. 1971. A conspicuous production theory of hospital behavior. *Southern Economic Journal* 38(1):48–58.

Long, M. F. 1964. Efficient use of hospitals. In S. Muskin, ed., *The Economics of Health and Medical Care*. Ann Arbor: University of Michigan Press.

McClure, W. 1976. The medical care system under national health insurance: Four models. *Journal of Health Politics, Policy and Law* 1(1):22–68.

McClure, W. 1981. Structure and incentive problems in economic regulation of medical care. *Millbank Memorial Fund Quarterly* 59(2):107–44.

Mechanic, D. 1974. *Politics, Medicine, and Social Science*. New York: Wiley-Interscience.

Mechanic, D. 1980. *Future Issues in Health Care: Social Policy and the Rationing of Medical Services*. New York: Free Press.

Miller, R. 1978. *Intermediate Microeconomics: Theory, Issues and Applications*. New York: McGraw-Hill.

Miller, A. E., and M. G. Miller. 1981. *Options for Health and Health Care: The Coming of Post-Clinical Medicine*. New York: John Wiley & Sons.

Morrisey, M. A., D. A. Conrad, S. M. Shortell, and K. S. Cook. 1984. Hospital rate review: A theory and an empirical review. *Journal of Health Economics* 3(1):25–47.

Morrisey, M. A., F. A. Sloan, and S. A. Mitchell. 1983. State rate setting: An analysis of some unresolved issues. *Health Affairs* 2(1):36–47.

Newhouse, J. P. 1970. A model of physician pricing. *Southern Economic Journal* 37(2):174–83.

Nyman, J., S. Levey, and J. Rohrer. 1987. RUGs and equity of access to nursing home care. *Medical Care* 25(5):361–72.

Pauly, M. V. 1980. *Doctors and Their Workshops: Economic Models of Physician Behavior*. Chicago: University of Chicago Press.

Pauly, M., and M. Redisch. 1973. The not-for-profit hospital as a physician cooperative. *American Economic Review* 63(1):87–99.

Penchansky, R., and G. Rosenthal. 1965. Productivity, price, and income in the physician's services market—a tentative hypothesis. *Medical Care* 3:240–44.

Perrow, C. 1961. The analysis of complex organizations. *American Sociological Review* 26(6):854–65.

Reder, M. 1965. Some problems in economics of hospitals. *American Economic Review* 56(2):472–80.

Rice, R. 1966. Analysis of the hospital as an economic organism. *The Modern Hospital* 106(4):88–91.

Roemer, M., and J. Friedman. 1971. *Doctors in Hospitals: Medical Staff Organization and Hospital Performance*. Baltimore, MD: Johns Hopkins University Press.

Rosko, M. D. 1982. *Hospital responses to prospective rate setting*. Unpublished doctoral dissertation, Temple University.

Rosko, M. D. 1984. Differential impact of prospective payment on hospitals located in different catchment areas. *Journal of Health and Human Resources Administration* 7(4):61–83.

Rosko, M. D., and R. W. Broyles. 1987. Strategic hospital marketing responses to prospective payment. *Journal of Hospital Marketing* 1(3/4):71–81.

Saltman, R. B., and D. W. Young. 1983. Hospital cost containment and the quest for institutional growth: A behavioral analysis. *Journal of Public Health Policy* 4(3):313–34.

Scanlon, W. J. 1980. A theory of the nursing home market. *Inquiry* 17(1):25–41.

Schroeder, S. A. 1980. Variations in physician practice patterns: A review of medical cost implications. In E. J. Carels, D. Neuhauser, and W. B. Stason, eds., *The Physician and Cost Control*. Cambridge, MA: Oelgeschlager, Gunn and Hain, pp. 23–50.

Schulz, R., and J. Rose. 1973. Can hospitals be expected to control costs? *Inquiry* 10(1):3–8.

Shalit, S. 1977. A doctor-hospital cartel theory. *Journal of Business* 59(1):1–20.

Shortell, S., and J. LoGerfo. 1981. Hospital medical staff organization and quality of care: Results for myocardial infarction and appendectomy. *Medical Care* 19(10):1041–55.

Simon, H. A. 1965. *Administrative Behavior*. New York: Macmillan.

Sloan, F. A., and B. Steinwald. 1980. *Insurance, Regulation, and Hospital Costs*. Lexington, MA: D.C. Heath & Co.

Ward, B. 1958. The firm in Illyria: Market syndicalism. *American Economic Review* 48(4):566–89.

Wennberg, J.E. 1984. Dealing with medical practice variations: A proposal for action. *Health Affairs* 3(2):6–32.

5

HOSPITAL OUTPUT MEASURES

The absence of homogeneous output measures for health care providers has hindered analysis in the areas of research, management and policy. As we will demonstrate in Chapter 7 and Chapter 8, the inability to control variations in product-mix with precision has threatened the validity of cost function estimates, production-function estimates, and the analysis of efficiency. As illustrated by Broyles and Rosko (1986), managers require homogeneous measures of output in order to effectively perform their planning, controlling and budgeting activities. Finally, well-defined measures of output will facilitate the development of sound payment and community health planning policies (Hornbrook 1982).

In this chapter, we examine the issues of output measures that are germane to the analysis of costs, production, and payment policy. Most of the recent work in this area has emphasized the development of isoresource groups (e.g., Diagnosis Related Groups) or case-mix severity adjustments. Accordingly, this chapter will focus on these areas; however, to facilitate evaluation of earlier studies or research efforts that, because of unavailability of required information or budgetary constraints, used less refined output measures, we will analyze some of the earlier measures. Measures of hospital output are analyzed in this chapter, to be followed by a chapter devoted to output measures employed in other sectors of the health care industry.

EARLY HOSPITAL OUTPUT MEASURES

It is commonly argued by economists that the final output of a firm is a good or service that yields satisfaction to the consumer. As hospitals have accelerated their efforts to diversify their businesses during the 1980s, it is clear that they produce services, and, to a lesser extent, goods for a variety of consumers. Nevertheless, the inpatient continues to be the most important consumer of hospital services. Accordingly, the primary output of the hospital should be defined in terms of the benefits that patients expect to receive as a result of their course of treatment in the hospital (i.e., improvement in health status or relief from pain and anxiety); however, formidable obstacles have precluded the measurement of the final output of the hospital. Accordingly, analysts of the hospital industry have relied on intermediate measures of output, including: (1) patient days, (2) cases treated, and (3) services provided.

We shall discuss each of these factors in turn.

Patient Days

The patient day has been the most commonly used measure of output in the hospital and nursing home industries. As summarized by Berki (1972), the problem with defining output in terms of patient days stems from the heterogeneity of services provided to patients who have different needs. Simply put— all patient days are not equal.

It is convenient to dichotomize the types of services provided by hospitals as stay-specific or diagnosis-specific. Stay-specific services include routine nursing care and the so-called "hotel services." The provision of stay-specific services varies directly with the length of stay and is reflected fairly accurately by the patient day. On the other hand, the mix of required diagnostic-specific or ancillary services, such as physical therapy, laboratory tests, surgical procedures or radiological examinations, depends, in part, on the patients' diagnoses. Further, the services required by patients who are assigned to the same diagnostic grouping may vary substantially according to the severity of illness (Horn, Horn, and Sharkey 1984). Therefore, it is clear that the patient day is a poor measure of output because it does not reflect the variation in patient needs associated with case-mix (i.e., distribution of patients by diagnostic grouping) or severity of illness (i.e., seriousness of illness within a diagnostic grouping).

In recognition of the limitations of defining output in terms of patient days, a number of researchers have attempted to estimate multiproduct cost functions for hospitals by entering patient days by category. These studies have used classification schemes associated with age (i.e., pediatric, adult, and geriatric patients) or broad diagnostic groupings (i.e., medical, surgical, OB/GYN, etc.). Although an improvement over the use of the unadjusted patient day as an output measure, these groupings fail to capture with precision the multiproduct nature of the hospital.

Cases Treated

Often defined as an inpatient admission or discharge, the case is another commonly used measure of hospital output. Conceptually, the discharge is more closely related to the economic definition of hospital output since it is possible to presume that the decision to release a patient is based, in part, on a professional assessment of the individual's health status. For example, the restoration of the patient's desired health status or a reduction in the presenting medical need that permits treatment in a less intensive setting represent factors that support the decision to release the individual. However, the case treated captures neither differences in stay-specific services (e.g., an episode of hospital care might be 2 days or 20 days), nor differences in diagnostic-specific services. Indeed, as we shall discuss later in this chapter, Diagnosis Related Groups (DRGs) were developed in response to these deficiencies.

Services Provided

In recognition of the variations in services provided associated with length of stay and diagnosis, output has been defined as the sum of weighted services. In one of the earliest studies that used the weighted measure, Cohen (1967) expressed output as:

$$S_k = \sum_{i=1}^{n} w_i Q_{ik} \qquad (5.1)$$

where S_k = service output of the kth hospital; Q_{ik} = quantity of the ith service in the kth hospital; and w_i = weight of the ith service.

Cohen used estimated average cost to weight the output, an approach that has two limitations. First, arbitrary methods are often used by hospitals to allocate costs. A commonly applied cost allocation formula considers the ratio of inpatient to outpatient charges to apportion costs among cost centers. Such an approach is valid if charges are systematically related to costs; however, many hospitals employ differential pricing to maximize revenues and transfer costs from one group of patients or payers to another (Ginsburg and Sloan 1984). Even though a possible bias is introduced, the weighted measure should provide at least a crude indication of the service-mix consumed by patients. The second weakness of Cohen's indicator of output is best evaluated in the context of the purpose for which the measure was constructed. Cohen used weighted services to examine the variation in the cost of the mix of care provided by different hospitals. In this context, we would expect a high degree of correlation between the dependent variable, total costs, and the independent variable, services weighted by costs, because he constructed a tautology. Although limited, it is clear that Cohen's measure reflects the multiproduct nature of hospitals much better than unweighted patient days or admissions.

Surrogate Measures

Recognizing the limitations of the early output measures, a number of researchers have used surrogate or proxy variables thought to be correlated with case-mix in their analysis of hospitals. In our review of these measures, we refer to Watts and Klastorin's (1980) research, which facilitates a comparison of the

Table 5.1
Explanatory Power of Surrogate Output Measures

Output Measure	Pearson Correlation Coefficient of Output Measure With Cost Per Case	Incremental Adjusted R^2 of Output Measure
Number of beds	.43	.05
Number of basic services (NBS)	.05	
Number of quality-enhancing services (NQS)	.17	.11[*]
Number of community services (NCS)	.55	
Number of complex services (NCXS)	.43	
Weighted index of facilities and services	.45	.07
Facility dummy variables	not given	.12
DRG index	.52	.17

Source: Watts, C.A., and T.D. Klastorin. 1980. The impact of case-mix on hospital
    cost: A comparative analysis. Inquiry 17 (4): 357 - 367.
[*] Incremental R^2 of NBS, NQS, NCS, and NCXS entered simultaneously into the equation.

explanatory power of a wide variety of case-mix measures. In their study, 11 cost functions were estimated on a common set of data, thereby allowing valid comparisons of the adjusted R^2 statistic. In each equation, the cost per case served as the dependent variable, and a different case-mix measure was added to three other independent variables (i.e., location, area wage index, and the hospital's outpatient volume). In Table 5.1, we summarize the Pearson correlations of the case-mix variables with cost per case and the incremental adjusted R^2 values calculated by Watts and Klastorin. The incremental adjusted R^2 values represent the increase in explanatory power resulting from the addition of the surrogate case-mix variables to the other three independent variables. For comparative purposes, summary statistics for a DRG index (weighted by cost) also are included in Table 5.1.

Observing that larger hospitals tend to have more sophisticated facilities and attract a complex (and costly) case-mix, Lave and Lave (1970) used the number of beds as a surrogate for case-mix. Using this approach, one erroneously assumes that institutional objectives or other factors do not affect case-mix. For example, proponents of this approach assume that a 400-bed suburban hospital without an internship or residency program has the same case-mix as a 400-bed university medical school hospital. However, it is well recognized that objectives (e.g., teaching) and environmental factors influence case-mix in a manner not reflected by the number of beds. This position is supported by Table 5.1, which indicates that the incremental explanatory power of beds in the cost equation is only .05. Further, the use of beds as a proxy for case-mix results in a parameter estimate that is confounded by the effects of scale on costs.

In response to the need to develop an indicator that measures case-mix more accurately than the number of beds, several analysts used variables that depict the scope of services that are available in a given hospital. Such an approach is predicated on the assumption that the distribution of patients, and hence, the case-mix of a given hospital, is influenced by differences in the scope of available services. For example, hospitals offering a specific component of care, such as open-heart surgery, are more likely to attract patients requiring the services than hospitals in which the procedure is unavailable. In addition, since the American Hospital Association compiles an annual listing of approximately 60 services and facilities that are available in member institutions, the construction of variables that depict differences in the scope of services is facilitated by the ease with which required data might be acquired.

The scope of services has been entered into cost equations in a number of ways. Carr and Feldstein (1967) used the total number of services offered by hospitals, an approach that might be criticized for assigning an equal weight to each service irrespective of its contribution to case-mix or costs. Berry (1970) attempted to rectify this deficiency by employing binary variables that represented the presence or absence of 40 services and facilities. The coefficients of the dummy variables were intended to capture the contribution of case-mix to the costs of each service. However, the reliability of the parameter estimates was reduced substantially by the presence of multicollinearity. In response to this problem, Berry used factor analysis to identify four groups that were relatively homogeneous with respect to costs. Independent variables depicting the number of facilities and services offered by the hospital were then developed for each of the groups. As shown in Table 5.1, these variables were identified as the number of basic services, the number of quality-enhancing services, the number of community services, and the number of complex services. Shuman, Wolfe, and Hardwick (1972) and Dowling, House, and Lehman (1976) used a panel of experts to develop subjective estimates of the costs of various services and programs. The estimates were used to calculate an index of facilities and services weighted by relative costliness. However, our examination of the rank ordering of services that were common to both studies reveals inconsistencies between the judgments of the two panels, a result that raises questions about the interrater reliability of this approach. In addition to the individual problems discussed above, each approach is based on the incorrect assumption that utilization is the same in every hospital that offers the service.

As indicated in Table 5.1, the use of either Berry's scope of service category variables or a weighted facility index results in a slightly higher R^2 than the use of the bed-size variable. None of the surrogates for case-mix, however, explains as much of the variation in costs as the scalar DRG index. The DRG index used by Watts and Klastorin (1980) was based on the first-generation DRG-classification system, which explains less variation in costs per case than the second generation DRGs currently used in the Medicare prospective payment system.

DIRECT MEASURES OF HOSPITAL CASE-MIX

The limitations of the surrogates, described in the previous section, have caused researchers to focus on diagnostic nomenclature in the development of direct measures of case-mix. Two major approaches have been employed—the formation of isoresource consumption groups and the creation of scalar case-mix indices. In the former, research focuses on a recognized disease classification system, typically a version of the International Classification of Diseases (ICD) (Commission on Professional and Hospital Activities 1978), and defines hospital-specific case-mix by a vector of case proportion in each category. Since the number of classifications in the ICD is unmanageable, attention has been focused on methods to reduce the number of categories. Aggregation procedures have reflected the objectives of the researchers. For example, Fetter, Mills, Riedel, and Thompson (1977) were interested in product-line management and emphasized reduction of variance in resource consumption while developing DRGs. In contrast, Gonnella (1981), a clinical professor of medicine, focused on the degree and extent of system involvement as he developed a staging protocol.

The other approach to case-mix measurement represents an extreme case of reducing the number of categories to a single-valued scalar index reflecting the output of the hospital. The scalar index is easily understood, and its use in regression equations avoids the problem of multicollinearity that is associated with the use of a vector of output measures (Berry 1970; Evans 1971).

International Classification of Diseases

All of the current direct measures of case-mix rely on diagnostic nomenclature. Accordingly, it is appropriate to begin our discussion of patient classification systems with a definition of a diagnosis and how it is translated into commonly recognized terminology and codes. This section will be followed by a description and an evaluation of patient classification systems.

A diagnosis is a hypothesis pertaining to the nature of a patient's illness. It contains four elements: etiology, manifestation, location, and severity (Gonnella 1981). Since physicians order tests and procedures for their patients on the basis of the diagnostic hypothesis, it is clear that the measurement of hospital output requires a classification system that can be used to aggregate patients on the basis of the similarities and differences in their diagnoses.

Considerations about reliability require that any patient classification system be based on nomenclature that is consistently applied irrespective of geographic location or physician specialty. Accordingly, all of the diagnosis-based classification systems have relied on the ICD; the most recent version of this system is the International Classification of Disease, 9th Revision, Clinical Modification (ICD-9-CM), which was implemented on January 1, 1979 (Fetter, Shin, Freeman, Averill, and Thompson 1980). This coding scheme, as well as its predecessors, was developed to classify conditions of morbidity and mortality for statistical reporting purposes. The ICD-9-CM contains 16 broad classes of disease and injury, which are shown in Table 5.2. Each of the classes is divided into specific clinical entities and residual groups resulting in 10,171 categories.

Coding schemes that are based on the ICD usually consist of a large number of categories, an outcome that reduces their usefulness for managerial and statistical purposes. Accordingly, the Commission on Professional and Hospital Activities (CPHA) developed an aggregated patient classification system that was called the *List A: Hospital Diagnosis Groups* (CPHA 1966). The List A, was based initially on 183 primary diagnosis groups and has been revised three times since its inception. Currently, List A consists of 398 mutually exclusive, primary diagnostic categories. In order to reduce the variance in length of stay within each diagnostic group, the categories were partitioned on the basis of the presence or absence of a secondary diagnosis, the presence or absence of any surgery, and five age categories (0–19, 20–34, 35–49, 50–64, 65+). The refinement resulted in 20 subcategories for each of the 398 primary diagnostic categories and a total of 7,960 patient classes. This system has been used extensively by Professional Standards and Review Organizations (PSROs) to establish length of stay guidelines that are used in their concurrent utilization review process (Fetter et al. 1980).

Although List A contains fewer groups than any of the ICD coding schemes, a classification system with 7,960 cells is too cumbersome for most applications. With a large number of cells, the frequency of cases in many categories is too small to be useful for analysis. Furthermore, entering these cells as a vector of case-mix proportions would entail the sacrifice of an excessive number of degrees of freedom. Indeed, to cope with this problem, List A has been converted into a scalar measure, the *Resource Need Index*, which is discussed later in this chapter.

In addition to the unwieldly number of groups, the List A–system has three disadvantages. First, each primary diagnostic category (except those pertaining to newborns) is divided into the same 20 subcategories. As the development of DRGs has demonstrated, however, the factors on which partitions are based (i.e., age, surgery and comorbidity) are not relevant indicators of the length of stay in many diagnostic categories. Hence, this classification system has many

Table 5.2
ICD-9-CM Disease and Injury Classes

1. Diseases of the nervous system and sense organs

2. Diseases of the respiratory system

3. Diseases of the circulatory system

4. Diseases of the digestive system

5. Diseases of the musculo-skeletal system and connective tissue

6. Diseases of the skin, and subcutaneous tissue

7 Endocrine, nutritional, and metabolic diseases and immunity disorders

8. Diseases of the genitourinary system

9. Complications of pregnancy, childbirth, and the puerperium

10. Certain conditions originating in the perinatal period

11. Diseases of the blood and blood-forming organs

12. Neoplasms

13. Infectious and parasitic diseases

14. Mental disorders

15. Injury and poisoning

16. Classification of factors influencing health status and contact with health service (supplementary classification)

Source: Commission on Professional and Hospital Activities. 1978. The International
Classification of Diseases, 9th revision, Clinical Modification, Volume 1, Diseases,
Tabular List. Ann Arbor, MI, p. XIX.

superfluous categories (Fetter et al. 1980). Further, in many diagnostic categories, more precise information is required to predict the length of stay or costs (Horn, Horn, and Sharkey 1984). A second disadvantage of the List A–system is its reliance on an endogenous factor, the performance of surgery, to group patients. Thus, this output measure is not independent of the inputs used in the treatment of patients. Finally, the categories defined by the List A are not independent of the skill of the physician in diagnosing comorbidity or to the level of effort devoted to recording comorbidity. For example, the presence of more than one diagnostic code on the discharge abstract fails to distinguish a true comorbidity (i.e., the presence of an unrelated pre-existing condition) from a complication of the primary diagnosis.

Diagnosis Related Groups

Diagnosis Related Groups (DRGs) were developed by a group of researchers at Yale University to identify a set of case types, each representing a class of patients with similar processes of care and receiving a predictable bundle of services (i.e., a product) from an acute care hospital. Although initially developed to assist hospitals with the management of product-lines, DRGs have gained most of their notoriety as a unit of payment in state and federal hospital rate regulation systems. As of 1988, two generations of DRGs have been used in prospective payment systems. In 1980, the State of New Jersey operated the first DRG-based, hospital rate regulation program. Under this system, prospective payment rates were established for 383 DRGs that were based on ICDA–8 (International Classification of Diseases, Adapted, 8th Revision) nomenclature. In 1983, the Medicare program implemented a prospective pricing mechanism based on a second generation DRG system that consists of patient categories and uses the ICD-9-CM diagnostic codes.

ICD-8-DRGs

The formation of the first generation of DRGs followed several steps. First, a panel of clinicians divided all diagnoses into 84 mutually exclusive and col-lectively exhaustive Major Diagnostic Categories (MDCs). These broad cate-gories, which were essentially subdivisions of the ICDA–8 codes, were designed to be consistent in terms of either their anatomic and physiopathologic charac-teristics, or the manner in which they were managed clinically.

The second step involved forming DRGs within each MDC in order to reduce the within-group variation in length of stay, subject to the constraint that the number of categories (i.e., DRGs) was manageable. In this phase of the research, discharge abstracts from three sources were examined: (1) 500,000 medical records from 118 hospitals in New Jersey; (2) 150,000 records from Yale–New Haven Hospital; and (3) 52,000 records from 50 hospitals in one region of South Carolina. A statistical program called Automatic Interaction Detector (AID) was used to identify variables that would be used to partition the MDCs into DRGs. The set of independent variables that was used in the classification algorithm was restricted to variables that were readily available from discharge abstracts. Subgroups were developed on the basis of empirical and subjective criteria. In general, a variable was used to create further subcategories if (1) it significantly reduced the variation in the length of stay, (2) it created groups that were homogeneous from a clinical perspective, and (3) it resulted in a subgroup that had at least 200 cases. This process defined 383 DRGs that were described by primary diagnosis, secondary diagnosis, surgical procedure, and age. Gender, which was found to be statistically insignificant in explaining variation in length of stay, was not used to form DRGs.

There are three notable problems associated with the formation of the first generation of DRGs. First, resource consumption was measured in terms of length of stay. This measure accounts for the stay-specific dimension of output but may not reflect costs that vary with the severity of illness. Second, the derivation of this set of DRGs depended on a data set that was not representative of all hospitals in the United States. Given the well-known regional variations in the patterns of medical care (Wennberg 1984), it is likely that the use of data from different areas would have created a different set of DRGs. Indeed, researchers who used data sets from Western Pennsylvania (Young, Swinkola, and Hutton 1980) and Cleveland (Doremus 1980) reported that an application of the classification algorithm on different sets of data produced a different number of DRGs that were based on different variables. Cameron and Knauf (1981) argued that Young et al. obtained different groups with the Western Pennsylvania data because different clinical judgments were used. This suggests the third limitation of the development of the first generation of DRGs. Specifically, these patient groupings were based on the subjective judgments of clinicians that were never articulated explicitly. Accordingly, it is likely that if a different clinical panel evaluated the same data set, a different set of patient groupings would have been defined.

ICD-9-DRGs

Unlike the first generation of DRGs, the second set was generated from a national, random sample of medical records. Applying a sampling rate of 0.285, approximately 400,000 discharge abstracts for 1979 were obtained from the CPHA. The sample was stratified on the basis of hospital size, region, population of the area, and the teaching status of the hospital.

In the new classification system, cases were first grouped into 23 MDCs, which were subsequently partitioned into 471 DRGs. As shown in Table 5.3, the MDCs were grouped according to system or organ involvement, an approach that is congruent with the organization of medical specialties. As illustrated by Figure 5.1, which shows the decision rules for partitioning MDC 16 (Diseases and Disorders of the Blood and Blood-Forming Organs), the formation of ICD-9-CM DRGs was based more on clinical decisions than statistical partitioning. Cases are assigned to an MDC on the basis of principal diagnosis. Before any statistical analysis is performed, the MDC is partitioned on the basis of the presence or absence of an operating room procedure. A surgical patient who had two separate operations is classified into the more resource intensive DRG. For example, a patient who had a splenectomy (DRG 392) and any other operation in the MDC (DRG 394) is assigned to DRG 392. Unlike the ICDA–8 DRGs, the new DRGs were formed by using specific significant complications and comorbidities as partitioning variables. Complications and comorbidities were defined as significant, and thus were included as possible partitioning variables, if their presence was likely to increase the length of stay by one day in 75 percent

Table 5.3

Major Diagnostic Categories of ICD-9-CM DRGs

Major Diagnostic Category	Number of DRGS	Major Diagnostic Category	Number of DRGS
1. Diseases and disorders of the nervous system	35	14. Pregnancy, childbirth, and the puerperium	15
2. Diseases and disorders of the eye	13	15. Newborns and other neonates with conditions originating in the perinatal period	7
3. Diseases and disorders of the ear, nose and throat	26	16. Diseases and disorders of the blood and blood-forming organs and immunity disorders	8
4. Diseases and disorders of the respiratory system	28	17. Myeloproliferative diseases and disorders and poorly differentiated malignancy and other neoplasms NEC	15
5. Diseases and disorders of the circulatory system	43	18. Infectious and parasitic diseases (systemic or unspecified site)	9
6. Diseases and disorders of the digestive system	45	19. Mental diseases and disorders	9
7. Diseases and disorders of the hepatobiliary system and pancreas	18	20. Substance use and substance induced mental disorders	6
8. Diseases and disorders of the musculoskeletal system and connective tissue	48	21. Injury, poisoning, and toxic effects of drugs	17
9. Diseases and disorders of the skin, subcutaneous tissue, and breast	28	22. Burns	5
10. Endocrine, nutritional, and metabolic diseases and disorders	17	23. Factors influencing health status and contact with health services	7
11. Diseases and disorders of the kidney and urinary tract	32		
12. Diseases and disorders of the male reproductive system	19		
13. Diseases and disorders of the female reproductive system	17		

Source: Federal Register. 1985. Part III. Medicare Program: Changes to the inpatient hospital prospective payment system and fiscal year 1986 rates; final rule. 50 (170): 35722 - 35735, Sept 3.

Figure 5.1
Major Diagnostic Category 16: Diseases and Disorders of the Blood and Blood-Forming Organs and
Immunological Disorders (CC = Comorbidity and/or Complication)

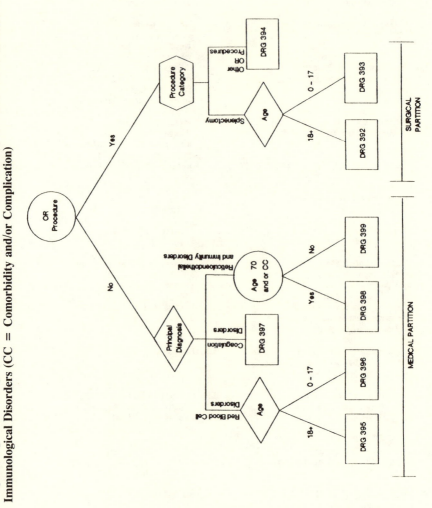

CC = Comorbidity and or Complication

of the cases. As Figure 5.1 illustrates, patients with reticuloendothelial and immunity disorders are partitioned into two DRGs. The assignment criteria for DRG 398 is age of 70 years or older with significant complications or comorbidities. If both of these criteria are not satisfied, the case is assigned to DRG 399. As illustrated by the DRGs comprising the medical subgroup of MDC 16, age may be used alone or in conjunction with complications and comorbidities to partition DRGs. Further, the age criteria when used to split DRGs may vary. Although 70 years of age is most commonly used, Figure 5.1 shows that 17 years of age is the cutoff point for DRG 396. The use of age as a criterion to form a DRG was determined on the basis of the judgment of clinical experts and on the basis of variance reduction.

The ICD-9-CM DRG classification system relies more on utilization factors (i.e., operating room procedures) than the original system. Thus, the new DRGs should be more homogeneous with respect to resource consumption than the original DRGs; however, similar to the ICDA–8 DRGs, the new DRGs were developed with average length of stay as a measure of resource consumption and were based on actual practice patterns rather than on the most appropriate treatment strategies.

Disease Staging

Researchers from Thomas Jefferson Medical College and Systemetrics Inc. have developed a disease-staging protocol that defines progressive levels of clinical severity (Gonnella and Goran 1975; Gonnella, Hornbrook, and Louis 1984). This system classifies diseases rather than health problems. For example, an infection is termed a health problem by clinicians because it is a general description of psychological-physiological structure and/or functioning. Diseases, on the other hand, are defined by clinicians in much more specific detail, including location of the problem, manifestations of the medical problem, cause of the problem, and severity of the problem.

Consistent with the clinical definition of disease and similar to the National Cancer Institute's staging protocol for oncology patients, stages of disease corresponding to the biological progression and complications of the disease were identified. In general, the four stages of disease (cancer has five) can be described in ascending order of severity:

Stage 1. Conditions with no complications or problems of minimal severity.

Stage 2. Problems limited to an organ or organ system with increased probability of complications.

Stage 3. Generalized systemic involvement, poor prognosis.

Stage 4. Death.

In order to avoid the expense of classifying all diseases, two criteria were used to select diseases for which a staging protocol would be developed. First, only the major diseases in each etiology-body system class should be staged. Second, the classification system should cover the majority of admissions to a typical short-term general hospital. Achievement of the first goal will result in a classification system that is useful to clinicians. On the other hand, attainment of the second goal will result in a classification system that serves the needs of hospital administrators, regulators, and researchers.

A panel of 23 medical consultants assisted in the specification of the disease-staging criteria. Each disease was assigned to two members of the panel who developed staging criteria independently. Although the panelists were instructed to divide each condition into at least four primary stages, they were allowed to specify an unlimited number of substages. The number of substages was constrained only by the requirement that each subsequent substage should place the patient at a significantly higher risk of morbidity or mortality than the previous substage.

The staging criteria were applied initially on a manual inspection of medical records. Since this may be too costly for widespread use in a payment system, a computerized version of staging was developed. A team of medical records technicians translated each stage and substage code, using the three primary disease classification systems: ICDA-8, Second Revision of Hospital ICDA (H-ICDA-2), and ICD-9-CM. Available computer software will classify patients into any of 420 diagnostic categories, which contain about 90 percent of all admissions to short-term general hospitals, and assign an ordinal stage within each category. With few exceptions, diseases are staged on the basis of principal diagnosis, secondary diagnosis and discharge status (i.e., alive or expired).

Johns Hopkins Severity of Illness Index

Researchers from Johns Hopkins University have developed the Severity of Illness Index (SII), which seems to reduce the intra-DRG heterogeneity of resource consumption due to variations in severity of illness (Horn 1981; Horn, Horn, and Sharkey 1984). The SII is an ordinal measure of patient severity consisting of four levels. The assessment of severity depends on the scores for the following seven variables:

1. Stage of the principal diagnosis
2. Complications of the principal diagnosis
3. Concurrent interacting conditions that affect the hospital episode of treatment
4. Dependency on the hospital staff
5. Extent of non–operating room procedures
6. Rate of response to therapy or rate of recovery
7. Residual impairment remaining after therapy for the acute aspect of the hospitalization

Horn and Horn (1986) argue that the first three variables relate to the burden of illness presented to the hospital. The fourth and fifth variables, dependency

and non–operating room procedures, are included for internal monitoring purposes only. The last two variables reflect the rate of response to hospital care.
The authors state that objective, disease-specific criteria are used to define each
of the four levels within each of the variables pertaining to dimensions of severity.
The overall SII value for a case is determined by assessing the pattern of the
seven dimensions. The overall severity rating is consistent with a "mode rule"
about 80 percent of the time, i.e., the evaluator selects an overall SII value that
is the same as the level common to four or more of the variables. If there is no
mode, the overall severity rating is based on the mean of the scores for the seven
dimensions. Since the different severity dimensions view medical needs from
several different but related perspectives, it is not surprising that for almost all
cases, the scores on all seven dimensions are within one level of each other
(Horn and Horn 1986).

SII raters, who may be physicians or nurses, require fairly extensive training
that begins with a three-day training session. Follow-up training is given during
the second and third months of the initial training sessions and quarterly thereafter. SII raters have been demonstrated to be reliable and valid in situations
where the rater does not have an incentive to place a patient in a higher severity
category (Horn, Chachich, and Clopton 1983; Horn and Horn 1986). When
viewed from the perspective of using the SII to adjust the prospective payment
rates for hospitals there is concern that the subjective aspects of the SII criteria
may result in inappropriate manipulation by the hospital. Further, since the SII
is based on information pertaining to the patients' entire stays in the hospital,
rather than their condition upon admission, there is concern that besides severity,
the SII may also reflect faulty clinical decisions or faulty execution (Muller 1983;
Schumacher, Parker, Kofie, and Munns 1987).

In response to concerns about the SII, the Computerized Severity Index (CSI)
has been developed (Horn and Horn 1986). In the CSI system, a patient is placed
in one of four ordinal categories of severity for each disease on the basis of
comorbidity, complications, and interactive effects of conditions. The CSI uses
information based on laboratory values, vital signs, radiologic findings, and
other clinical information found in the medical record but not summarized in
current discharge abstract forms. Computer software for this system was developed in 1986.

Patient Management Categories

Researchers from Blue Cross of Western Pennsylvania utilized 50 disease-
specific panels, composed of specialist and generalist physicians, to develop
approximately 800 Patient Management Categories (PMCs) (Young 1984b).
Unlike the development of DRGs, which emphasized a statistical approach to
aggregation, Young, Swinkola, and Zorn (1982) attempted to develop categories
that represented clinically distinct patient types, each requiring a different clinical
and diagnostic strategy for effective care. Once explicit categories, or PMCs,

were specified by physician panels, ICD-9-CM diagnostic codes were mapped to the categories to facilitate the assignment of patients to PMCs by computer. The categorization software can be applied to any database compatible with the Uniform Hospital Discharge Data Set (UHDDS). Since most third-party payers require the use of the UHDDS, this software is readily exportable.

The PMC protocol relies primarily on diagnosis and secondarily on clinical procedures. Age and gender serve as additional classification criteria for only a few PMCs. Recognizing that physicians treat symptoms and suspected conditions that may not be suggested by the principal diagnosis, the PMC system also relies on the admitting diagnosis and secondary diagnoses to classify patients. This system also recognizes that patients with multiple diagnoses can be dichotomized as those who are (1) subject to a single disease process, and (2) comorbid.

Severity of illness is implicitly recognized by the assignment of the case into a PMC. For example, patients with acute myocardial infarction (AMI), who would be classified into DRG 121 in the current Medicare system, could be placed in any of eight PMCs pertaining to AMI (Young 1984a). Severity of illness of these different AMI categories can be determined, in an economic sense, by their relative costliness.

The clinical orientation of the development of PMCs allowed Young (1984a) to establish relative cost weights for each category on the basis of clinical norms rather than empirical criteria. More specifically, in the process of defining PMCs, the physician panels also specified the types and the amounts of services required for the effective management of a typical patient in each PMC. Incorporated in the management strategy are diagnostic and treatment components of care, as well as expected length of stay in special care units and in routine nursing units. By using data that depict the inputs required to produce services and factor prices, it is possible to determine the costs of the required (i.e., clinically indicated) services per case rather than the costs of services rendered per case. The latter measure reflects the inappropriate provision or omission of services. The former measure may be biased by inaccurate specifications by the physician panel.

EVALUATION OF PATIENT CLASSIFICATION SYSTEMS

The evaluation of any patient classification system requires a specification of desired attributes. Although different criteria have been established, depending upon the perspective of the evaluator, the consensus of opinion suggests that any patient classification should have the following properties (Ament, Kobrinski, and Wood 1981; Hornbrook 1982; Pettengill and Vertrees 1982):

1. The classification system must be based on information that is reliable.
2. Patients who consume resources of relatively equivalent values should be grouped together.
3. The number of categories should be manageable.

4. The classification system must be clinically meaningful to physicians.

5. Information used to classify patients must be easily accessible at a reasonable cost.

Reliability

Reliability refers to the extent to which a measuring instrument produces the same results on multiple applications to the same phenomenon. For example, if two patients, who present identical symptoms and problems, are treated the same way, a reliable patient classification system will group them in the same category. Since all of the current case-mix systems, except the Severity of Illness Index, use a computerized algorithm to classify patients, the primary threats to reliability are processing errors (i.e., accidentally entering the wrong codes into the computer), observer errors by physicians who may assign an incorrect diagnosis to a case, and classification errors by medical records technicians who may assign an incorrect code to a diagnosis. According to the Institute of Medicine (1980), the principal diagnosis has been miscoded as frequently as 60 percent of the time for certain diseases. However, this percentage has declined as hospitals have responded to the Medicare prospective payment system by improving the documentation of medical records (Ginsburg and Carter 1986).

Kerlinger (1973) states that interrater reliability (agreement between raters) and intrarater reliability (consistency by a rater over time) can be adversely affected by imprecise or unclear criteria for assigning a phenomenon a score or to a category. The diagnostic nomenclature on which all case-mix systems rely has been criticized with respect to precision and clarity. As noted by Gertman and Lowenstein (1984), the "International Classification of Diseases" is still based on an anatomic approach to disease developed in the late nineteenth century. Although this classification system has been updated decennially, it was never intended to accommodate the precision required for a payment system. The central flaw in the ICD-9-CM system is that there are no clear rules for determining when a patient has a particular problem that fits the ICD-9-CM code.

Two studies have assessed the reliability of ICD coding. In a study of 50 hospitals, the Institute of Medicine (1980) reported that the principal diagnosis on reabstracted medical records disagreed with the condition reported on the original abstract 36.6 percent of the time. In a similar study, Doremus and Michenzi (1983) found that errors and discrepancies in the listing of the principal diagnosis occurred over 20 percent of the time. With respect to processing errors and diagnostic misclassification, none of the current patient classification systems enjoys a relative advantage since all of them rely on the ICD-9-CM nomenclature and classification rules. However, the Severity of Illness Index (SII) is the only system that relies on detailed chart review and subsequent manual classification based upon judgment. Consequently, the reliability of SII scores has been subject to the most scrutiny.

The reliability of the SII has been assessed by comparing the severity ratings performed by regular raters with those of experts who conducted blind reratings from patient charts. In a study of 18 hospitals, the level of agreement between the two severity ratings was 93.5 percent (Horn and Horn 1986). These results are slightly better than the 90 percent agreement reported in an earlier study, conducted in four hospitals (Horn, Chachich, and Clopton 1983). A more recent study (Schumacher et al. 1987), however, found that the SII had an agreement rate among raters of 73 percent (Kappa statistic $=0.41$) and concluded that this instrument may be too unreliable to be used in a payment system. Further, Schumacher et al. found that the SII exhibited better reliability in the extremes of severity: the rater agreement was reliable among level #1 (71 percent) and level #4 patients (83 percent); but it was unreliable among level #2 (34 percent agreement) and level #3 patients (25 percent agreement). Schumacher and associates attribute the low reliability scores to a rigorous (but realistic) study environment characterized by time pressures and the lack of cues or feedback from colleagues. Indeed, they note that in the artificial training settings, similar to those found in the studies by Horn and associates, their raters had agreement rates consistently above 80 percent.

In response to concerns that the reliability and validity of the SII might be adversely affected by the subjective manual ratings, researchers at Johns Hopkins developed the Computerized Severity Index (CSI). In this system a sixth digit reflecting severity of illness is added to the five-digit, ICD-9-CM code. Severity will be ordinally ranked from 1 to 4, and will be defined in terms of objective signs and symptoms, laboratory values, radiological values, etc. (Horn and Horn 1986).

Homogeneity

It is commonly agreed that patient groupings should be homogeneous with respect to resource consumption. From the perspective of rate regulation, heterogeneous patient groups are undesirable because they cause variations in net income earned by treating patients who have different resource requirements but generate the same revenue. This disparity creates an incentive for the provider to implement a differential admission policy that favors those patients whose treatment is expected to generate net income (Broyles and Rosko 1985).

From a research perspective, heterogeneous output measures are undesirable because they can confound economic analysis. For example, in the absence of precise case-mix information it is difficult to determine whether investor-owned hospitals are less expensive because they practice "cream-skimming," as commonly alleged, or because they are more efficient.

Young (1984a) distinguishes between required and observed resource utilization. From a theoretical perspective, required resource utilization is a preferred criterion to evaluate the homogeneity of output measures. For example, observed data may reflect the use of unnecessary inputs and unnecessary services, outcomes that reduce efficiency, diminish effectiveness and may fail to improve the quality of the product. Unfortunately, the determination of required services for each distinct patient category and the mix of resources per service is expensive and a subjective process. Accordingly, many case-mix systems, including DRGs, have relied on observed resource utilization.

The DRG patient classification system has been criticized for using hetero-geneous patient categories. Smits, Fetter, and McMahon (1984) suggest that the heterogeneity within DRGs is due to a number of factors. First, as discussed in the section on reliability, many cases have been assigned to an incorrect category because of coding errors. Second, variations in physician practice, unrelated to the patient's condition, have affected resource consumption. Third, the decision to limit DRGs to a manageable number has led to the formation of broad "catch-all" categories (i.e., diagnoses not elsewhere covered by a DRG in the MDC) that contain heterogeneous subgroups. Fourth, there are variations in severity of illness among patients classified in the same DRG. With the exception of var-iations in severity these sources of heterogeneity are either self-correcting or affect a relatively small number of cases. For example, hospitals have responded to the Medicare DRG system by improving coding practices (Ginsburg and Carter 1986) and by taking actions to reduce variations in physician practice that are not justified clinically (Spiegel and Kavaler 1986). Further, although hospital responses have not been rigorously evaluated, the Medicare pricing mechanism provides incentives for the more efficient production of hospital services (Broyles and Rosko 1985).

Variations in the severity of illness within DRGs continue to be subject to much controversy and confusion. The latter has been caused by conflicting definitions of severity of illness. Economists, rate regulators and managers tend to view severity of illness from the perspective of costliness. For example, each of two 50-year-old patients who have the principal diagnosis, *diabetes mellitus*, would be assigned to DRG 294 even though one patient had no complications and had a treatment cost of $1,700, while the other patient's condition was accompanied by acidosis resulting in a longer hospital stay with more services and costing $2,700. From the economic perspective, the more expensive patient would be considered to be more severely ill.

Physicians view severity of illness from the perspective of increased risk of morbidity or mortality. In the example above, they would agree with the econ-omist that the diabetic patient with acidosis was more severely ill; however, if a third patient with *diabetes mellitus* was admitted to the hospital and shortly thereafter expired before extensive services were performed, the physician would view the third patient as most severely ill, while the economist would classify this patient as the least severely ill of the three because his treatment consumed the fewest resources.

Before examining the homogeneity of DRGs and other hospital patient clas-sification systems, it is appropriate to mention some of the factors that confound our analysis. First, all of the classification systems have been in a state of evolution. Thus, two different studies that compared the performance of DRGs and the Severity of Illness Index (SII) may have examined different versions of each system. Second, different criteria have been used to evaluate the case-mix systems. The measures of resource consumption have included length of stay, expenses, and charges. Statistical tests or measures of homogeneity have included reduction in variance, the coefficient of variation, the F-statistic for analysis of variance, and the coefficient of multiple correlation (R^2). Third, the units of empirical observation have ranged from the individual case to the hospital. Since aggregation at the hospital level dampens variation, the R^2 statistic for equations in which the level of observation is the individual case will tend to be much smaller than the R^2 for equations in which more aggregated data are used. For example, in a study of 15 hospitals, the R^2 for regression equations based on individual cases was 0.28, while the R^2 in the aggregated analysis was 0.75 (Horn, Sharkey, Chambers, and Horn 1985). Finally, different data sets were employed. As we suggested earlier, factors exogenous to the classification system (e.g., variations in physician's practice or efficiency) can affect the measured homogeneity. Thus, comparisons between data sets, which do not control these confounding influences, are not valid. In light of the confounding influences of these problems, we will not discuss some of the earlier (and less relevant) studies (Ament, Dreachslin, Kobrinski, and Wood 1982; Horn and Sharkey 1983; Horn, Sharkey, and Bertram 1983), which analyzed the first generation of DRGs.

Pettengill and Vertrees (1982) conducted the first assessment of the homogeneity of ICD-9 DRGs in a national data base ($n = 5,071$ hospitals). They estimated regression equations for the average cost per case, aggregated at the hospital level, with cross-sectional data for 1979. About 30 percent of the variation in the cost per case was explained by an equation that used the Medicare case-mix index, a scalar measure of the relative costliness of a hospital's distribution of patients by DRG, as the only independent variable. In an equation in which other factors (size, wage index, teaching activities, urban location) thought to affect costs were included with the Medicare case-mix index, the adjusted R^2 increased to 0.72. Using the case as the level of aggregation, Calore and Iezzoni (1987) reported that DRGs accounted for 17 percent of the variation in the cost per case of patients in Michigan hospitals.

Frank and Lave (1985) demonstrated that the homogeneity of ICD-9 DRGs varies substantially by broad clinical categories (i.e., surgical, medical, or psychiatric). They reported that the average coefficient of variation for each of three measures of resource consumption (i.e., length of stay, costs, and charges) by surgical DRGs was significantly ($p < .05$) less than that of psychiatric DRGs. For each resource consumption measure, the variability of medical DRGs was greater than surgical DRGs but less than psychiatric DRGs. However, the surgical/medical differences were significant for all three measures of consumption while the medical DRGs had a coefficient of variation significantly less than that of psychiatric DRGs only for length of stay. Further support for the differences in homogeneity between surgical and medical DRGs was provided by Calore and Iezzoni (1987) who reported that the variation in costs explained by surgical DRGs was 34 percent, while medical DRGs explained only 6 percent. Frank and Lave argued that the surgical DRGs were more homogeneous than medical DRGs because the former were created on the basis of both diagnoses and specific treatment procedures, whereas the latter are grouped only on the basis of diagnoses. Corroboration of the conclusions pertaining to the heterogeneity of psychiatric DRGs is provided by Taube, Lee, and Forthofer (1984) who reported an R^2 equal to 0.03 from an application of analysis of variance (ANOVA) to the length of stay of psychiatric patients.

From the perspective of rate regulation, the observed heterogeneity of patients within DRGs might be acceptable if variations in patient severity are distributed randomly among hospitals so that losses incurred in the provision of services to "high-cost" patients are offset by profits earned by treating "low-cost" patients. Critics of the Medicare prospective payment system however, have argued that, due to heterogeneity, the use of DRGs to determine rates of compensation will result in inequitable payments to innercity hospitals, which treat a disproportionately larger number of patients who are severely ill because of their socioeconomic environment (Broyles and Rosko 1985).

The absence of widely used severity measurements makes it difficult to assess the impact of variations in illness severity on equitable payments. Anderson and Lave (1986) replicated part of the analysis that was performed by the Health Care Financing Administration (HCFA) to identify factors that might be used to make adjustments in the rates of compensating hospitals (Pettengill and Vertrees 1982). To the original HCFA cost per case equation, they added the percentage of hospital patients that were nonpaying or Medicaid recipients. This variable was included as a proxy for patients who are more severely ill. Since the coefficient of this variable was positive and highly significant, Anderson and Lave concluded that the Medicare payment mechanism penalizes hospitals that have a more severely ill patient mix.

Horn et al. (1985) used a direct measure, the SII, to examine the severity of illness within DRGs. In a study of 15 hospitals, using the case as the level of aggregation, they reported that ICD-9-CM DRGs explained 28 percent of the variability in the cost per case while DRGs adjusted by the SII explained 61 percent of the variability in cost per case. Further, Horn et al. calculated that if hospitals were paid on the basis of severity adjustments to DRGs, payment would vary by as much as 35 percent. The latter finding, while not identifying the type of hospital that is likely to suffer under the Medicare prospective payment system, indicates that severity of illness is not symmetrically distributed in all hospitals, a pattern which could lead to inequitable payments.

In a companion study, Horn, Horn, Sharkey, and Chambers (1986) assessed the ability of the SII to explain the variability of resource use within each of the 470 ICD-9 DRGs. The data set included over 106,000 discharges. Operating costs per case, adjusted for medical education and area wage levels, were used as a measure of resource consumption.

The SII explained more than 20 percent of the variation in cost per case in 94 percent of the DRGs, which contained 97 percent of the patients, and more

Table 5.4

Reduction of Variance in Charges: A Comparison of DRGs with the Severity of Illness Index

Method	Reduction Of Variance In Charges
DRGs	33%
Severity of Illness Index	49%
Severity of Illness Index applied in Major Diagnostic Categories	57%
Severity of Illness Index applied in DRGs	69%

Source: Horn, S., R. Horn, and P. Sharkey. 1984. The Severity of Illness Index as a severity
     adjustment to diagnosis related groups. Health Care Financing Review (Annual Supplement)
     : 38, Figure 5.

than 50 percent of the variation in the cost per case in 36 percent of the DRGs. The researchers also found that the coefficient of variation in severity adjusted DRGs was 39 percent smaller than that of the unadjusted DRGs. Although there is no standard for determining what is "too large" a value for the coefficient of variation (C.V.), a value of one or more is not consistent with a normal distribution. Almost 43 percent of the unadjusted DRGs had a C.V. exceeding 1.0, while only 4 percent of the severity adjusted DRGs had a C.V. greater than 1.0.

In recognition of the variations of illness severity within DRGs a number of researchers have assessed the feasibility of incorporating direct severity of illness measures (i.e., staging or the SII) or a proxy (age) in the DRG system to reduce heterogeneity. Horn, Horn, and Sharkey (1984) assessed the ability of the Severity of Illness Index (SII) to reduce the heterogeneity within DRGs. In a study of 19,000 cases from one university teaching hospital, the researchers examined the relative reduction of variance in charges by four classification systems. With the number of categories in parentheses, the systems assessed were SII adjusted for procedures (12), SII in major diagnostic categories (233), SII in DRGs (1,425) and DRGs (436). As indicated by Table 5.4, the use of the SII in conjunction with DRGs resulted in groupings that were substantially more homogeneous than DRGs alone. The other two classification systems also reduced more variance than DRGs.

In a recent pilot study, Conklin, Lieberman, Barnes, and Louis (1984) examined the effects of combining disease staging with the DRG system in the predictions of the costs incurred in the treatment of individual patients. The study was based on over 32,000 Medicare patient abstracts from Maryland and New Jersey. For analytical purposes, DRGs were aggregated into "Adjacent DRGs," which were formed by combining individual DRGs that were partitioned on the basis of age and/or the presence of complications or comorbidities. For example, the Adjacent DRG, *diabetes mellitus,* was created by merging DRG 294 and DRG 295, categories that split diabetic patients into two categories on the basis of age. A total of 10 Adjacent DRGs, common to the Medicare population, were analyzed. General linear models were used to assess the variance explained by DRG splits and partitions based on stage of illness, age, and unrelated comorbidity. A monotonically increasing relationship between costs and stage was observed in the first three stages. In the analysis of two adjacent DRGs, however, patients in stage 4 had lower costs than those in stage 3. This was expected because stage 4 patients (deceased) may expire early in their course of treatment before many resources are consumed. Regarding the other variables that were analyzed, the existence of unrelated comorbidities was positively and significantly related to costs, while age failed to exert a consistent impact on costs. In the regression analysis of four Adjacent DRGs, the R^2 in equations based on staging splits always exceeded the R^2 of equations based on DGR splits. Further, the F-values of the variables reflecting staging were highly significant ($p < 0.001$) in each of the four Adjacent DRGs; the presence/absence of unrelated comorbidity was highly significant in all but one patient grouping; and age was significant in only one instance.

Coffey and Goldfarb (1986) examined the homogeneity of length of stay within patient groupings that were formed by different classification schemes including DRGs, disease staging, and combinations of the two. The analysis was based on 378,000 Medicare discharges from Maryland hospitals during the period 1979–1981. Table 5.5 presents a summary of the percent reduction in the sum of the squared deviations and the coefficient of variation for length of stay for patients grouped by one of the following: DRGs; principal staged disease category (SDC), which is assigned an integer value of 1 to 4; principal staged disease category disaggregated by substages (SDC-stage), which reflect increasing degrees of severity; DRGs disaggregated by SDCs; and DRGs disaggregated by SDC-stage. As Table 5.5 indicates, the coefficients of variation for DRGs and SDCs are almost identical. Further reductions in heterogeneity may have been offset by increases in the number of categories and were achieved by the use of more disaggregated classification schemes. Recognizing the disadvantages of using a large number of categories, Coffey and Goldfarb suggest the Medicare prospective payment system could be refined by introducing disease staging only in DRGs that exhibit an excessive degree of heterogeneity.

Calore and Iezzoni (1987) found results that weaken Coffey and Goldfarb's argument for the use of severity adjusters to modify DRG payments. Calore and Iezzoni evaluated the explanatory power of DRGs, staging and patient management categories (PMCs) in a study that employed a data base of 300,122 dis-

Table 5.5
Homogeneity of Length of Stay within Patients Grouped by Alternative Classification Schemes

Classification Scheme	Number of Groups	Percent Reduction in Sum of Squared Deviations	Coefficient of Variation Within Groups
Ungrouped	1	Reference Category	109.2
DRG	396	16.5	93.2
SDC	299	8.6	93.8
SDC - stage	692	10.8	91.7
DRG - SDC	1615	18.9	84.8
DRG - SDC - stage	2587	20.5	83.4

Source: Coffey, R., and M. Goldfarb. 1986. DRGs and disease staging for reimbursing Medicare patients. Medical Care 24 (9): 821.

charges from Michigan hospitals in 1982. Using cost per case as the dependent variable, regression analysis found that DRGs explained 17 percent of the variation in cost, while PMCs ($R^2 = .15$) and staging ($R^2 = .10$) exhibited less explanatory power.

Since the results suggested that staging or PMCs should not replace DRGs as a payment mechanism, Calore and Iezzoni examined the feasibility of using these severity measures as DRG-modifiers. Given budget constraints, their analysis was restricted to two tracer conditions, pneumonia and prostatic disease, common to Medicare beneficiaries. Using stepwise regression, they entered DRGs as the first independent variable and, in alternate equations, entered staging or PMCs in the second equation and compared the increments in explanatory power. For the pneumonia cluster, the assignment of patients to seven possible DRGs explained 9.7 percent of the variation in costs. Staging increased the R^2 to .109, while PMCs increased the R^2 to .108. For the prostatic disease cluster, the assignment of cases to nine DRGs resulted in an R^2 of .135, while the use of DRGs with staging resulted in an R^2 of .155, and the use of DRGs with PMCs yielded an R^2 of 0.144.

Johansen (1986) compared the homogeneity of DRGs with that of the prospective individualized reimbursement (PIR) model. The PIR model is similar to the DRG system except that it does not split groups on the basis of age. Instead age is treated as a continuous variable that is used to adjust prospective payment rates within patient groupings. Thus, the 471 DRGs are collapsed into 377 patient groups. Using a random sample of 10,000 patients who were treated in Maryland hospitals in 1983, Johansen reported that DRGs explained 38.1 percent of the variation in length of stay, while the PIR model explained 44.1 percent of the variation. Further, in analysis of the ten largest DRGs, the average difference between actual charges and charges established by the rate-setting commissions was $426 with DRGs and $262 when the PIR model was used.

The results of this study should be viewed cautiously because of its limited sample size and restriction to a single state. Further, the reported statistical significance of age is at odds with the finding that in the DRG classification system, age alone, in the absence of comorbidities or complications, has little effect on costs or length of stay (DesHarnais, Chesney, and Fleming 1988) and that among staged cases age does not affect resource consumption (Conklin et al. 1984).

If the PIR is valid, however, it may be a useful refinement to DRGs because it appears to reduce heterogeneity by applying a simple procedure that relies on objective information—age—which is already reported on most discharge abstracts. Since the age distribution of hospital patients varies by region as well as local catchment area, the PIR model appears to address a possible source of inequity that results from the methods of determining rates of prospective payment to hospitals.

McNeil, Kominski and Williams-Ashman (1988) suggest that the current DRG classification system should be modified by splitting DRGs into more homogeneous subgroups. With a panel of clinical experts they identified 41 DRGs that were believed to be heterogeneous. Using a national data set, they found that 24 of these DRGs exhibited significant differences ($p \leq .05$) in standardized charges between the modified DRG and the original DRG. Further, in 16 of the DRGs, one or more modified DRG had an average standardized charge that differed from the mean value of the original DRG by more than 10 percent.

Although the research by McNeil et al. (1988) suggests that the development of a relatively small number of additional DRGs can increase the homogeneity of this patient classification system, their failure to measure reductions in variance precludes an assessment of the trade-off between the increased number of categories and the reduction of heterogeneity.

Although the establishment of criteria for an acceptable level of homogeneity must be arbitrary, the relatively low degree of explanatory power of DRGs combined with the apparent systematic variations in illness severity, not explained by DRGs, suggests that this classification system is not sufficiently homogeneous to be used for either payment or research purposes. However, some pilot studies have suggested that DRGs can be augmented with severity measures to achieve a substantially higher degree of homogeneity with respect to resource comsumption within DRGs. As discussed next, however, the gains in heterogeneity reduction may be offset by increases in the number of categories, as well as increases in costs.

Clinical Validity

In order to control the use of resources within their hospitals, managers must be able to communicate standards of performance to the attending physicians. Hence, the ability of administrators to influence the behavior of physicians is enhanced by a classification system that is clinically valid (i.e., meaningful to physicians). Wood, Ament, and Kobrinski (1981, p. 249) conclude:

Medical meaningfulness is defined as the extent to which knowledge of a patient's case type alone—without other information about the individual patient—conveys clinical expectations and enables clinicians to exchange information about those expectations . . . regarding the natural history of the disease, the appropriate ways to manage the case, the prognosis, the likelihood of complications of specific kinds, and the risk of death.

As this definition implies, the determination of medical meaningfulness is a subjective process that is best accomplished by a consensus of physicians.

In the absence of a comprehensive assessment by physicians, our evaluation of clinical meaningfulness is based primarily on the degree and extent of physician involvement in the development of patient classification systems. However, we are able to supplement our evaluation with some information from a panel of physicians who evaluated the PMC and staging systems (Thomas, Ashcraft, and Zimmerman 1986).

In general the panel of physicians felt that the staging concept is based on an appropriate premise—i.e., the biological progression of disease tends to result in increasing levels of involvement and poorer prognosis if the patient is untreated. The panel was concerned, however, that each disease stage is not adjusted for the presence of comorbidities. Thus, although the stages reflected differences in severity within a particular disease category, the staging system does not reflect well the overall severity of patients' illnesses.

The panel rated the content validity of PMCs as strong. They felt that the logic of assigning a patient to a PMC is clinically reasonable and understandable; however, the panel did not believe that all of the categories were homogeneous with respect to patient severity. Finally, the panel expressed reservations about the reliance of PMCs and staging on ICD-9-CM codes. They were concerned about the imprecision of this code and the opportunity for error in translating a patient's condition from the medical record into ICD-9-CM codes. Accordingly they felt that too many patients would be assigned to an incorrect group (Thomas, Ashcraft, and Zimmerman 1986).

DRGs and the SII were not evaluated by this panel of physicians; however, physicians were heavily involved in the development of each. Unlike the ICD-8 DRGs, which emphasized statistics in the formation of DRGs, clinical judgment was relied on more extensively to develop ICD-9-CM DRGs. Nevertheless, none of these systems are likely to receive the universal acceptance or approval of physicians. For example, Dr. Alan Brewster, the developer of the proprietary Medical Illness Severity Grouping System (MEDISGRPS) classification system, stated that DRGs are neither clinically based nor easily understood by physicians (McIlrath 1985). Despite the protests of a few vocal physicians, neither DRGs nor the other classification systems have been vigorously opposed by large numbers of physicians.

Manageable Number of Categories

The patient classification system should result in a manageable number of categories. If a large number of groups is used, the frequency of cases in some categories will be too small for patterns of central tendency to emerge. Hospital managers are unable to detect stable patterns of behavior if the number of admissions in specific categories is small, an outcome that impairs their ability to develop appropriate cost-containment strategies. Further, except for studies with an extremely large number of observations, the existence of a large number of categories would preclude the use of a vector of case-mix proportions for each category in regression analysis because an excessive number of degrees of freedom would be sacrificed.

Table 5.6 summarizes the number of patient groups in each of the classification systems reviewed in this chapter. The values in this table are based on our judgment of the most frequent use of these systems. For example, in some analyses of the SII, Horn has used as few as 12 categories (i.e., 4 severity levels

Table 5.6
Number of Categories in Hospital Patient Classification Systems

Classification System	Number of Primary Categories	Number of Partitions or Subcategories	Total Categories
Diagnosis Related Groups (Federal Register 1985)	468	-	468
Severity of Illness Index with DRGs (Horn and Horn 1986)	468	4	1872
Disease Staging (Conklin et al. 1984)	420	4	1680
Patient Management Categories (Young 1984a)	800	-	800
Prospective Individualized Reimbursement (Johansen 1986)	337	-	337
CPHA List A (CPHA 1978)	398	20	7960

× 3 procedure categories); however, the SII is more likely to be used to complement the DRG classifications; thus we list 1872 categories (468 DRGs × 4 severity levels).

As indicated in Table 5.6, there is a substantial range in the number of categories in patient classification systems. The CPHA List A scheme was developed for utilization review monitoring and clearly consists of too many categories for payment purposes. Although there are 800 PMCs, a number that might be unmanageable, most patients are assigned to a much smaller number of categories. About 75 percent of discharges are classified in the 117 largest PMCs; and 287 PMCs describe 90 percent of the caseload of a typical hospital (Young 1984b). Although severity-adjusted DRGs and disease-staging systems yield substantially more categories than the 468 DRGs, severity levels or stages can be viewed as qualitative adjustments to the primary category. Thus, the total number of categories for these systems may be misleading and thus it is more appropriate to consider the primary categories that are equal to or less than the number of DRGs.

Accessibility and Acquisition Cost of Data

In order for a patient classification system to be economically feasible for large-scale application, patient categories should be defined by information that is easily and inexpensively obtained. In recognition of the importance of this criterion, all of the patient classification systems reviewed in this section, except Horn's SII, rely on information available from the Uniform Hospital Discharge Data Set (UHDDS). The restriction to these data, however, has reduced the reliability, clinical validity, and homogeneity of the patient classifications.

SCALAR MEASURES

Although most of the patient classification systems that we evaluated in the last section can be used for a number of purposes, including rate regulation, internal planning, control, and quality assurance, each of them contains a large number of categories, a feature that prevents their use in estimating cost or production functions. Accordingly, researchers have collapsed patient groupings into a single-valued scalar measure. In this section we will discuss three of the most commonly used diagnosis-based scalar output measures—the information theory index, the Resource Need Index (RNI) and the Medicare Case-Mix Index (MCMI).

Each of these indices can be represented by the general formula:

$$CM_j = \left[\sum_{i=1}^{n} w_i\, p_{ij} \right] \div \left[1/N \sum_i \sum_j w_i\, p_{ij} \right] \tag{5.2}$$

where CM_j represents the case-mix index for the jth hospital; w_i represents the weighting factor for the ith category; p_{ij} represents the proportion of cases in the ith category in hospital j; and N represents the number of hospitals. An inspection of equation 5.2 shows that scalar output indices can be differentiated by:

1. functional form (e.g., linear or nonlinear)
2. weighting criteria (e.g., costs or length of stay)
3. patient categories (e.g., DRGs or CPHA List A)

In the following sections, we will describe how the scalar output measures vary with respect to these three dimensions.

Information Theory Case-Mix Index

Evans and Walker (1972) used information theory (Theil 1967) to describe inequalities in the distribution of case types within the hospital system of British Columbia and within individual hospitals. Case-mix proportions (i.e., p_{ij}) were calculated by grouping patients into 98 broad diagnostic categories based on the ICDA-7 patient classification system. Information theory was used to generate complexity weights (w_i) for each category.

The complexity weights were inversely related to the commonality of cases among hospitals. Implicit in this weighting scheme is the assumption that patients with a rare diagnosis have a complex problem that tends to be treated by a relatively small number of hospitals with extensive facilities and sophisticated staff. Conversely, simple and less expensive cases tend to be treated by all hospitals. Thus, they argue that the degree of concentration of a case type across hospitals can be used as a measure of its complexity.

Using information theory, Evans and Walker defined the complexity of a diagnostic category as the difference in the expected information received from two sets of probabilities (i.e., prior and posterior) that patients in a given category will be discharged from any particular hospital. Depending on the type of information available, the prior probability might equal $1/H$, where H is the number of hospitals in the province, or P_i/P, where P_i is the number of patients discharged from the ith hospital, and P is the sum of patients discharged from each hospital in the province.

A brief example will illustrate their approach. Assume that hospital i, which accounts for 1 percent of all patients discharged in the province (i.e., the prior probability equals 0.01), discharges 1.05 percent of all simple appendectomy patients in the province (i.e., the posterior probability of the event equals 0.0105). The information gained by learning the posterior probability for this diagnosis at this hospital is small. If patients with this diagnosis are similarly distributed (i.e., prior and posterior probabilities are approximately the same, at all the other hospitals in the region), a low complexity value will be computed for a simple appendectomy. In contrast assume that this hospital has a posterior probability of discharging a patient with *cellulitis* equal to 0.20. Since no other information has changed, the hospital maintains a prior probability equal to 0.01 of admitting a patient in this category. Assuming that patients with *cellulitis* are bunched into a small number of other hospitals, a high complexity value would be assigned for this diagnosis.

Evans and Walker maintained that their case-mix complexity measure had comparative validity because it was strongly correlated ($r = 0.44$) with educational activity which, in turn, is correlated with case-mix complexity. They attempted further validation of their measure by observing which diagnoses and hospitals had high and low complexity scores. In general, the expected patterns (e.g., teaching hospitals and high-cost diseases had high complexity scores) were found. Further, their average cost regression equations contained estimates of the information theory case-mix variable that were positive and very reliable ($p < 0.01$).

Barer (1982) performed analysis similar to that of Evans and Walker on the same group of Canadian hospitals with a more recent data set. In each of the cross-section estimates of the cost per case for the period 1966–1973, a positive and significant ($p < 0.05$) coefficient was estimated for the case-mix complexity variable. However, the magnitude of the estimated coefficients, as well as the *t*-statistic, was much smaller than those reported by Evans and Walker (1972).

In addition to the Canadian studies, the information theory approach has been used by Schumacher, Horn, Solnick, Atkinson, and Cook (1979), Horn and Schumacher (1979), and Watts and Klastorin (1980) to study the case-mix complexity of hospitals located in the United States. Horn and Schumacher assessed the validity of an information theory case-mix index in a study of 45 Maryland hospitals. The first generation of 383 DRGs was used to form patient categories; however, the complexity index based on information theory resulted in logically inconsistent weights for 167 DRGs. To remove this problem, the DRGs with the inappropriate weights were collapsed into a new set of 56 DRGs by eliminating DRG-splits that were based on age, surgery, or presence of comorbidity. Using empirical criteria, Horn and Schumacher established 0.75 as the cutoff value for high and low complexity, resulting in the classification of 80 (27 percent) DRGs as highly complex. To validate their complexity index, Horn and Schumacher examined the relationship between the information theory characterization of complexity with a clinically related definition of complexity. A high degree of interrater reliability (*Kappa* $= .42$, $Z = 700$, $p < .001$) between the classifications from the two assessment techniques was found. Further, the two major teaching hospitals in the sample had the highest complexity scores, a result consistent with a priori expectations.

Although the authors concluded that information theory is a useful way to construct a case-mix complexity index, it is not without problems. In 46 of 97 DRGs that were classified by clinicians as high mortality/high complexity, the value of the complexity index was less than 0.75, the cutoff point for complex cases. These misclassified cases included a number of DRGs (e.g., acute myocardial infarction or diabetes with amputation of an extremity) that are expensive and dispersed among most hospitals.

In a comparison study, Schumacher et al. (1979) entered case-mix complexity as an explanatory variable in a regression equation that was used to predict the cost per case. In an analysis of all ($n = 45$) Maryland hospitals reporting complete data, the complexity variable was positive and significant ($p < 0.04$). In regression equations for 16 rural hospitals, however, the complexity variable was negative and significant ($p < .01$). Schumacher et al. attributed this unexpected result to the treatment in rural hospitals of a higher proportion of high cost patients with high clinical complexity, but with low information-theory complexity numbers.

Watts and Klastorin (1980) also provide results that weaken the support for the use of information theory to construct a case-mix index. In this study, a case-mix index, based on information theory and using DRGs as the patient classification system, was entered as an independent variable into a cost per case equation. In their first analysis, the case-mix variable based on information theory was positive and significant, but its contribution to the explanatory power of the basic cost equation was small ($R^2 = 0.03$). In a second analysis in which medical school affiliation was added to all equations, the coefficient of the information theory index became insignificant ($p > .10$). This result was due to a strong correlation ($r = 0.53$) between medical school affiliation and the information theory complexity index in this data set. The introduction of a teaching activity variable caused a reduction in the reliability of the information-theory index variable in the study conducted by Schumacher et al. (1979). In five regression equations without a teaching activity variable, the probability value for the coefficient of the complexity variable ranged from .002 to .0001. When the teaching variable was added, however the probability value of the complexity coefficient increased to .04, which is still very respectable but certainly much higher than in the other equations.

Resource Need Index

The Resource Need Index (RNI), a scalar diagnosis-based output measure, has been used more frequently in cost function studies than any other case-mix measure. The RNI takes on the general functional form expressed by equation 5.2. It is based on the 3,490 cells derived from the 20 subcategories of the 349 broad disease categories classified by the CPHA List A. The weights for the RNI are computed from the average charge per case for each cell, and are based on a sample of over 2 million patient records collected from 50 hospitals that participated in the CPHA's Survey of Charges during 1971 and 1976. If a hospital has a case-mix identical to the average hospital in the data base, the institution is assigned an RNI value equal to 1.0. A hospital with a case-mix that is more costly than the average hospital will have an RNI value greater than 1.0.

The RNI has exhibited strong predictive power. In cost equations, the estimated coefficient of RNI has been positive and significant ($p < .01$) (Becker and Sloan 1985; Sloan and Becker 1981; Sloan, Feldman, and Steinwald 1983; Watts and Klastorin 1980). The positive association between the value of the RNI and teaching activities has been cited as evidence of its predictive validity. Becker and Steinwald (1981) reported a monotonically increasing relationship between three binary independent variables representing increasing levels of teaching commitment (i.e., hospital with a residency program, hospital with a medical school affiliation, and hospital with membership on the Council of Teaching Hospitals) and the RNI, which served as the dependent variable. In a univariate analysis, Ament, Kobrinski, and Wood (1981) reported that the value assigned to the RNI of teaching hospitals was significantly larger than that of non–teaching hospitals. Similar results were reported by Sloan, Feldman, and Steinwald (1983). Further support of the validity of the RNI is its strong correlation ($r = 0.97$) with a DRG index based on case weights developed from New Jersey hospitals (Watts and Klastorin 1980).

Medicare Case-Mix Index

The Medicare Case-Mix Index (MCMI) is calculated by following a procedure similar to that described for the RNI. The major differences between the two indexes are (1) the MCMI is based on DRG categories, while the RNI is based on CPHA List A categories, and (2) the MCMI is weighted by costs, standardized for indirect teaching costs and local wages, while the RNI is weighted by charges. The weights of the MCMI were calculated in a study that collected observations from 1.93 million cases treated in 5,947 hospitals during 1979. The MCMI has been a reliable predictor of the cost per case. Anderson and Lave (1986) estimated six specifications of equations for Medicare cost per case. In each, the MCMI had a parameter estimate that was positive and highly significant ($p < 0.001$). Pettengill and Vertrees (1982) reported similar results from an equation that also estimated Medicare cost per case. They also reported that the MCMI was strongly correlated with two surrogate measures of case-mix, the number of beds ($r = 0.54$), and the ratio of interns and residents per bed ($r = 0.36$).

Although the RNI and the MCMI are relatively easy to construct and are reliable predictors of the cost per case, they share a number of problems that may compromise their validity. First, the weighting factors of DRGS and RNIs are observed costs and charges, respectively. Ideally, the weights should be based on the total costs of appropriately managed cases in hospitals that were operated efficiently and were of the optimum scale. As is well known, charges per case may not be representative of costs per case, since hospitals establish charge schedules to maximize reimbursement. Further, case weights, based on actual costs, will be biased if the distribution of patients in case-mix categories is systematically related to size or inefficiency.

Second, the charge or cost weights of the RNI and MCMI have not been

recalculated with sufficient frequency to reflect changes in factors, such as technological or medical changes, that affect the costs of efficiently treating patients
requiring different services.

Third, scalar indexes lose substantial amounts of information via the aggregation process. For example, two hospitals may have the same index value even
though they treat a significantly different distribution of patients. Thus, this type
of measure can not be used to measure or reflect the potential efficiencies gained
through the joint production of outputs (i.e., economies of scope) or the ability
to more easily monitor and control the activities of physicians whose patients
are concentrated into a more dense distribution of case-types. Finally, scalar
indexes share the strengths and weaknesses of the patient classification system
upon which their categories are based.

In summary, two types of scalar-indexes of hospital output have been evaluated. The information theory approach has relied exclusively on statistical
considerations to determine category weights. Although indexes based on information theory have been shown to be reliable predictors of hospital costs, the
main premise of the approach is not conceptually strong. Specifically, information theory assigns a high case weight to cases that are concentrated in a
smaller number of hospitals and a lower weight to cases common to most hospitals. The implicit assumption is that rarer cases represent more complicated
illnesses requiring the sophisticated and expensive services of tertiary care hospitals. Horn and Schumacher (1979), however, reported that there are many
high-cost patients (e.g., acute myocardial infarction) that are incorrectly assigned
a lower case-mix weight by the information theory approach.

Other case-mix indexes, i.e., the RNI and the MCMI, have been weighted
according to actual charges or costs. This approach is faulted for the possible
lack of correspondence between observed costs or charges and costs incurred by
an efficient hospital. Both approaches suffer information loss through the aggregation procedure; however, this may be a necessary price to pay to reduce
multicollinearity in certain studies. In some instances, for example, the investigation of cost structures such as economies of scope or economies of scale,
the multiproduct nature of the hospital cannot be captured by a single variable.
This issue will be discussed in more detail in the chapters devoted to production
functions and cost functions. Before we discuss these subjects, we describe
classification schemes that have been developed for patients requiring nursing
home care and other types of services.

SUMMARY

In this chapter we described and evaluated a number of hospital output measures, including the early surrogate measures and the more recently developed
direct case-mix measures. Although the state of the art has increased dramatically
during the last decade, the measurement of the outputs of hospitals has remained
a perplexing problem for researchers, regulators and hospital managers. It is

clear that DRGs are not very homogeneous with respect to resource consumption; however, even though DRGs can be augmented with severity of illness measures, it is not clear that reductions in heterogeneity are worth the increases in patient categories and costs. Although case-mix measures may require modifications to improve potentially inequitable hospital payments, we are certain that advances in hospital output measurement have led to more precise estimation of the determinants of hospital costs, a subject explored in Chapter 8.

REFERENCES

Ament, R. P., E. J. Kobrinski, and W. R. Wood. 1981. Case mix complexity differences between teaching and nonteaching hospitals. *Journal of Medical Education* 56(11):894–903.

Ament, R. P., J. L. Dreachslin, E. J. Kobrinski, and W. R. Wood. 1982. Three case-type classifications: Suitability for use in reimbursing hospitals. *Medical Care* 20(5):460–67.

American Hospital Association. 1986. *AHA Guide to the Health Care Field, 1986 Edition.* Chicago, IL: American Hospital Association.

Anderson, G. F., and J. R. Lave. 1986. Financing graduate medical education using multiple regression to set payment rates. *Inquiry* 23(2):191–99.

Barer, M. L. 1982. Case-mix adjustment in hospital cost analysis: Information theory revisited. *Journal of Health Economics* 1(1):53–80.

Becker, E. R., and B. Steinwald. 1981. Determinants of hospital case mix complexity. *Health Services Research* 16(4):439–58.

Becker, E. R., and F. A. Sloan. 1985. Hospital ownership and performance. *Economic Inquiry* 23(1):21–36.

Berki, S. 1972. *Hospital Economics.* Lexington, MA: Lexington Books.

Berry, R. E. 1970. Product heterogeneity and hospital cost analysis. *Inquiry* 7(1):67–75.

Broyles, R. W., and M. D. Rosko. 1985. A qualitative assessment of the medicare prospective payment system. *Social Science and Medicine* 20(11):1185–90.

Broyles, R. W., and M. D. Rosko. 1986. *Planning and Internal Control Under Prospective Payment.* Rockville, MD: Aspen Publishers.

Calore, K. A., and L. Iezzoni. 1987. Disease staging and PMCs: Can they improve DRGs? *Medical Care* 25(8):724–37.

Cameron, J. M., and R. A. Knauf. 1981. DRGs: An assessment of the assessment. *Medical Care* 19(2):243–45.

Carr, W. J., and P. J. Feldstein. 1967. The relationship of cost to hospital size. *Inquiry* 4(2):45–65.

Coffey, R., and M. Goldfarb. 1986. DRGs and disease staging for reimbursing Medicare patients. *Medical Care* 24(9):814–29.

Cohen, H. A. 1967. Variations in cost among hospitals of different sizes. *Southern Economic Journal* 34(1):355–72.

Commission on Professional and Hospital Activities (CPHA). 1966. *Length of Stay in Short-Term General Hospitals (1963–1964).* New York: McGraw-Hill.

Commission on Professional and Hospital Activities (CPHA). 1978. *The International Classification of Diseases, 9th Revision, Clinical Modification*, Vol. 1, Diseases, Tabular List. Ann Arbor, MI: CPHA.

Conklin, J. E., J. V. Lieberman, C. A. Barnes, and D. Z. Louis. 1984. Disease staging: Implications for hospital reimbursement and management. *Health Care Financing Review* 5 (Annual Supplement):13–22.

DesHarnais, S. I., J. D. Chesney, and S. T. Fleming. 1988. Should DRG assignment be based on age? *Medical Care* 26(2):124–31.

Doremus, H. D. 1980. DRGs may be raising false expectations. *Hospitals* 54(15):47–51.

Doremus, H., and E. Michenzi. 1983. Data quality: An illustration of its potential impact upon a diagnosis-related group's case mix index and reimbursement. *Medical Care* 21(10):1001–11.

Dowling, W. L., P. J. House, J. M. Lehman et al. 1976. *Evaluation of Prospective Reimbursement of Hospitals in Downstate New York*. University of Washington: Center for Health Services Research.

Evans, R. G. 1971. Behavioral cost functions for hospitals. *Canadian Journal of Economics* 4(2):198–215.

Evans, R. G., and H. D. Walker. 1972. Information theory and the analysis of hospital cost structure. *Canadian Journal of Economics* 5 (3):398–418.

Federal Register. 1985. Part III. Medicare Program: Changes to the inpatient hospital prospective payment system and fiscal year 1986 rates; final rule. 50(170):35722–35, September 3.

Fetter, R. B., R. E. Mills, D. C. Riedel, and J. D. Thompson. 1977. The application of diagnostic specific cost profiles to cost and reimbursement control in hospitals. *Journal of Medical Systems* 1(2):137–49.

Fetter, R. B., Y. Shin, J. C. Freeman, R. F. Averill, and J. D. Thompson. 1980. Case mix definition by diagnosis-related groups. *Medical Care* 18(2):1–53.

Frank, R. G., and J. R. Lave. 1985. The psychiatric DRGs: Are they different? *Medical Care* 23(10):1148–55.

Gertman, P. M., and S. Lowenstein. 1984. A research paradigm for severity of illness: Issues for the diagnosis-related group system. *Health Care Financing Review* 5 (Annual Supplement):79–90.

Ginsburg, P., and G. Carter. 1986. The Medicare case-mix index increase. *Health Care Financing Review* 7(4):51–66.

Ginsburg, P. B., and F. Sloan. 1984. Hospital cost shifting. *New England Journal of Medicine* 310(14):893–98.

Gonnella, J. S. 1981. Patient case mix: Implications for medical education and hospital costs. *Journal of Medical Education* 56(7):610–11.

Gonnella, J. S., and M. J. Goran. 1975. Quality of patient care—A measurement of change: The staging concept. *Medical Care* 13(6):467–73.

Gonnella, J. S., M. Hornbrook, and D. Louis. 1984. Staging of disease: A case-mix measurement. *Journal of American Medical Association* 251(5):637–44.

Horn, S. 1981. Validity, reliability and implications of an index of inpatient severity of illness. *Medical Care* 19(3):354–62.

Horn, S. D., B. Chachich, and C. Clopton. 1983. Measuring severity of illness: A reliability study. *Medical Care* 21(7):705–14.

Horn, S. D., and D. N. Schumacher. 1979. An analysis of case-mix complexity using information theory and diagnostic related grouping. *Medical Care* 17(4):382–9.

Horn, S. D., G. Bulkley, P. D. Sharkey, A. F. Chambers, R. A. Horn, and C. J.

Schramm. 1985. Interhospital differences in severity of illness. *New England Journal of Medicine* 313(1):20–24.

Horn, S. D., and P. D. Sharkey. 1983. Measuring severity of illness to predict patient resource use within DRGs. *Inquiry* 20 (4):314–21.

Horn, S. D., P. D. Sharkey, A. F. Chambers, and R. A. Horn. 1985. Severity of illness within DRGs: Impact on prospective payment. *American Journal of Public Health* 75(10):1195–9.

Horn, S. D., P. D. Sharkey, and D. A. Bertram. 1983. Measuring severity of illness: Homogeneous case mix groups. *Medical Care* 21(1):14–25.

Horn, S. D., and R. A. Horn. 1986. Reliability and validity of the severity of illness index. *Medical Care* 24(2):159–69.

Horn, S. D., R. A. Horn, and P. D. Sharkey. 1984. The Severity of Illness Index as a severity adjustment to diagnosis related groups. *Health Care Financing Review* (Annual Supplement):33–45.

Horn, S. D., R. A. Horn, P. D. Sharkey, and A. F. Chambers. 1986. Severity of illness within DRGs: Homogeneity study. *Medical Care* 24(3):225–35.

Hornbrook, M. C. 1982. Hospital case mix: Its definition, measurement and use: Part II. Review of alternative measures. *Medical Care Review* 39(2):73–123.

Institute of Medicine. 1980. *Reliability of National Hospital Discharge Survey Data*, Pub. No. 10M 80–02. Washington, DC: Institute of Medicine.

Johansen, S. 1986. Comparison of two prospective rate-setting models: The DRG and PIR models. *Health Services Research* 21(4):547–59.

Kerlinger, F. N. 1973. *Foundations of Behavioral Research*, 2nd ed. New York: Holt, Rinehart and Winston.

Lave, J., and L. Lave. 1970. Hospital cost functions. *American Economic Review* 60(3):379–95.

McIlrath, S. 1985. Review systems based on illness severity. *American Medical News* 28(2):2, 17, 18.

McNeil, B., G. Kominski, and A. Williams-Ashman. 1988. Modified DRGs as evidence for variability in patient severity. *Medical Care* 26(1):53–61.

Muller, C. 1983. Paying hospitals: How does a severity measure help? *American Journal of Public Health* 73(1):14–15.

Pettengill, J., and J. Vertrees. 1982. Reliability and validity in hospital case-mix measurement. *Health Care Financing Review* 4(2):101–28.

Schumacher, D. N., B. Parker, V. Kofie, and J. M. Munns. 1987. Severity of Illness Index and the Adverse Patient Occurrence Index: A reliability study and policy implications. *Medical Care* 25(8):695–704.

Schumacher, D. N., S. D. Horn, M. F. Solnick, G. Atkinson, and J. Cook. 1979. Hospital cost per case: Analyses using a statewide data system. *Medical Care* 17(10):1037–47.

Shuman, L. J., H. Wolfe, and C. P. Hardwick. 1972. Predictive hospital reimbursement and evaluation model. *Inquiry* 9(2):17–33.

Sloan, F. A., and E. R. Becker. 1981. Internal organization of hospitals and hospital costs. *Inquiry* 18 (3):224–39.

Sloan, F. A., R. D. Feldman, and A.B. Steinwald. 1983. Effects of teaching on hospital costs. *Journal of Health Economics* 2(1):1–28.

Smits, H. L., R. B. Fetter, and L. F. McMahon. 1984. Variation in resource use within diagnosis-related groups: The severity issue. *Health Care Financing Review* 5 (Annual Supplement):71–78.

Spiegel, A. D., and F. Kavaler. 1986. *Cost Containment and DRGs: A Guide to Prospective Payment*. Owings Mills, MD: National Health Publishing.

Taube, C., E. S. Lee, and R. N. Forthofer. 1984. DRGs in psychiatry: An empirical evaluation. *Medical Care* 22(7):597–610.

Theil, H. 1967. *Economics and Information Theory*. Amsterdam: North-Holland Publishers.

Thomas, J. W., M. L. Ashcraft, and J. Zimmerman. 1986. An Evaluation of Alternative Severity of Illness Measures for Use by University Hospitals, Vol. II: Technical Report. University of Michigan School of Public Health.

Watts, C. A., and T. D. Klastorin. 1980. The impact of case mix on hospital cost: A comparative analysis. *Inquiry* 17(4):357–67.

Wennberg, J. 1984. Dealing with medical practice variations: A proposal for action. *Health Affairs* 3 (2):6–32.

Wood, W. R., R. P. Ament, and E. J. Kobrinski. 1981. A foundation for hospital case mix measurement. *Inquiry* 18(3):247–54.

Young, W. W. 1984a. Incorporating severity of illness and comorbidity in case-mix measurement. *Health Care Financing Review* 5 (Annual Supplement):23–46.

Young, W. W. 1984b. Patient management categories. Paper presented at Annual meeting of American Public Health Association, Anaheim, CA, November 14, 1984.

Young, W. W., R. B. Swinkola, and M. A. Hutton. 1980. Assessment of the AUTOGRP patient-classification system. *Medical Care* 18(2):228–44.

Young, W. W., R. B. Swinkola, and D. M. Zorn. 1982. The measurement of hospital case mix. *Medical Care* 20(5):501–12.

6

LONG-TERM CARE AND OTHER PATIENT CLASSIFICATION SYSTEMS

In this chapter we examine systems that have been developed for classifying patients who receive care in long-term care facilities, psychiatric units, and ambulatory settings. Relative to acute inpatient hospital classification systems, the development and evaluation of grouping schemes for other types of patients have not received much attention. Consequently, we are not able to provide the detailed assessment presented in the previous chapter. We emphasize long-term care patient classification systems because they have been the focus of a substantial amount of attention in recent years. Further, as the "graying of America" continues its inevitable course, we expect an increase in the importance of developing patient classification systems for the purpose of compensating long-term care facilities.

LONG-TERM CARE PATIENT CLASSIFICATION SYSTEMS

Several systems of classifying long-term patients for the purpose of determining rates or levels of prospective payment have been proposed. In contrast to the hospital DRG system, most of the classification systems developed for the long-term care industry rely on measures of physical, mental, and social disorders to form groups of patients who are expected to consume a similar mix of resources. Perhaps the most commonly used measure of case mix is the Index of Independence in Activities of Daily Living, developed initially by Katz, Ford, Moskowitz et al. (1963). Typically, the index of independence is based on the ability to eat, bathe, dress, walk, transfer to and from bed, use toilet facilities, and communicate. Activities of daily living (ADLs) have been used in conjunction with service characteristics in Illinois, Maryland, Ohio, and West Virginia to determine a case-severity measure for each patient, from which rates of compensation are determined (Adams and Schlenker 1986). The collection of the data on which these measures are based, however, requires lengthy instruments that are expensive and unreliable (Smits 1984). Further, the severity index used to establish rates of compensation in Illinois was based on several subjectively determined components, and hence fell victim to manipulation by nursing homes that attempted to maximize income (Walsh 1979).

Currently, the focus of patient classification systems is on the development of isoresource groups. In general, these mechanisms are derived from objective data and require information that is available in most facilities or might be assembled inexpensively. Among those frequently cited as a potential basis for developing prospective rates of compensation are the Resource Utilization Groups (RUGs), developed by Fries and Cooney (1985), the RUG-II System developed by Schneider, Holden, and Fries (1985), the classification system developed by Cameron (1985), and the nursing resource use system proposed by Arling, Nordquist, Brant, and Capitman (1987).

These systems share a number of common features. First, the development of the patient classification schemes was guided by the requirement for the formation of patient groups which are statistically stable, clinically meaningful, limited in number, and generalizable to other long-term care facilities. In addition, previous studies employed AUTOGRP, an interactive statistical program, to identify categories of patients that were similar with respect to resource consumption or cost, thus forming the basis for developing prospective rates of compensation.

Cameron's Classification System

The classification scheme proposed by Cameron (1985) was based on the level of functioning and the mix of services consumed by 1,151 individuals residing in 23 long-term care facilities. Data assembled for each patient depicted general attributes, demographic characteristics, diagnostic condition, medications, independence in the performance of ADLs, behavioral or social function, and dependence on special treatments or procedures. The dependent variable examined by Cameron measured the value of direct patient care provided to each individual. This variable was based on the standard mix of nursing personnel required to provide each service and the average wage rate for each category of labor. Expert opinion or subjective judgment was used to derive standard times for each component of service.

The formation of patient groups was guided by four criteria that were defined in terms of statistical stability, clinical meaningfulness, limitation on the number of categories and generalizability among long-term care facilities. Further, the partitioning of patients into isocost groups was governed by the general rule that the medical diagnosis constituted the primary variable for forming clusters, followed by variables depicting control of urinary function, independence in the performance of ADLs and, finally, the use of therapeutic services.

The presence or absence of severe neurologic impairment constituted the basis

Table 6.1
Cameron's Long-Term Care Classification System

Patients with diagnoses indicating severe neurologic impairment.

1. Requiring tube feeding

2. Continent, not requiring catheter

3. Incontinent, without mobility

4. Incontinent, with mobility

5. Requiring catheter, without mobility

6. Requiring catheter, with mobility

Patients without diagnoses indicating severe neurologic impairment.

7. With decubitus ulcers,
   Stage II, III, or IV

8. Requiring catheter

9. Incontinent, totally dependent
   for feeding

10. Incontinent, not totally dependent
    for feeding

11. Continent, dependent walking

12. Continent, independent walking,
    with special treatment

13. Continent, independent walking,
    without special treatment

Source: Cameron, J.M. 1985. Case-mix and resource use in long-term care. Medical Care
       23 (4): 296-309.

for dividing the study population into two groups. Employing AUTOGRP, the interactive statistical system, the two sets of patients were formed into the 13 groups summarized in Table 6.1. The number of patients in each category ranged from 18 to 286. Further, the groups were relatively homogeneous, as evidenced by the ratio of the mean value of resource consumption to the standard deviation, which ranged from 2.70 to 8.06. Finally, the 13 groups explained 68.5 percent of the total variance in resource consumption per patient, a finding that is of particular importance when evaluating the desirability of basing rates of compensation on this classification scheme.

Resource Utilization Groups

Similar to the classification scheme developed by Cameron, the approach proposed by Fries and Cooney (1985) assigns patients to one of several Resource Utilization Groups. Applying criteria used to develop DRGs and Cameron's system, RUGs were intended to be clinically meaningful, homogeneous with respect to resource consumption, and statistically stable.

The initial development of RUGs was based on a sample of 1,469 patients who were selected from five long-term care facilities. The dependent variables consisted of subjective estimates of the direct staff time required to provide care to each patient. The independent variables consisted of items such as primary diagnosis, the number of coexisting diagnoses, and variables depicting independence in the performance of ADLs.

Focusing on each variable in the data set, AUTOGRP was employed to develop the first partition. Only two of the variables depicting diagnosis, both representing neurological problems, resulted in a statistically significant ($p \le .05$) reduction in variance. In contrast to the maximum variance reduction of 1.85 percent achieved by the two diagnostic conditions, nine variables depicting physical functioning individually resulted in more than a 20 percent reduction of variance when they were used to form the first partition. As a consequence, the initial development of RUGs was based on physical functioning rather than medical diagnosis.

Appearing in Table 6.2 are the nine patient groups that were identified by Fries and Cooney. The first partition was based on the ability to dress; while the ability (inability) to feed or walk without assistance and the need for monitored intake/output of fluids formed subsequent divisions. With the exception of the need to monitor fluids, all partitions were based on variables depicting independence in the performance of ADLs. These findings are consistent with earlier studies that found that indices of ADL variables are the most important determinants of resource consumption by nursing home patients (Skinner and Yett 1973; Parker and Boyd 1974; Flagle, Young, McKnight et al. 1977; Swearingen, Schwartz, and Fisher 1978; Cavaiola and Young 1980). The nine patient groups explained 37.8 percent of the variation in the dependent variable, staff estimates of resource consumption by each patient. Similar to the groups developed by Cameron, each of the nine RUGs was found to be relatively homogeneous, as evidenced by the coefficients of variation for the groups that ranged from 0.15 to 0.46.

Essentially two methodological limitations in the initial development of RUGs were identified. First, rather than objective and verifiable information, the data

Table 6.2
Resource Utilization Groups

Group 1: Able to dress without
help or with supervision.

Group 2: Able to dress only with
help; walks without help or
with supervision.

Group 3: Able to dress only with
help; walks only with help
or confined to bed/chair.

Group 4: Requires total care for
dressing; eats independently
or with supervision; walks
without help.

Group 5: Requires total care for
dressing; eats independently;
walks only with help.

Group 6: Requires total care for
dressing; eats independently;
confined to bed/chair.

Group 7: Requires total care for
dressing; eats only with help.

Group 8: Requires total care
for dressing and feeding; no
monitoring of intake/output
of fluids.

Group 9: Requires total care for
dressing and feeding; has
monitored intake/output.

Source: Fries, B.E. and L.M. Cooney. 1985. Resource utilization groups: A
patient classification system for long-term care. Medical Care
23 (2): 110-122.

that were used to measure resource consumption were derived from subjective estimates or opinions of nurses and nurses aides. In addition, the information used in the initial analysis was obtained from skilled nursing facilities located in only two counties in Connecticut.

Recognizing the limitations that were inherent in the initial study, Cooney and Fries (1985) attempted to validate previous findings by performing similar analyses on separate sets of data that were collected by Battelle Human Affairs Research Center in the course of two studies during 1974 and 1977 (McCaffree, Winn, and Bennett 1976; McCaffree, Baker, Perrin et al. 1979). The two sets of data contained direct measures of staff time required to provide service to long-term care (LTC) patients. Further, the set of data assembled in 1974 was derived from 1,615 patients residing in 12 nursing homes that were located in five states, while the information compiled in 1977 was obtained from 1,261 patients of 16 facilities that were located in three states.

Using AUTOGRP, Cooney and Fries created seven RUGs from the 1974 data and eight RUGs from the data assembled in 1977. The RUGs derived from the 1974 data explained 34 percent of the variance in aide time while those formed from the set of data assembled in 1977 explained 53.8 percent of the variance in aide time. Since three sets of data were examined, the analysis was expected to yield different groups. Cooney and Fries attempted to validate their approach by demonstrating that the same patients were grouped together in each classification system. The test of validity consisted of an evaluation of the extent to which each individual was assigned to the same RUG. The proportion of agreement ranged from .88, when the initial RUGs were compared with those formed from the 1974 Battelle data, to .97 when the accuracy of pairings obtained from the two Battelle sets of data was measured. The index of agreement was statistically significant ($p \leq .001$) in each case (Cooney and Fries 1985).

RUG-II

In a more recent study, Schneider, Holden, and Fries (1985) used information depicting services provided to 3,400 patients by 52 long-term care facilities located in New York to develop the RUG-II classification system, which would be used to set prospective payment rates for Medicaid patients. The facilities were selected so that the sample was representative of size, ownership status (proprietary vs. nonprofit), sponsorship (hospital-based vs. free-standing), level of care, and staffing patterns. The system of classification was derived from 277 elements of data, including the amount of time required to provide direct patient care, demographic attributes of patients, diagnostic mix, symptoms, ADLs, psychosocial functioning, behavioral problems, services, treatments, and comments concerning patients requiring special care.

A two-stage process was used to form the RUG-II groups, which are listed in Table 6.3. In the first stage, clinical judgment was the basis for forming five groups that were identified as special care, rehabilitation, clinically complex,

Table 6.3
Resource Utilization Groups II

Category*	ADL Index
Special care: Very heavy care; functional level very low	
1. A	5-7
2. B	8-10
Rehabilitation: PT or OT ≥ 5 days per week	
3. A	3-4
4. B	5-10
Clinically complex: acute medical problems or extensive medical needs	
5. A	3
6. B	4-6
7. C	7-8
8. D	9-10
Severe behavioral problem: high frequency or severe level behavior problems	
9. A	3
10. B	4-7
11. C	8-10
Reduced physical functioning: reduced ADL functioning	
12. A	3
13. B	4
14. C	5-7
15. D	8
16. E	9

Source: Schneider, D.P., F. Holden and B.E. Fries. 1985. DRG and
RUG interactions in resource allocation. Paper presented at
AHPA/VA conference, December, 1985.
* Patients are grouped within major categories on the basis of their
scores on the ADL index.

severe behavioral problems, and reduced physical functioning. In the second stage, AUTOGRP was used to divide the five clinical groups into 16 patient categories that were distinguished by the level of physical functioning as defined by the ADL Index. Using the patient as the level of aggregation, RUG-II groups explained 2 percent of the overall variation in resource consumption. The variance explained on a facility level would be much higher than the patient level reported here because the broader level of aggregation dampens variations in the dependent variable.

Nursing Resource Use

In a recent pilot study, Arling et al. (1987) developed a system of classifying patients into groups on the basis of use of nursing resources. The intensity of resource consumption was defined as the amount of time devoted to direct patient care by RNs, LPNs, aides, and other nursing staff. The predictor variables in the study were impairment in the performance of ADLs, conditions resulting in a dependence on special care (e.g., wounds or lesions, quadriplegia, coma) and potential for physical rehabilitation.

The analysis was based on 558 Medicaid patients residing in 12 Virginia nursing homes. Data on resource use were obtained from a set of self-reports submitted by the nursing staff and validated by concurrent work sampling. A standardized instrument completed by the nursing staff yielded assessments concerning the health and functional status of patients.

Patients were initially grouped by their need for specialized care. Those that required specialized care were split into two subgroups based on the presence or absence of a catheter/ostomy. Those without specialized care requirements were split into four subgroups based on ADL impairment scores and need for assistance in eating. This approach explained 53 percent of the variance in nursing resource use.

Evaluation of Nursing Home Patient Classification Systems

The suitability of the measures of case-mix for payment purposes is evaluated next by considering a number of criteria that we used in the previous chapter to assess patient classification systems developed for the hospital industry. First, the patient classification system should result in patient groups that are homogeneous with respect to resource consumption. Greater homogeneity in resource consumption reduces the incentive to implement a selective admissions policy and lessens the variation in nursing home solvency that is attributable to differences in case-mix. The percentage of variation in resource consumption explained by patient classification systems ranged from 34 percent when RUGs were applied to the 1974 Battelle data set to 68 percent in Cameron's analysis. However, direct comparisons between these patient classification systems are not possible since different sample sizes and variables were employed, thus affecting the percentage of variation explained by the cluster analysis. Furthermore, none of these studies examined the percentage variation in costs explained by nursing home patient classification systems.

Any benchmark level for an acceptable level of variance explanation must be arbitrary. By way of comparison, however, at the patient level of aggregation, DRGs explain approximately 16 percent of the variation in length of stay (Coffey and Goldfarb 1986), an amount that is substantially less than the explanatory power of the four nursing home patient classification systems discussed in this chapter. As a result, the measures of case-mix appear to create less incentive to implement a selective admissions policy and less potential for adverse effects on the fiscal position of nursing homes than the Medicare hospital pricing system. However, external regulation of nursing homes specifies minimum levels of staffing and service availability. When payment is tied to the minimum service level, as it is in many states, available services and staff time are constrained to a maximum as well as a minimum level. Services tend to be more homogeneous, suggesting that differences in the explanatory power of DRGs and RUGs may be overstated.

Second, the patient classification system should result in a manageable number of patient categories. If a large number of groups are used, the frequency of cases in some categories may be too small for patterns of central tendency to emerge. In addition, administrators of nursing homes may not be able to detect stable patterns of behavior if the number of patients in specific categories is small, a problem that prevents the development of appropriate cost containment strategies. In contrast to the 471 DRGs that are used in the Medicare prospective payment system, nursing home patient classification systems have resulted in a relatively small number of patient groups, ranging from the 6 patient categories developed by Arling et al. (1987) to the 16 groups in the RUG-II grouping system. Although the number of categories in long-term care patient classification schemes is relatively small, some of the groups still contained only a few patients. For example, there were no patients in 4 of the 9 original RUGs in several of the Connecticut nursing homes. The other studies did not provide a distribution of patients by facility. However, several of Cameron's groups contained less than 2 percent of the entire sample. Similarly, 4 of the 16 RUG-II groups each contained less than 2 percent of the entire sample.

Third, the classification system should be based on objective information in order to prevent the institution from increasing the compensation level by reassigning patients to groups that yield higher payments. Most measures of case-mix rely on information pertaining to diagnoses, services provided, and level of functioning. Diagnoses that are based on objective criteria are least subject to provider manipulation. For this reason, principal diagnosis was selected as the most important criterion for classifying patients into DRGs. Unfortunately, diagnosis has been shown to be a poor predictor of consumption of long-term care services, since nursing home residents often present multiple and interrelated problems (Schneider, Holden, and Fries 1985). As with the DRG classification systems for psychiatric patients, whose treatment is also characterized as open-ended and is subject to substantial discretion by practitioners, the predictive power of a diagnosis-based classification system for nursing home patients is likely to result in heterogeneous patient groupings (Taube, Lee, and Forthofer 1984).

Although not as desirable as diagnosis, service characteristics have been used to define patient groups in long-term care and acute care settings. For example, the presence or absence of a surgical procedure performed in an operating room is used to classify hospital patients into different DRGs. As Smits (1984) notes, however, there are important differences between surgery and the types of services used to develop case-mix systems for nursing home patients. In the hospital, surgical decisions are made by physicians who typically are not employed by the hospital. Thus, their decisions are based more on the efficacy of treatment and incentives imbedded in the physician compensation system than on incentives created by hospital payment mechanisms. In contrast, although the physician must prescribe care for long-term care patients, the services are usually performed by nursing home employees. Further, the initiation of these services often results from negotiations with nurses who must manage the patients for long periods in the absence of the physician. Consequently, the nurse may effectively control the negotiations regarding patient treatments. Thus, in contrast to the decision to perform surgery, which is made by a physician who is independent of the hospital, the decision to provide nursing home services is influenced strongly by nursing home employees.

The potential of a service-based payment mechanism to induce perverse behavior is exacerbated by the discretionary nature of many components of nursing home care. For example, Smits (1984) points out that a urinary catheter, one of the services used to develop the classification scheme proposed by Cameron, is a convenient method of dealing with chronic incontinence; however, the decision to use a catheter for this purpose is based on subjective criteria. Similarly, although a number of patients might be hand-fed with patience and coaxing, tube feeding is a medical necessity for others. Thus, the use of service to form patient groups that constitute the basis for developing a payment system may result in inappropriate manipulation and undesirable provider behavior.

A service-based payment mechanism induces providers to increase revenue by maximizing the number of patient days requiring heavy resource consumption. If catheterization and incontinence generate higher levels of compensation, there is no incentive to rehabilitate bowel and bladder function, an outcome that is unfortunate for two reasons. First, failure to rehabilitate the patient prevents an improvement in the individual's quality of life. Second, providers are induced to avoid the large outlays that initially reduce short-run profitability, an outcome that may prevent the realization of cost savings that result from rehabilitation and occur after the passage of time.

Several of the existing nursing home patient classification systems satisfy several well-accepted criteria. As our evaluation suggested, however, none of the classification systems is without serious flaws. Therefore, further research must be conducted to allow the formation of patient groups on the basis of more objective data that is less subject to manipulation by the nursing home operators. It must be emphasized that, given the poor discriminatory power of objective information such as diagnosis, a nursing home patient classification scheme will inevitably be forced to rely on some subjective information such as that required to construct the ADL index. Accordingly, it will be necessary to impose controls with enforceable sanctions, which will preclude manipulation of patient classifications. These controls, however, are the subject of another discussion.

AMBULATORY CARE PATIENT CLASSIFICATION SYSTEMS

The development of classification systems for ambulatory care patients has not matched the progress achieved in the areas of inpatient care or long-term care. Although a number of grouping systems, such as "Diagnosis Clusters" (Schneeweis, Rosenblatt, Cherkin, Kirkwood, and Hart 1983), "Episodes of Care" (Johnson, Vogt, and Penn 1984), and "Ambulatory Visit Groups" (Fetter, Averill, Lichtenstein, and Freeman 1984) have been developed, we will discuss only the last because it has been applied in most studies.

Ambulatory Visit Groups (AVGs) (formerly called Ambulatory Patient Groups) were developed in order to classify ambulatory patients into groups that are homogeneous with respect to patterns of services and required quantities of resources. Using data from the National Ambulatory Medical Care Survey (National Center for Health Statistics 1982), a group of researchers from Yale University created 154 AVGs from 14 Major Ambulatory Categories (MACs) (Fetter et al. 1984). These categories were created using the Automatic Interaction Detector to assign patients to groups that were homogeneous with respect to the dependent variable, time spent with the physician. The variables on which the partitions were based are these:

1. presenting problem as defined by chief complaint

2. primary diagnosis

3. secondary diagnosis

4. age of patient

5. type of visit (e.g., initial visit versus follow-up visit)

6. type of care provided (e.g., adult, pediatric, prenatal, postnatal, postoperative, or other)

7. referral status

8. psychotherapy visit

Recognizing that the patient classification system derived from the National Ambulatory Medical Care Survey data base was restricted to hospital outpatient departments, a group of researchers from Yale University developed a set of revised AVGs in 1986 (Schneider, Lichtenstein, Fetter et al. 1986). The new system developed patient clusters while using data collected from 13 different types of ambulatory care settings (Spiegel and Kavaler 1986).

In the revised AVG system, the first partition is based on whether or not the reason for the visit is linked to a body system. If not, the type of visit is classified as prevention, treatment (e.g., social problem counseling, rehabilitation, surgical aftercare, or desensitization to allergens), medico-legal problems (i.e., rape, abused child exam, or psychiatric exam), administrative (e.g., physical exams), and other problems not classified elsewhere.

Visits related to a body system are classified into one of 19 Major Ambulatory Diagnostic Categories (MADCs), which follow the ICD-9-CM classification scheme, except that eight Major Diagnostic Categories are collapsed into four MADCs. In the next partition, MADCs are split into medical visit clusters or procedure visit clusters on the basis of the performance of a significant clinical procedure. Subsequent partitions were based on the type of patient (i.e., new patient or a revisit) and diagnosis. At this time, 571 revised AVGs have been developed (Schneider, Lichtenstein, Fetter, Freeman, and Newbold 1986) but the revised AVG classification system has not been subject to a comprehensive evaluation. In a pilot study conducted at hospital outpatient departments and neighborhood health centers in Boston and New York City, Lion, Malbon, and Bergman (1987) attempted to classify 10,145 visits into AVGs. Due to missing data, only 88 percent of the visits were classified. Analysis revealed that in over half of the AVGs the coefficient of variation for direct costs per visit exceeded 1.0, indicating that AVGs are not very homogeneous with respect to resource consumption. Consistent with this finding, Karen Schneider (1986), project director of the Yale AVG study group, stated that this patient classification is best suited for internal management controls and quality review. She also noted that AVGs need further evaluation and refinement before she would recommend their use as a unit of payment.

PSYCHIATRIC DRGs

Under the ICD-9-CM system, all patients with a principal diagnosis of an alcohol abuse, drug abuse, or mental health condition are grouped into one of 15 psychiatric care DRGs. Many analysts are troubled by the large degree of heterogeneity within psychiatric DRGs. In light of a recent supplemental issue of *Medical Care* (Jencks, Horgan, Goldman, and Taube 1987), devoted to an analysis of classification systems for psychiatric patients and an assessment of policy issues pertinent to the use of prospective payment to compensate psychiatric facilities, we will provide only a brief analysis of these subjects.

Taube, Lee, and Forthofer (1984) reported that DRGs explained only about 3 percent of the variation in length of stay among psychiatric patients. Using data collected from a 20 percent sample of Medicare patients hospitalized in 1981 and deleting "outliers" (i.e., those with costs or length-of-stay more than three standard deviations from the means), Frank and Lave (1985) concluded that the psychiatric DRGs are not homogeneous with respect to resource consumption. The coefficient of variation for standardized costs exceeded 0.9 for all but one of the DRGs. A similar pattern was found for length of stay (Frank and Lave 1985). Using a different data set, English et al. (1986) reported similar results. A review (Horgan and Jencks 1987) of recent published and unpublished studies reported that with one exception (i.e., an R^2 of .15), psychiatric DRGs explained from 2 percent to 8 percent of the variation in resource use.

Recognizing the deficiencies of psychiatric DRGs, Taube, Lee and Forthofer (1984) developed alternate DRGs (ADRGs) for psychiatric inpatients. Using a data base containing information on 12,618 discharges from psychiatric units of general hospitals ($n = 4,611$), private psychiatric hospitals ($n = 5,437$), and public hospitals ($n = 2,570$), the Automatic Interaction Detector (AID) was used to place 35 diagnostic groups into 5 categories. Using ability to explain variation in length of stay as the classification criterion, these 5 groups were expanded into 10 groups that were more clinically meaningful. Next the AID program partitioned these groups into 22 more homogeneous (with respect to length of stay) subcategories (i.e., ADRGs) on the basis of age, type of treatment received, marital status, receipt of prior mental health care, and referral status.

Analysis of variance (ANOVA) models of length of stay were compared to assess the homogeneity of ADRGs relative to DRGs. When used without other variables, ADRGs explained 11.8 percent of the variation in length of stay, an amount that exceeded the explanatory power of DRGs $(R^2 = 0.032)$. However, when the ANOVA model was expanded to include binary variables representing two of the three types of hospitals that were sampled in this study, the difference in explanatory power between ADRGs $(R^2 = 0.207)$ and DRGs $(R^2 = 0.172)$ diminished. In a review of published and unpublished studies, Horgan and Jencks (1987) reported that, with one exception, alternate patient classification systems explained from 2.6 percent to 18.1 percent of the variation in resource consumption. They wrote that the use of the Severity of Illness Index, which was not able to classify 15 percent of the patients studied, had an R^2 equal to .34 in a study of 10 hospitals.

The lack of homogeneity within psychiatric DRGs is not surprising. Similar to the situation in long-term care, many psychiatrists have pointed out that diagnosis alone is not a good indicator of future treatment (Williams 1979; Goldman, Pincus, Taube, and Regier 1984). Unlike the systems developed for long-term care, however, we are not sanguine about prospects for the development of homogeneous groupings of psychiatric patients. A consensus of psychiatrists who researched disease staging, severity of illness, and patient management categories agreed that none of these alternatives were clearly superior to psychiatric DRGs (Freiman 1985). A more recent evaluation of these and other patient classification systems developed especially for mental health disorders concluded that the classification systems do not perform strongly (Horgan and Jencks 1987).

OTHER DRGs

The limitation of the Medicare prospective payment system to hospital inpatient services has reduced its ability to control health care costs. Accordingly HCFA has considered the advisability and feasibility of paying for physicians' inpatient services and skilled nursing facility services on the basis of the same DRG classification currently being used for Medicare inpatient hospital care. In the following sections we will discuss the limited evidence pertaining to "physician DRGs" and "nursing home DRGs."

Physician DRGs

The term *physician DRG* is a misnomer because it suggests that it pertains to a case-mix classification system, such as AVGs, that has been developed expressly for physician services. Rather, what is usually meant by physician DRGs, is a prospective payment system for physicians' inpatient services, similar to the Medicare hospital payment mechanism. In such a system, two DRG payment rates would be calculated for each Medicare inpatient admission. One would be calculated for hospital services, while the other would be calculated for the bundle of physician services (e.g., administration of anesthesia, radiological procedures, consultations, etc.) that are associated with each inpatient admission.

Mitchell (1985) evaluated physician DRGs in a study that relied on a data base comprised of 904,596 hospital stays in four states during 1982. Homogeneity of physician DRGs was assessed by examining the coefficient of variation of physician payments for individual DRGs, and the percentage of the cost variation explained by physician DRGs. Simulated costs were computed at the individual patient level by summing all payments for physician services provided while the patient was hospitalized.

Although all 467 DRGs were analyzed, Mitchell only presented results for ten high-volume medical and surgical DRGs. Similar to the findings of Frank and Lave (1985), surgical DRGs were quite homogeneous, with coefficients of variation ranging from 0.18 to 0.34, while the coefficients of variation for the medical DRGs ranged from 0.70 to 1.11. The analysis of the variance exhibited by the data, which excluded outliers, yielded a similar pattern. The amount of variation in physician costs accounted for by DRGs ranged from 58 percent to 70 percent in surgical DRGs, and from 6 percent to 18 percent in medical DRGs.

These results suggest that medical DRGs are heterogeneous and should not be used to determine payment rates for physicians. Mitchell points out that potential inequities are exacerbated by training systems that refer more severely ill patients to specialists. For example, if general practitioners treated cases of mild, uncomplicated acute myocardial infarction (AMI), and cardiologists treated severe AMI cases that require monitoring in a special care unit, a physician DRG payment rate that was not adjusted for severity would discriminate against the specialists and might deter them from treating Medicare patients.

In addition to physician DRGs, which can be viewed as ''inpatient condition packages,'' Mitchell, Cromwell, Calore, and Stason (1987) have proposed the following physician payment packages: collapsed procedure, office visit, special procedure, and ambulatory condition. Physician payment packages are intended to encourage physicians to take a broader view of the patient care process and create incentives to reduce the number of procedures from which the patient receives little or no benefit. Physician payment packages are in an early stage of development and the homogeneity of only two packages has been assessed by Mitchell et al. (1987). The coefficient of variation (C.V.) of the collapsed procedure package ranged from .6 to .7, while the C.V. of the office visit package exceeded 1.5. Both values are large and suggest that a substantial amount of heterogeneity exists within the physician package. Mitchell et al. describe the following issues that must be resolved before the Medicare Program can implement physician payment packages.

1. Who will receive the package payment?
2. What services should be included in the package?
3. How should the packages be priced?
4. Will packaging work if assignment remains voluntary?

These issues are complex as well as controversial and will be difficult to resolve.

Nursing Home DRGs

Cotterill (1986) has suggested three reasons why DRGs should be used as the basis for developing a prospective payment system for the Medicare skilled nursing facility (SNF) program. First, since the Medicare SNF benefit is restricted to skilled convalescent or rehabilitation care that follows a hospital stay of at least three days, it seems appropriate to classify the SNF stay in the same terms as the hospital stay. Further, it appears that Medicare SNF patients differ from other nursing home patients in ways that are consistent with the focus of the Medicare program on short-term skilled care (Shaughnessy, Kramer, Schlenker, and Polesovsky 1985). Second, the use of DRGs to classify hospital and SNF patients would greatly facilitate the eventual development of an inclusive payment mechanism involving both types of care. Third, administration of a Medicare SNF prospective payment system would be less costly if each SNF patient could be assigned to a DRG prior to admission to the SNF.

Cotterill evaluated the feasibility of DRG-based payment for Medicare SNF patients by examining the explanatory power of a SNF case-mix index (CMI), which he developed for this study. The SNF CMI is a scalar index, similar to those discussed in Chapter 5, in which the 66 most frequent DRGs of Medicare patients treated by SNFs served to define the patient categories. Charges were used to weight the index.

Using a data base consisting of over 220,000 SNF stays in 5,157 nursing homes in 1980, several cost equations were estimated. Although the coefficient of the SNF CMI variable was positive and significant in most equations, it added little incremental explanatory power to the regression equations. The SNF CMI often had an estimated coefficient well in excess of unity, suggesting a disproportionately large increase in costs with measured increases in case-mix. These large positive elasticities suggest that payments based on Cotterill's SNF CMI could result in nursing homes developing policies that would deter the admission of Medicare patients with heavy care needs because payment for such patients would be less than costs. As a consequence, the study suggests that the index is not well suited for payment purposes.

In recognition of the limitations of DRGs for Medicare SNF patients, a new system of RUG-II classifications is under development for this patient population. Preliminary results indicate that a RUG-II type classification developed for Medicare SNF patients can achieve as much as 55.5 percent reduction in variance of per diem SNF costs (Fries, Schneider, Foley, and Dowling 1986).

SUMMARY

In this chapter we described and evaluated a variety of patient classification systems proposed as the basis of compensating general nursing home services, inpatient psychiatric care, ambulatory care, bundles of inpatient physician services (i.e., physician DRGs), and Medicare skilled nursing care.

Although deficient with respect to some of our criteria, several nursing home patient classification systems achieved substantial reductions in the heterogeneity of resource consumption. Indeed, the State of New York recognized the high degree of refinement in the RUG-II system and incorporated it as the basis of compensation in the Medicaid prospective payment system. In contrast to nursing home classification systems, the grouping protocols for other types of patients require substantial development before they will be suitable for payment purposes.

REFERENCES

Adams, E. K., and R. E. Schlenker. 1986. Case-mix reimbursement for nursing home services: Simulation approach. *Health Care Financing Review* 8(1):35–46.
Arling, G., R. H. Nordquist, B. A. Brant, and J. A. Capitman. 1987. Nursing home case mix: Patient classification by nursing resource use. *Medical Care* 25(1):9–19.
Cameron, J. M. 1985. Case-mix and resource use in long-term care. *Medical Care* 23(4):296–309.

Cavaiola, L. J., and J. P. Young. 1980. An integrated system for patient assessment and classification and nurse staff allocation for long-term care facilities. *Health Services Research* 15(3):281–306.

Coffey, R. M., and M. G. Goldfarb. 1986. DRGs and disease staging for reimbursing Medicare patients. *Medical Care* 24(9):814–29.

Cooney, L. M., and B. E. Fries. 1985. Validation and use of resource utilization groups as a case-mix measure for long-term care. *Medical Care* 23(2):123–32.

Cotterill, P. 1986. Testing a diagnosis-related group index for skilled nursing facilities. *Health Care Financing Review* 7(4):75–85.

English, J., S. Sharfstein, D. Scherl, B. Astrachan, and S. Muszynski. 1986. Diagnosis related groups and general hospital psychiatry: The APA study. *American Journal of Psychiatry* 143(2):131–39.

Fetter, R. B., R. F. Averill, J. L. Lichtenstein, and J. L. Freeman. 1984. *Ambulatory Visit Groups: A Framework for Measuring Productivity in Ambulatory Care*. New Haven, CT: Yale University.

Flagle, C., J. P. Young, E. McKnight et al. 1977. Health services in long-term care. The Johns Hopkins University and the Hospital Association of New York State. Report of US PHS Grant 5-R18-H501250, November.

Frank, R. G., and J. R. Lave. 1985. The psychiatric DRGs: Are they different? *Medical Care* 23(10):1148–55.

Freiman, M. P. 1985. DRG and alternative classification methods. In L. J. Morrison, ed., *A Study of Patient Classification Systems for Prospective Rate Setting for Medicare Patients in General Hospital Psychiatric Units and Psychiatric Hospitals*. Contract No. NIMH–278–84–0011 (DB), October 31, 1985.

Fries, B. E., and L. M. Cooney. 1985. Resource utilization groups: A patient classification system for long-term care. *Medical Care* 23(2):110–22.

Fries, B. E., D. P. Schneider, W. Foley, and M. Dowling. 1986. A classification system for medicare patients in skilled nursing facilities. Paper presented to the Annual Meeting of the APHA, Las Vegas, 1986.

Goldman, H. H., H. A. Pincus, C. A. Taube, and D. A. Regier. 1984. Prospective payment for psychiatric hospitalization: Questions and issues. *Hospital and Community Psychiatry* 35(5):460–69.

Horgan, C., and S. Jencks. 1987. Research on psychiatric classification and payment systems. *Medical Care* 25(9) Supplement: S22-S36.

Jencks, S. F., C. Horgan, H. H. Goldman, C. A. Taube. 1987. Bringing excluded psychiatric facilities under the Medicare prospective payment system: A review of research evidence and policy options. *Medical Care* 25(9), supplement.

Johnson, R. E., T. M. Vogt, and R. L. Penn. 1984. An episode approach to the care and costs of obesity. *Journal of Ambulatory Care Management* 7(1):47–60.

Katz, S., A. B. Ford, R. W. Moskowitz et al. 1963. Studies of illness in the aged: The index of ADL. *Journal of American Medical Association* 195:914.

Lion, J., A. Malbon, and A. Bergman. 1987. Ambulatory visit groups: Implementation for hospital outpatient departments. *Journal of Ambulatory Care Management* 10(1):56–69.

McCaffree, K., J. Baker, E. B. Perrin et al. 1979. Long-term care case-mix compared to direct care time and costs. Final Report, Contract No. HRA–230–76–0285. Battelle Human Affairs Research Center.

McCaffree, K., S. Winn, and C. A. Bennett. 1976. Final report of cost data reporting system for nursing home care. Seattle, WA: Battelle Human Affairs Research Center.

Mitchell, J. B. 1985. Physician DRGs. *New England Journal of Medicine* 313(11):670–75.

Mitchell, J., J. Cromwell, K. Calore, and W. Stason. 1987. Packaging physician services: Alternative approaches to Medicare Part B reimbursement. *Inquiry* 24(4):324–40.

National Center for Health Statistics. 1982. Series 13, No. 66, The National Ambulatory Medical Care Survey, United States, 1979 Summary. Hyattsville, MD: U.S. Department of Health and Human Services.

Parker, R., and J. Boyd. 1974. A comparison of a discriminant versus a clustering analysis of a patient classification for chronic disease care. *Medical Care* 12(11):944–57.

Schneeweiss, R., R. A. Rosenblatt, D. C. Cherkin, C. R. Kirkwood, and L. G. Hart. 1983. Diagnosis clusters: A new tool for analyzing the content of ambulatory care. *Medical Care* 21(1):105–22.

Schneider, D. P., F. Holden, and B. E. Fries. 1985. DRG and RUG interactions in resource allocation. Presented to AHPA/VA Conference, December 1985.

Schneider, K. 1986. Ambulatory care DRGs: Yes? No? Maybe so? *Hospitals* 60(4):70.

Schneider, K., J. Lichtenstein, R. Fetter, J. Freeman, and R. Newbold. 1986. The new ICD-9-CM ambulatory visit groups classification scheme: Definitions manual. New Haven, CT: Yale University School of Organization and Management.

Shaughnessy, P. W., A. W. Kramer, R. E. Schlenker, and M. B. Polesovsky. 1985. Nursing home case-mix differences between medicare and non-medicare and between hospital-based and freestanding patients. *Inquiry* 22(2):162–77.

Skinner, D. E., and D. E. Yett. 1973. Debility index for long-term care patients. In R. L. Berg, ed., *Health Status Indexes*. Chicago, IL: Hospital Research and Educational Trust.

Smits, H. L. 1984. Incentives in case-mix measures for long-term care. *Health Care Financing Review* 6(2):53–59.

Spiegel, A. D., and F. Kavaler. 1986. *Cost Containment and DRGs: A Guide to Prospective Payment*. Owings Mills, MD: National Health Publishing.

Swearingen, C., D. Schwartz, and J. Fisher. 1978. A methodology for finding, classifying, and comparing costs for services in long-term care settings, ABT Associates.

Taube, C., E. S. Lee, and R. N. Forthofer. 1984. DRGs in psychiatry: An empirical evaluation. *Medical Care* 22(7):597–610.

Walsh, T. J. 1979. Patient-related reimbursement for long-term care. In V. LaPorte and J. Ruben, eds. *Reform and Regulation in Long-Term Care*. New York: Praeger.

Williams, P. 1979. Deciding how to treat: The relevance of psychiatric diagnosis. *Psychological Medicine* 9:197–205.

7

PRODUCTION FUNCTION ANALYSIS

The rising costs of health care have prompted concerns about the efficiency of the participants in the industry. In this chapter, we will demonstrate that efficiency can be measured directly by the analysis of production relationships or indirectly by the analysis of cost relationships. Although economic analysis in the health care sector has focused on costs, an examination of production relationships provides a useful understanding of factors that can cause costs to vary between organizations.

In this chapter, we first discuss the nature of the production function and its relationship to the cost function. This is followed by a technical analysis of the problems associated with the estimation of production functions, including the definition and measurement of inputs and outputs, as well as the specification of the functional form. The next sections provide a discussion of the uses of production function analysis in which we review studies that have examined economies of scale, input substitution, and efficiency. The chapter concludes with a summary and recommendations for future research.

The term production function refers to the physical relationship between an organization's input of productive resources and its output of goods or services per unit of time. The production function can be represented:

$$Q = f(X_1, X_2, \ldots X_n) \qquad (7.1)$$

where Q is the quantity of output obtainable per period of time from specific combinations of inputs $X_1, X_2, \ldots X_n$.

A number of assumptions are made about the production function. First, depending on the period of analysis, some of the inputs may be fixed. If so, the production function is more properly called a short-run production function. Conversely, if all inputs are variable, the production function measures the relation between inputs and outputs after long-run adjustments have occurred. In this regard, it is difficult to estimate economies of scale from cross-sectional data since all organizations may not have implemented proper adjustments and employed an optimal combination of inputs.

Second, the production function is a technical specification of the relationship between inputs and outputs, which indicates the maximum quantity of production, Q^*, that is obtainable from any combination of inputs. That the maximum quantity is produced is an appropriate assumption for cost-minimizing firms, such as those postulated to exist in perfect competition; however, given the departures from the competitive norm in the health care industry (Arrow 1963), the assumption of cost-minimization is subject to question.

The third assumption states that the production process can be represented by a smooth and continuous function in which inputs can be varied by small amounts, resulting in a gradual change in outputs. While it is true that a hospital can hire part-time employees, many items of capital equipment are available in a limited number of capacities. Thus, a smooth and continuously variable production process can be achieved only if the firm wishes to partially utilize its equipment. Given the substantial initial fixed outlays for some types of specialized medical equipment, this "indivisibility" may result in an inverse relationship between volume of output and unit costs, depending on the nature of variable costs.

DUALITY THEORY

As indicated in the introduction to this chapter, the duality theory (Diewert 1974) posits a relationship between production functions and cost functions in which the specification of one implies the specification of the other. Accordingly, given certain assumptions, the structure of production (e.g., economies of scale) can be studied empirically by estimating a production function or a cost function.

We will now use isoquant analysis to illustrate the dual relationship between production and cost functions. In addition, isoquants will be used to illustrate the concept of scale economies. A more detailed treatment of production theory and isoquant analysis is provided in any intermediate microeconomics textbook. For an example, see Thompson (1985).

Illustrated in Figure 7.1 are isoquants Q_i and budget lines TC_i. The isoquants, which are derived from a production function, show different combinations of inputs that will produce the same level of output. For example, letting K and L represent the inputs capital and labor, an inspection of Figure 7.1 indicates that an output of 1,200 units per period of time can be produced by using any of the input combinations represented by isoquant Q_1, including the input combinations at point A (L_1, K_3), point B (L_2, K_2) or point C (L_3, K_1).

Figure 7.1 also includes isocost lines (labeled TC_1), which indicate the combinations of inputs that can be purchased for a given level of expenditure. The isocost line can be expressed symbolically:

Figure 7.1
Optimal Input Combination to Minimize Cost Subject to a Given Level of Output

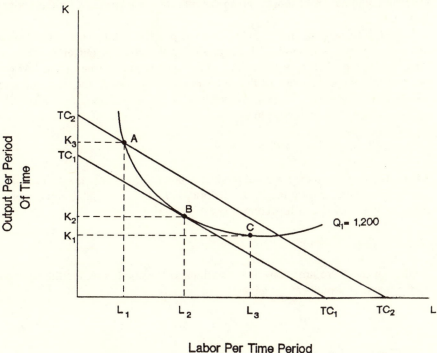

Labor Per Time Period

$$TC = P_L L + P_K K \qquad (7.2)$$

where TC represents total costs; P_L, P_K represent the price of labor and capital, respectively; and L, K represent the quantity of labor and capital. Rearranging terms, equation 7.2 can be expressed:

$$K = TC/P_K - (P_L/P_K) L \qquad (7.3)$$

In equation 7.3, the ratio TC/P_K is the intercept and indicates the quantity of capital that might be acquired with a given level of expenditure if no labor is employed while the ratio $-P_L/P_K$ is the slope of the isocost line and measures the market rate of substitution between capital and labor. This graph indicates that 1,200 units of output can be produced at a total cost of TC_1 if the input combination represented by point B, which is the point of tangency between Q_1 and TC_1, is chosen; or at a higher cost if the firm chooses to operate at point A where TC_2 intersects isoquant Q_1.

If the target output is 1,200 units, the firm will minimize costs by selecting input combination $K_2 L_2$ at point B. Thus, although all the possible input combinations on isoquant Q_1 are technically efficient (i.e., represent a maximum output for a given combination of inputs), only point B represents an economically efficient combination of inputs, given the ratio of prices implied by the budget line TC_1.

Indeed, it is easily verified (Thompson 1985 p. 219) that the cost of producing any target output is minimized by operating at the point of tangency between the isoquant representing the desired level of output and an isocost line. At the point of tangency, the slope of the isoquant (which is termed the marginal rate of technical substitution) is equal to the slope of the isocost line, the market rate of substitution. This can beexpressed:

$$MRTS_{LK} = -MP_L/MP_K = -P_L/P_K \qquad (7.4)$$

where MP_L represents the marginal product of labor, MP_K represents the marginal product of capital, and P_L and P_K are the prices of labor and capital. Rearranging terms, Equation 7.4 can be expressed:

$$MP_L/P_L = MP_K/P_K \qquad (7.5)$$

Further, when there are more than two inputs, the conditions for the optimal employment of inputs can be generalized:

$$MP_1/P_1 = MP_2/P_2 = \ldots = MP_n/P_n \qquad (7.6)$$

Our brief review of production theory has prepared us to examine the dual relationship between production and cost functions. We will first demonstrate the equivalence of the goals of maximizing output, subject to a given budget constraint, and minimizing cost, subject to a given level of output. Next, the structure of production (i.e., nature of scale economies) can be illustrated by isoquants, which are derived from the firm's production function, or from the long-run average cost curve, which is derived from the firm's cost function.

Earlier, we stated the well-known economic axiom that to minimize the cost of producing a desired level of output, the firm must employ the mix of inputs such that (as labeled in Figure 7.1) the isocost line, TC_1, is tangent to the isoquant, Q_1, representing the target output, satisfying the condition $MP_L/P_L = MP_K/P_K$. The dual to cost minimization, subject to a given output, is output maximization subject to a budget constraint. An inspection of Figure 7.2 shows that, given a budget constraint implied by isocost line TC_1, output is maximized at point E where TC_1 is tangent to Q_1, which is the same as the solution to the cost minimizing problem. Note that at point F, where the optimality rule is violated, a smaller output (Q_o) is possible while the financial resources required to obtain the inputs needed to produce 1,700 units (i.e., Q_2) exceed the budget constraint TC. A more formal treatment of this dual relationship is available in most intermediate microeconomics textbooks (e.g., see Thompson 1985, pp. 184–

Figure 7.2
Optimal Input Combination to Maximize Output Given a Budget Constraint

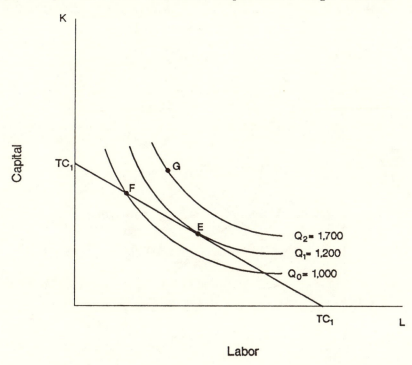

Labor

241). An advanced mathematical proof of this relationship is provided by Shephard (1970).

We will now illustrate that the nature of returns to scale can be derived from the production information (i.e., isoquants) or from the cost information (i.e., long-run average cost curve). The concept of returns to scale pertains to the character of changes in output when all resource inputs are changed proportionally. Therefore, the ray OZ drawn in Figure 7.3 can be called a scale line because its constant slope assures that the ratio of inputs (i.e., capital/labor) remains in the same proportion as the firm moves along this ray. By observing changes in output as we vary inputs proportionally along the scale line, we can determine the structure of the production function. As implied by the equal spacing of the isoquants in Figure 7.3, moving from point F to point G to point H requires the same increments to inputs while the resulting increment to output increases. Since the change in output is more than proportional to the change in inputs, the production process over this range of output is characterized as increasing returns to scale. Going from point H to point I to point J, constant returns to scale are said to occur because the change in output is proportional to the change in inputs. Going from point J to point K, the structure of production is said to

Figure 7.3
Returns to Scale

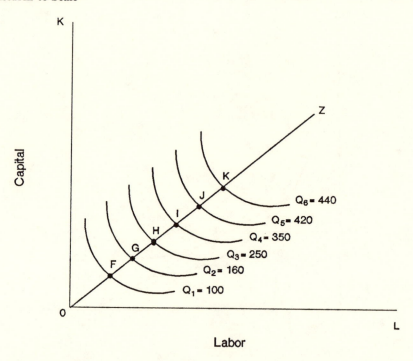

Labor

be decreasing returns to scale because the change in output is less than proportional to the change in inputs.

A cost curve can be derived from the production structure, implied in Figure 7.3, by dividing the quantity of output associated with each output by the costs associated with each relevant isocost curve (which are not shown in order to avoid clutter in the graph). The reader can verify that in the region characterized by increasing returns to scale, average costs are declining; in the region of constant returns to scale, average costs are constant; and, in the region of decreasing returns to scale, average costs are increasing. Thus, we can see that the commonly hypothesized "U-shaped" long-run average cost curve (LAC), which is shown in Figure 7.4, is due to the varying nature of returns to scale. Furthermore, we have shown that the nature of the production function can be inferred from either a cost curve, which is derived from a cost function, or from a series of isoquants, which are derived from a production function.

ESTIMATING PRODUCTION FUNCTIONS

The decision to examine the structure of production directly by estimating a production function or indirectly by estimating a cost function should be influ-

Figure 7.4
Long-Run Average Cost Curve

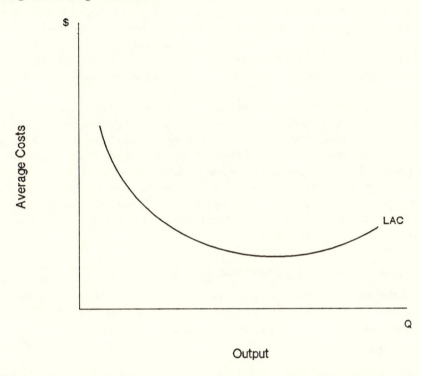

Output

enced by statistical considerations as well as by the research objectives of the study.

The most important statistical consideration is whether the duality relationship between cost and production functions exists in the health care industry. Walters (1963) has demonstrated that if firms are not cost minimizers, it becomes very difficult to derive the duality relationship between cost and production functions. A number of reasons why hospitals may not minimize costs are summarized by Berki (1972). First, many health care organizations have goals (see Chapter 4) such as conspicuous production (Lee 1971) that conflict with the goal of cost minimization. Second, as mentioned earlier, inputs such as beds or specialized staff are difficult to adjust to cost-minimizing levels in the short-run. Third, the absence of required information may preclude some organizations from implementing the most technically efficient production process. Finally, institutional, social, legal, and professional influences may constrain the ability of the organization to use more efficient combinations of inputs.

Concerns about simultaneity bias also guide the choice of direct or indirect analysis of the structure of production. If the inputs are not exogenous with respect to the outputs, the estimation of a production function by ordinary-least-squares regression will result in a simultaneity bias because the residual will be dependent on the input levels. Since this is likely to be the case in the health care industry, it may be advisable to estimate a cost or a production function by a more costly simultaneous equations technique such as two-stage least squares. Concerns about simultaneity bias have been allayed by studies (Hoch 1958; Konijn 1959; Griliches 1963; Reinhardt 1972) that conclude that the use of ordinary-least-squares to estimate production functions results in only a small bias.

The objectives of the study will also determine whether cost functions or production functions will be estimated. For example, Goldman and Grossman (1983, p. 5) stated: "the estimation of average cost functions allows us to incorporate the impact of indivisibilities, randomness of demand and complexities of large-scale operations which are not fully reflected in the production function." Furthermore, since the topic of rising costs has been very important among policy analysts, hospital executives and politicians, it is not surprising that more emphasis has been placed on the estimation of cost functions, a topic that we examine in the next chapter.

Issues in Constructing Production Functions

In this section we will discuss three issues which must be resolved before production functions can be estimated: (1) model specification, (2) definition and measurement of the output, and (3) definition and measurement of inputs.

Model Specification

The two most common models used in the estimation of hospital production functions have been the Cobb-Douglas and the transcendental logarithmic (translog). In a simple case involving two inputs, the Cobb-Douglas production function can be expressed as:

$$Q = AL^{\alpha} K^{\beta} \tag{7.7}$$

where Q represents output; A is a constant term; L represents the quantity of labor; K represents the quantity of capital; and, α and β represent the output elasticities of labor and capital, respectively. As summarized by Walters (1963), the properties of the Cobb-Douglas function are these:

(1) The function is homogeneous of degree $\alpha + \beta$. If $\alpha + \beta$ exceeds unity, there are increasing returns to scale;
   if $\alpha + \beta = 1$, there are constant returns to scale;
   if $\alpha + \beta < 1$, there are decreasing returns to scale.
(2) Marginal physical productivity of labor declines if
   $\alpha < 1$ as the labor input is increased. Specifically, if
   $\alpha < 1$, then $\partial^2 Q / \partial L^2 = \alpha(\alpha - 1)Q/L^2$ and is negative.
(3) The elasticity of input substitution is unity.

The translog function is a logarithmic expansion of a Taylor series (Brown, Caves, Christensen 1979). As demonstrated by Christensen, Jorgenson, and Lau (1975), the translog function is a very general form that can be used to estimate any arbitrary function. A representative specification of a translog model for p inputs was developed by van Montfort (1981):

$$\ln Q = a_o + \sum_{i=1}^{p} a_i \ln X_i + \sum_{i \leq j} b_{ij} \ln X_i \ln X_j \qquad (7.8)$$

where Q represents output; a_o is a constant term; a_i represents the output elasticity of the ith input; and b_{ij} is the substitution elasticity between the ith and jth inputs.

In the translog model (equation 7.8), the substitution elasticities and the output elasticities are dependent on the level of input utilization. In contrast, the Cobb-Douglas model is based on a less realistic assumption that output elasticities are independent of the level of inputs. Most of the recent hospital production functions and their duals (i.e., cost functions) have been estimated with the use of the translog form, a result attributable to the greater realism and flexibility of this functional form.

Hellinger (1975) compared results of estimated production functions using not only the translog and Cobb-Douglas specifications but also other well-known production functions such as the constant elasticity of substitution (CES), Uzawa, and Sato. However, since these latter functions are infrequently used in studies of the health care industry, we will omit them from our discussion. Hellinger reported that the coefficient of multiple determination (R^2), adjusted for degrees of freedom, ranged from 0.64 in the translog model to 0.08 in the Cobb-Douglas model. These results were very robust, changing very little as different measures of inputs and output were used. Further, the results of the F-test for the suitability of the restrictions imposed by the Cobb-Douglas specification indicated that the estimated coefficients of this form were significantly different from those estimated with the translog functional form. Thus, Hellinger concluded that the restrictions of the Cobb-Douglas function are too constraining. Similar conclusions were advanced by Feldstein (1968), van Montfort (1981), Jensen and Morrisey (1986a), and McGuire (1987).

Contradictory results were given by Pauly (1980), who found almost identical parameter estimates and coefficients of multiple determination in the regression equations based on the translog and Cobb-Douglas production functions. These results, however, were obtained from a study of small rural hospitals and may not be generalizable to a broader cross-section of hospitals. Further, the "translog form" used by Pauly was not fully specified because it excluded all two-way interactions.

Frank and Taube (1987) also compared the performance of these two specifications using the criteria of conformance of coefficient estimates with theory, mean square error of estimated models and forecast error. In evaluating econometric models of the production of mental health services, Frank and Taube found that the Cobb-Douglas model performed as well as the translog production function in one dimension of performance (i.e., mean square error) and slightly better in the other two performance areas. These results, however, may reflect a simple production technology used in freestanding outpatient mental health clinics and, thus, should not be generalizable to inpatient hospital settings.

Definition and Measurement of the Output

The primary output of hospitals and other health service organizations is the improvement of the health status of their patients. Since it is difficult if not impossible to measure changes in health status, economic studies of hospitals have used intermediate output measures such as discharges, patient days or services. In recognition of the multiproduct nature of the hospital, it has been necessary to adjust these measures of output. Indeed, Jensen and Morrisey (1986a) observed estimates of the marginal product of physicians that were larger when output was adjusted for case-mix than for an unadjusted surrogate. These findings suggest that the absence of case-mix adjustment results in biased estimates of the hospital production function.

Feldstein (1968) dealt with the output heterogeneity problem in two ways. First, relative costliness was used to weigh the output measure, hospital discharges. Second, Feldstein included independent variables for the proportion of patients in various diagnostic categories. Goldman and Grossman (1983) adopted similar procedures to estimate translog production functions for community health centers. Output was measured by the sum of patient care encounters with primary care physicians, specialist physicians, midlevel practitioners and nurses, weighted by the relative costliness of the staff member who made the encounter. Their right-hand-side output adjustment consisted of a vector of case-mix variables. In the absence of diagnostic information, Goldman and Grossman were forced to use age group variables as surrogates for case-mix. None of the age category variables exerted an influence that approached conventional levels of statistical significance as the most reliable coefficient had a t-value of 1.06.

With the exception of Pauly (1980), who defined output as the number of admissions, all of the other production function studies reviewed in this chapter used relative costliness to measure output. Only Goldman and Grossman included direct case-mix variables, however. Jensen and Morrisey (1986a) used the relative costliness of DRGs to weight their output measure. Hellinger (1975) defined output as a cost weighted combination of patient days of routine services, Xrays, laboratory procedures and operations. The weight given to a particular service was based on the average cost of all hospitals in the sample. A similar procedure was used by van Montfort (1981), who based the service weights on charges established by a regulatory agency rather than on average costs.

Although most of the production function studies attempted to reflect the multiproduct nature of the hospital, it is doubtful that the output adjustments were adequate. For example, most of the studies used weighted discharges. As demonstrated by Horn, Horn, and Sharkey (1984), there is likely to be substantial heterogeneity within case-mix measures, even refined ones such as DRGs. Further, variations in case-mix are likely to be systematically related to size (Watts and Klastorin 1980) which results in biased estimates of economies of scale.

Definition and Measurement of Inputs

Factor inputs in a service industry such as health care can be classified as labor, capital, and supplies; however, these are broad aggregates that may not reflect the mix of inputs used by different organizations. For example, two hospitals might each employ 200 full-time equivalent personnel (FTEs) in the nursing department. However, one hospital might use a primary care nursing approach in which all nursing personnel are registered nurses (RNs), while the other hospital's nursing department might include a mix of RNs and nurses aides. Since it is likely that the productivity of RNs and nurses aides will differ, it is appropriate to disaggregate nursing personnel by skill level. Similarly, it may be preferable to disaggregate other types of personnel, as well as capital and supplies. However, as this review will show, most inputs have been entered in very broad categories. Consequently, the estimated coefficients on these resources represent averages in input categories. Further, to the extent that the mix of inputs within categories varies with volume, a bias has been introduced.

The broad labor input category can be subclassified as physicians, nurses, other professional staff, and nonprofessional staff. Since few would deny the importance of physicians in the production of hospital services, it is surprising that physician inputs have been omitted from hospital production functions (Hellinger 1975) or entered as a broad aggregate (Feldstein 1968; van Montfort 1981). Jensen and Morrisey (1986a) employed the most precise specification of physician input and included variables for the number of physicians on the hospital's medical staff in six mutually exclusive specialty categories. Further, recognizing that many physicians divide their time between hospitals, they included a variable for the number of hospital appointments per physician. Although the Jensen-Morrisey specification of physician inputs represents an improvement over those in earlier studies, it still suffers from the omission of data that indicates the number of hours spent by the physician at each hospital. Given the well-recognized variations in physician practice patterns, it is difficult to interpret the meaning of this coefficient.

Capital is another variable that has been difficult to measure. The number of beds has been used frequently as a surrogate for capital. This measure has a number of obvious problems. First, the number of beds does not reflect the level and mix of other capital inputs such as specialized equipment or facilities. Second, the number of beds does not reflect the mix of beds in terms of use (i.e., special care unit beds) or layout (i.e., private rooms versus wards). In recognition of this problem, Hellinger (1975) used depreciation costs to measure capital in one of his production function specifications. Of course, depreciation costs may not be an accurate reflection of the amount of capital employed because of differences in methods of evaluating depreciation between hospitals. The most accurate measure of hospital capital was developed by van Montfort (1981) who used beds as well as a facility index that reflected the diversity of other types of capital employed by the hospital.

Finally, with the exception of van Montfort's, previous specifications of the production function ignored the contributions of supplies and skilled paramedical personnel in the provision of hospital services. Certainly the use of aggressive physical therapy, inhalation therapy or other services performed by allied health personnel can lead to an earlier discharge of patients, thereby allowing the hospital to treat more patients per year. Similar expectations are realistic for more aggressive chemotherapy and other drugs. Consequently, the omission of variables pertaining to allied health personnel, drugs and supplies constitutes a serious specification error.

EMPIRICAL RESULTS: INPUT AND OUTPUT ELASTICITIES

Production functions can be used to estimate and measure the following: (1) output elasticities from which scale effects can be derived, (2) elasticities of input substitution, and (3) efficiency. In this section we discuss results from production function studies that are pertinent to the first two characteristics of the production process. This is followed by a section on efficiency in which we integrate a discussion of the previously reviewed production function studies with those that used linear programming to examine the efficiency of operations in health care organizations.

Output Elasticities and Scale Effects

As mentioned in the introductory section of this chapter, the nature of scale effects has important implications for planners and policy analysts. The type of returns to scale characteristic of a firm or industry can be ascertained by summing the coefficients of output elasticity for each input. A sum greater than one indicates increasing returns to scale; a sum equal to one reflects constant returns to scale; and a sum less than one indicates decreasing returns to scale.

As discussed previously, most of the examinations of scale economies in the health care sector have employed the cost function approach, which is discussed in the next chapter. Two hospital studies that estimated production functions reported similar results. Pauly's (1980) study of hospitals located in rural portions of the United States found constant returns to scale, while van Montfort (1981), who studied hospitals in Holland, reported very small increasing returns to scale.

In addition to hospitals, scale effects have been examined in a number of ambulatory care settings. Goldman and Grossman (1983) found constant returns to scale in community health centers, while Frank and Taube (1987) reported that the production of outpatient mental health services was characterized by decreasing returns to scale. Kimbell and Lorant (1977) found increasing returns to scale in solo or small group practices and decreasing returns to scale in large group practices characterized by multiple specialties. Their results suggest that the most efficient scale of operation is about seven physicians.

It is more difficult to interpret individual output elasticities than their sum because strong intercorrelations among the independent variables have reduced the reliability of the individual parameter estimates even though a bias has not been introduced. For example, in Pauly's data set, the number of beds was highly correlated ($r = 0.91$) with the number of personnel. Consequently, the production function estimate of the beds coefficient (0.086) was much smaller than expected and statistically insignificant ($p > 0.05$) in many equations. Similar problems were reported by Feldstein (1968). In consideration of the problems created by multicollinearity, we will restrict our discussion of estimated output elasticities to results that are statistically significant and intuitively realistic. In contrast to the low estimates by Pauly and Feldstein, van Montfort estimated that hospital beds had the largest output elasticity coefficient (0.64), followed by nonphysician staff (0.34), drugs (0.04), and specialist physicians (0.02). The low coefficient for specialist physicians may reflect their ability to attract a more severe case-mix with a longer length of stay, rather than their relative productivity.

Jensen and Morrisey (1986a) present results for the marginal product of inputs, a measure that indicates the change in the level of output associated with a one unit increase in an input, holding all other factors constant. In contrast, output elasticities relate the percentage increase in output (e.g., admissions) attributed to a 1 percent increase in an input, holding other factors constant. Evaluated at the mean, specialists in OB/GYN and pediatrics have the largest admissions marginal products. Hospital-based specialists (i.e., anesthesiologists, pathologists, and radiologists) and primary-care physicians have smaller but positive marginal products, while surgeons and other specialists have small negative marginal products. Although the marginal product of surgeons was low, an inspection of the interaction terms in the production function reveals that surgeons have a large positive influence on the productivity of hospital-based physicians. This result reflects the reliance of surgeons on the services of anesthesiologists and pathologists. The coefficients of the other interaction terms suggest that pediatricians, hospital-based medical staff, and primary-care physicians enhance the productivity of beds, a result that is due, in part, to the shorter average stays associated with patients admitted by these types of physicians.

Pauly (1980) conducted the only other study that examined the contribution to hospital productivity by physicians in different specialties. His classification of specialties differed from that of Jensen and Morrisey. For the specialties common to both studies (i.e., surgery and primary care), however, Pauly estimated higher marginal products. Pauly's results should be viewed as less credible because he did not adjust for differences in case-mix and used a functional form, the Cobb-Douglas, which may not be appropriate for hospitals. Since both produce biased estimates, we will not elaborate further on these findings.

The estimates of the physicians' admissions marginal product raise some interesting policy issues. First, assuming that current rates of surgical intervention are appropriate, is the high cost of training surgeons justified by their low marginal product? Second, is it prudent to emphasize the training of primary-care practitioners, who, contrary to commonly held expectations, increase hospital admissions and, consequently, total health system expenditures?

Elasticity of Input Substitution

It is important for planners and policy analysts to know whether two inputs are complements or are substitutes. For example, if beds and nurses are complements, increasing demand for hospital admissions creates a derived-demand for each of these inputs. In the unlikely event that these two inputs are perfect substitutes, the increased demand for hospital admissions could be satisfied by increasing only one of these inputs.

The sign of the coefficient of input substitution indicates whether inputs are complements (positive coefficient) or substitutes (negative coefficient). Further, the magnitude of this coefficient measures the ease with which one input can be replaced with another, holding constant the rate of output and the levels of other inputs. For two inputs, labor (L) and capital (K), the elasticity of input substitution can be interpreted as the percent change in the ratio of L to K for a 1 percent change in the marginal rate of substitution of the two factors.

Jensen and Morrisey (1986a) derived estimates of the coefficient of input substitution from their production function and reported that, in producing admissions, physicians in specialties other than primary care tend to be substitutes for each other and complements for primary-care physicians. Given that family practice physicians can admit patients but seldom have surgical privileges (Geyman 1979; Clinton, Schmitting, Stern, and Black 1981) and are often required to obtain consultations from other specialists (Warburton, Babula, and Wolff 1981), this result is consistent with observed practices. The input substitution elasticities also indicate that hospital-based physicians are substitutes for physicians in most other specialties. Jensen and Morrisey speculate that hospital-based physicians relieve admitting physicians of many inhospital tasks such as patient education and preparation for clinical procedures. As expected, they found a high degree of complementarity between OB/GYN specialists and pediatricians. Obviously, obstetrical admissions create subsequent demand for pediatricians.

Regarding the nonphysician inputs, Jensen and Morrisey found that nurses are strong complements with beds and other staff in producing admissions. Further, nurses are strong complements to primary-care physicians and weak complements to pediatricians; however, they are weak substitutes for physicians in the other categories. This result undoubtedly reflects the differences in treatment patterns and intensity of nursing care associated with patients of different case-types.

In a companion article, Jensen and Morrisey (1986b) reported that teaching and nonteaching hospitals had different production functions. This result was attributed to the use of a different input, resident physicians, by teaching hospitals. The researchers also found that residents reduce the marginal product of other inputs, a finding that suggests that nurses and staff physicians devote time to instruct residents.

Two policy implications can be drawn from the analysis conducted by Jensen and Morrisey (1986b). First, the small marginal admissions product of residents indicates, that under the Medicare prospective pricing mechanisms, the marginal revenue product of residents is well below the marginal costs they generate. Therefore, the extra payments made by Medicare to teaching hospitals (i.e., those for indirect medical education expenses) can be viewed as offsetting the teaching related costs not covered by the contributions of residents to output. Thus, if indirect medical expense payments were discontinued, it is likely that some residency positions would be eliminated.

The second policy implication derived from the research of Jensen and Morrisey pertains to the role of physicians in the hospital during a period characterized by a surplus of physicians and a shortage of registered nurses. Estimates provided by Jensen and Morrisey also indicate that physicians substitute for the services of registered nurses, thereby mitigating some of the problems associated with a shortage of nurses.

EFFICIENCY MEASURES

Economists typically examine two types of efficiency—technical and allocative. The former measures the extent to which the amount of output produced from a given set of resources is congruent with a technically constrained maximum defined in engineering terms. For example, the production function $Q = 4L^{.5}K^{.5}$ implies that the input combination $L = 4$, $K = 1$ will result in, at most, eight units of output. If the firm uses the combination of inputs and produces only six units of output, its efficiency rating is 6/8 or 0.75. Allocative efficiency measures the extent to which a firm is minimizing the cost of producing a desired level of output. From a production theory perspective, allocative efficiency measures the extent to which the optimal combination of inputs is employed by considering the relative marginal productivity and costs of the inputs. For example, given a simple two input situation, allocative efficiency occurs when the ratio of the marginal product of capital to the price of capital equals the ratio of the marginal product of labor to the price of labor. This is equivalent to operating at the point of tangency between the isocost line and the isoquant (e.g., point B in Figure 7.1). Accordingly, our review of efficiency studies will be divided into these two concepts of efficiency. The production function studies we have reviewed in previous sections have emphasized an analysis of allocative efficiency, while some other recent studies have used mathematical programming techniques to study technical efficiency in health care organizations.

Technical Efficiency

Data envelopment analysis (DEA) has been proposed as a technique for evaluating the efficiency of "decision-making units" (DMUs,) producing similar outputs (Charnes, Cooper, and Rhodes 1981). Pareto-Koopnass Efficiency, which is derived from the well-known social welfare criterion of Pareto Optimality, is used to define efficiency. This notion of efficiency is referenced from input and output orientations:

(a) Input orientation: A DMU is not efficient if it is possible to decrease any input without augmenting any other input and without decreasing any output.

(b) Output orientation: A DMU is not efficient if it is possible to augment any output without increasing any input and without decreasing any other output.

A DMU is characterized as efficient if, and only if, neither (a) nor (b) applies (Charnes, Cooper, and Rhodes 1981).

Two published studies (Nunamaker 1983 and Sherman 1984) have assessed the utility of DEA as a technique to examine hospital efficiency. Since the methods and conclusions of the two studies were similar, we will focus on Nunamaker's study, which had a larger sample size. In Chapter 12 we briefly review findings from an unpublished study (Hogan, Chesney, Wroblewski, and Fleming 1987) that used DEA to examine the impact of the Medicare prospective payment system on the technical efficiency of hospitals. Using data from 17 hospitals classified as producing similar services, Nunamaker (1983) applied DEA to measure the efficiency of producing routine nursing services. A linear programming technique was used to estimate the coordinates of the production frontier (i.e., maximum attainable outputs). After this was accomplished, the relative efficiency of each DMU was computed. Four DMUs were located on the production frontier and thus, had an efficiency rating of 1.0. The least efficient DMU had an efficiency rating of 0.72. Nunamaker compared the efficiency ratings with the routine cost per day to validate his techniques. Strong correlations between efficiency and costs were found in the 1978 data set ($r = -0.76$) and in the 1979 data set ($r = -.90$). Nunamaker also demonstrated how DEA could be used for cost containment purposes and calculated that, if each of the 12 inefficient hospitals moved to the production frontier, annual savings of $4 million would be achieved.

Although Nunamaker demonstrated the utility of employing DEA to obtain efficiency measures for hospitals, the study contained a number of flaws that may limit the applicability of his results. First, the input and output measures need to be refined. Inputs were measured by a single variable, inpatient routine costs. Although Nunamaker implies this is a self-weighting variable in which different mixes of inputs are adjusted by monetary information, it is clear that the value of inputs, such as capital, are distorted by arbitrary accounting conventions. Several output measures were used, including routine aged days, routine pediatric days, routine maternal days and all other routine days. It is obvious that these output classifications will not result in homogeneous groupings. However, the crudeness of the output measures was mitigated by the use of a subsample of hospitals that were clustered in the same peer group by the hospital rate-setting commission in Wisconsin.

Second, the most efficient DMUs may be inefficient, resulting in a poor "reliability yardstick." Given the well-known divergences of the health care industry from the competitive norm (Arrow 1963), this is a very serious concern.

Finally, the application of DEA analysis is based on two assumptions that may not be very realistic: (a) each DMU exhibits constant returns to scale over all ranges of output; and, (b) the constructed efficient production frontier is linear and continuous, implying that all points along the efficient surface are feasibly attainable production possibilities. The latter assumption is not realistic but can be avoided with the application of nonlinear mathematical programming techniques. We suggest that these be applied and compared with results based on linear programming to assess the restrictiveness of this assumption. As indicated earlier in this chapter, the former assumption that pertains to a homeothetic production process appears to be invalid for hospitals.

Grosskopf and Valdmanis (1987) and Register and Bruning (1987) examined hospital efficiency by using a linear programming technique, pioneered by Farrell (1957) and closely related to DEA, to identify the "best practice production frontier." In each study, an index of technical efficiency was calculated for each hospital by comparing the observed input/output ratios with the best practice production frontier. We will focus on the study by Register and Bruning, who not only examined the utility of the Farrell-technique, but also examined some interesting policy questions.

Register and Bruning (1987) used their technical efficiency index as the dependent variable in a regression equation that included independent variables for hospital size, the degree of competition and ownership status. Recognizing the multiproduct nature of hospital output, they attempted to reduce the impact of an underspecification bias, due to the absence of case-mix variables, by limiting their sample to medium-sized (i.e., 100 to 250 beds), nonteaching hospitals located in the 100 largest SMSAs of the United States. It was hoped that these restrictions would result in a sample of hospitals that produced a relatively homogeneous set of products.

The parameter estimates suggest that larger hospitals, in the 100 to 250 bed range of the sample, are more efficient than smaller hospitals. Ownership and the degree of competition did not exert effects that were significant ($p \leq .05$). These results cannot be generalized beyond a restrictively defined sample of hospitals. Further, the reliability and validity of the parameter estimates may be affected by an underspecified model that explained only 10 percent of the variation in the dependent variable. Finally, given the not-for-profit orientation of hospitals, the best practice production frontier may not coincide with the technically efficient production frontier.

Wilson and Jadlow (1982), who studied 922 nuclear medicine facilities, also defined inefficiency in terms of the distance between actual output (Q) and the output attainable on the production frontier (Q^*). Their measure of inefficiency, called the index of divergence (D), is expressed for the jth hospital:

$$D_j = (Q_j^* - Q_j) / Q_j^* \qquad\qquad (7.9)$$

Assuming production is characterized by a Cobb-Douglas form, Wilson and Jadlow used linear programming techniques to estimate a production frontier. Based on the theoretical work of Aigner and Chu (1968), which was later implemented by Timmer (1971), Wilson and Jadlow constrained observed hospitals' outputs to lie on or below the estimated production frontier such that $Q_j \leq A L_j K_j$ for the jth hospital. This method treats the largest output value for each observed input combination as the maximum attainable output for that combination of resources. Thus, the parameter estimates obtained in this manner describe a deterministic production surface for a set of 100 percent efficient firms.

Wilson and Jadlow followed Timmer's (1971) approach and estimated a probabilistic production frontier, an approach that involved discarding observations from outliers in order to avoid a distorted estimate of the production frontier. Once the production frontier was estimated, it was possible to compute the index of divergence.

Wilson and Jadlow used their inefficiency measure to study the impact of competition and hospital characteristics on the technical efficiency of producing nuclear medicine services. Applying a standard two-input, Cobb-Douglas production function, the researchers required data for labor, capital, and output. The labor input was defined in terms of FTE nuclear medical technologists, who constitute the primary labor input in this industry; however, radiologists, who also are required to produce nuclear medicine services, were not used to estimate the location of the production surface. Further, results from a recent cost-function study (Hosek and Palmer 1983) suggest that radiology residents contribute to the productivity of other inputs used to produce nuclear medicine services. Consequently, the labor inputs in this model may be misspecified.

Capital input was measured by the sum of the quantity of each type of nuclear medicine equipment weighted by the current market price for that type of equipment. This measure avoids the problems associated with arbitrary accounting conventions, which are used to determine a historical value of capital equipment.

Nuclear medicine facilities are multiproduct firms or divisions of hospitals that produce as many as 58 diagnostic and therapeutic procedures. Consequently, in order to represent the multiproduct nature of nuclear medicine, a weighted output measure was used. This was expressed:

$$Q_j = \sum_{i=1}^{58} P_i Q_{ij} \qquad\qquad (7.10)$$

where Q_j represents the weighted output of the jth hospital; P_i is a statewide price index for the ith procedure; and Q_{ij} represents the number of procedures in the ith category for the jth hospital.

Three interesting empirical results were obtained from this study. First, the sum of the output elasticities ($\alpha + \beta = 1.13$) indicates increasing returns to scale. Second, inefficiency, as measured by the index of efficiency divergence, was positively associated with the degree of hospital competition in the area. This result may be attributed to service competition in the hospital industry which, in this case, results in underutilized nuclear medicine facilities. Third, relative to community not-for-profit hospitals, nuclear medicine services tend to be produced more efficiently in investor-owned hospitals but less efficiently in government hospitals. These results may be attributed to the varying profit incentives in these types of hospitals.

This study shared three of the problems with Nunamaker's (1983) study of technical efficiency: (1) use of the Cobb-Douglas production function, (2) use of data from hospitals, which might be inefficient, to estimate a technically efficient production function, and (3) misspecification of independent variables.

Allocative Efficiency

Parameter estimates from production functions can be used to determine if firms are using the optimal mix of inputs. Any departure from this mix is termed allocative inefficiency. Although others (Reinhardt 1972; Pauly 1980) have examined optimal input combinations in health care organizations, we will focus on Goldman and Grossman's study (1983) of community health centers (CHCs) because they conducted the most comprehensive analysis of allocative efficiency in the health care industry.

Relying on the standard economic theory of production, Goldman and Grossman used information about local input prices and production function estimates to derive an index of inefficiency. As suggested in the section in which isoquants were discussed, a community health center that employs two inputs, physicians (P) and aides (A), can minimize the costs of producing a given level of output by selecting a combination of P and A such that the marginal rate of technical substitution of P for A, represented by the slope of the isoquant, equals the market rate of substitution, given by the slope of the isocost curve. A combination of inputs which causes a deviation from this equality represents allocative inefficiency. Recognizing this, Goldman and Grossman computed an index of inefficiency in the use of aides relative to physicians (EPA) which was expressed as:

$$EPA = MRTS_{PA} - 1/PR_{PA} \tag{7.11}$$

where the price ratio PR_{PA}' represents P_P divided by P_A' and $MRTS_{PA}$ corresponds to the marginal rate of technical substitution of P for A. Since the optimal employment of inputs occurs when $MRTS_{PA} = PR_{PA}'$ an increase in the value of EPA indicates less efficient input combinations.

A similar index of the inefficiency in the use of other personnel relative to physicians (labeled *EO*) was also constructed. Focusing on the results of an analysis based on these indices, Goldman and Grossman concluded that CHCs underutilize physician aides relative to physicians (*EPA* = 1.64) and overutilize other personnel relative to physicians (*EO* = 0.554). In other words, the same output could be produced at a lower cost by raising the ratio of physician aides to physicians and by lowering the ratio of other personnel to physicians. These results are consistent with the findings from Reinhardt's (1972) seminal study and those of Frank and Taube (1987), which concluded that physician aides are underused. Reinhardt suggested a number of reasons why physicians do not use more aides to enhance their productivity. First, some physicians may not be aware of the effectiveness of auxiliary staff. Second, physicians may wish to avoid the administrative burdens associated with a larger staff. Finally, physicians may fear that extensive reliance on physician assistants may affect the real or perceived quality of services rendered by their practices.

Goldman and Grossman tested a number of hypotheses pertaining to the determinants of allocative efficiency. Most CHCs are funded on an annual basis but received additional income from third-party payers. Their results show that, as third-party payments increased, which reduced the rigor of the prospectively determined annual budget, economic inefficiency increased, a finding that is consistent with the theoretical expectations.

The researchers also hypothesized a "U-shaped" relationship between inefficiency and volume of medical encounters. As volume increased, inefficiency was expected to be reduced because variations in demand would become smaller. At some point, however, coordination problems would emerge, offsetting the gains derived from a more predictable demand. These expectations were confirmed, and the authors concluded that the forces associated with the complexity of operations dominated those associated with the variability of demand throughout the range of observed output.

In other investigations of the determinants of efficiency, Reinhardt (1972) found that practice mode affected productivity. Holding other factors constant, he estimated that physicians, in group practice, produced 4.5 to 5.1 percent more visits than solo practitioners. Corroborating evidence is provided by Kimbell and Lorant (1977). Frank and Taube (1987) reported that county owned clinics produce 15 percent fewer visits than their privately owned counterparts. This result, however, might be biased by uncontrolled differences in case-mix. Held and Pauly (1983) reported that for-profit dialysis firms are more productive than their not-for-profit counterparts in areas where competition is low (i.e., high Herfindahl index value). In competitive areas, profit orientation did not affect efficiency. Held and Pauly argue that this result is consistent with the view that the for-profit form of organization leads to greater production efficiency, but that in response to competitors these gains are transferred to consumers in the form of higher levels of amenity. Since the level of amenity may systematically vary with competition, it is possible that an amenity bias may be present in production function estimates. Indeed, Held and Pauly found that estimated returns to scale were greater in the less competitive areas, where less amenities are likely to be provided, than in the more competitive areas.

SUMMARY

In this chapter we presented a technical discussion of production function studies as well as a summary of results from studies that attempted to analyze the structure of production in hospitals, physician office practices, and community health centers. The estimation of production functions has been hampered by the heterogeneous measures of output. Consequently, a study that reports that hospitals experience decreasing returns to scale may actually be confusing changes in product-mix with the size of facilities. Another technical problem is that the unit of observation in hospital production function studies may be too large. Since the hospital is a multiproduct firm, it would be more useful for planners to know the structure of production within the different entities or departments within the organization. Thus, although information from a limited number of production studies suggests that hospitals exhibit constant returns to scale, it is possible that these results reflect the offsetting effects of increasing and decreasing returns to scale in different departments as the hospital increases its overall capacity.

Finally from a policy perspective, it is noteworthy that only one attempt has been made to measure directly the impact of prospective payment on the efficiency of hospital production. This is ironic because many of the proponents of prospective payment have argued that this mechanism induces hospitals to reduce costs by increasing efficiency. Thus, although a substantial body of evidence, which we review in Chapter 12, has shown that prospective payment has constrained cost increases, we have little or no evidence of its impact upon efficiency. The emphasis on cost analysis is attributed, in part, to the ease of conducting behavioral cost function studies relative to structural studies of production and costs, a topic which we will discuss in the next chapter.

REFERENCES

Aigner, D. J., and C. F. Chu. 1968. On estimating the industry production function. *American Economic Review* 58(4):827–33.

Arrow, K. J. 1963. Uncertainty and the welfare economics of medical care. *American Economic Review* 53(4):941–73.

Berki, S. 1972. *Hospital Economics*. Lexington, MA: Lexington Books.

Brown, R. S., D. W. Caves, and L. R. Christensen. 1979. Modelling the structure of cost and production for multiproduct firms. *Southern Economic Journal* 46(1):256–73.

Charnes, A., W. W., Cooper, and E. Rhodes. 1981. Evaluating program and managerial efficiency: An application of data envelopment analysis to program follow through. *Management Science* 27(6):668–97.

Christensen, L. R., D. W. Jorgenson, and L. J. Lau. 1975. Transcendental logarithmic utility functions. *American Economic Review* 65(3):367–83.

Clinton, C., G. Schmitting, T. L. Stern, and R. R. Black. 1981. Hospital privileges for family physicians: A national study of office based members of the American Academy of Family Physicians. *Journal of Family Practice* 13(3):361–71.

Diewert, W. E. 1974. Applications of duality theory. In M.D. Intriligator and D. A. Kendrick, *Frontiers of Quantitative Economics*, vol. II. Amsterdam: North-Holland Publishing Co., pp. 106–206.

Farrell, M. 1957. The measurement of productive efficiency. *Journal of the Royal Statistical Association* Series A:253–90.

Feldstein, M. S. 1968. *Economic Analysis for Health Service Efficiency*. Chicago: Markham Publishing Co.

Frank, R., and C. Taube. 1987. Technical and allocative efficiency in production of outpatient mental health clinic services. *Social Science and Medicine* 24(10):843–50.

Geyman, J. P. 1979. Hospital practice of the family physician. *Journal of Family Practice* 8(5):911–12.

Goldman, F., and M. Grossman. 1983. The production and cost of ambulatory medical care in community health centers. *Advances in Health Economics and Health Services Research* 4:1–56.

Griliches, Z. 1963. Estimates of the aggregate agricultural production function from cross-sectional data. *Journal of Farm Economics* 45(2):105–29.

Grosskopf, S., and V. Valdmanis. 1987. Measuring hospital performance: A non-parametric approach. *Journal of Health Economics* 6(2):89–107.

Held, P. J., and M. V. Pauly. 1983. Competition and efficiency in the end stage renal dialysis program. *Journal of Health Economics* 2(2):95–115.

Hellinger, F. J. 1975. Specification of a hospital production function. *Applied Economics* 7(3):149–160.

Hoch, I. 1958. Simultaneous equation bias in the context of the Cobb-Douglas production function. *Econometrica* 26(4): 566–78.

Hogan, A. J., J. Chesney, R. Wroblewski, and S. Fleming. 1987. The impact of the Medicare prospective payment system on hospital efficiency: A data envelopment analysis. Paper presented to the American Economic Association Annual Meetings, Chicago.

Horn, S. D., R. A. Horn, and P. D. Sharkey. 1984. The Severity of Illness Index as a severity adjustment to diagnosis-related groups. *Health Care Financing Review* 5 (Supp.):33–46.

Hosek, J. R., and A. R. Palmer. 1983. Teaching and hospital costs: The case of radiology. *Journal of Health Economics* 2(1):29–46.

Jensen, G. A., and M. A. Morrisey. 1986a. Medical staff specialty mix and hospital production. *Journal of Health Economics* 5(3):253–76.

Jensen, G. A., and M. A. Morrisey. 1986b. The role of physicians in hospital production. *Review of Economics and Statistics* 68(3):432–42.

Kimbell, L. J., and J. H. Lorant. 1977. Physician productivity and returns to scale. *Health Services Research* 12(4):367–79.

Konijn, H. S. 1959. Estimation of an average production function from surveys. *Economic Record* 35(1):118–25.

Lee, M. L. 1971. A conspicuous production theory of hospital behavior. *Southern Economic Journal* 38(1):48–58.

McGuire, A. 1987. The measurement of hospital efficiency. *Social Science and Medicine* 24(9):719–24.

Nunamaker, T. R. 1983. Measuring routine nursing service efficiency: A comparison of cost per patient day and data envelopment analysis models. *Health Services Research* 18(2):183–205.

Pauly, M. V. 1980. *Doctors and their Workshops*. Chicago, IL: University of Chicago Press.

Register, C. A., and E. R. Bruning. 1987. Profit incentives and technical efficiency of hospital care. *Southern Economic Journal* 53(4):899–914.

Reinhardt, U. 1972. A production function for physician services. *Review of Economics and Statistics* 54(1):55–66.

Shephard, R. W. 1970. *Theory of Cost and Production Functions*. Princeton: Princeton University Press.

Sherman, H. D. 1984. Hospital efficiency measurement and evaluation. *Medical Care* 22(10):922–35.

Timmer, C. P. 1971. Using a probabilistic frontier to measure technical efficiency. *Journal of Political Economy* 79(4):776–94.

Thompson, A. 1985. *Economics of the Firm: Theory and practice*, 4th Ed. Englewood Cliffs, NJ: Prentice-Hall.

van Montfort, G. 1981. Production functions for general hospitals. *Social Science and Medicine* 15C:87–98.

Walters, A. A. 1963. Production and cost functions: An econometric survey. *Econometrica* 31(1–2):1–66.

Warburton, S. W., J. A. Babula, and G. T. Wolff. 1981. Hospital privileges of family physicians in North Carolina. *Journal of Family Practice* 12(4):725–8.

Watts, C. A., and T. D. Klastorin. 1980. The impact of case mix on hospital cost: A comparative analysis. *Inquiry* 17(4):357–67.

Wilson, G. W., and J. M. Jadlow. 1982. Competition, profit incentives, and technical efficiency in the provision of nuclear medicine services. *Bell Journal of Economics* 13(2):472–82.

8

COST FUNCTION ANALYSIS

An understanding of the determinants of the costs of operating health care organizations is essential for the formulation of public policy as well as for the development of organizational strategies. For example, if increasing (or decreasing) returns to scale exist, those concerned with cost containment would propose policies or incentives designed to increase (or decrease) the size of the health care facility. In another context, it is necessary to determine how variations in case-mix affect hospital costs in order to develop an equitable payment mechanism that allows for the fiscal viability of efficient organizations.

In this chapter we will review studies that have examined the determinants of costs in health care organizations. Our analysis will focus on the hospital, which has been the most frequent subject of cost function studies conducted in the health care industry. However, we will also examine the available literature pertaining to nursing homes. The chapter is organized as follows. The next section provides an introduction to theoretical cost functions in which the major determinants of hospital costs will be specified. Empirical studies pertaining to the major determinants of hospital costs will be reviewed in the following sections. Our survey will emphasize articles published after 1980, since the earlier literature has been reviewed extensively by Lave (1966), Mann and Yett (1968), Hefty (1969), Berki (1972), Feldstein (1974), and Cowing, Holtmann, and Powers (1983). Where relevant, the early literature will be discussed briefly. After the determinants of hospital costs have been reviewed, the analysis will be repeated for nursing homes. The chapter will conclude with a summary and implications for future research.

ISSUES IN COST FUNCTION ANALYSIS

In classical economic theory, a cost function describes the relationship between costs, quantities, mix of outputs a firm produces, and the input prices it pays.

Health care cost-function studies have extended the basic cost-function model to include internal characteristics, such as ownership and teaching orientation, as well as environmental factors, such as location and extent of regulatory activities.

Model Specification

Grannemann, Brown, and Pauly (1986) use a continuum to classify the wide variety of models that have been used to estimate hospital cost functions. At one end of the continuum are what Evans (1971) termed behavioral cost functions, which are based on a standard short-run model of hospital decision making (Sloan and Steinwald 1980a). In these models, the hospital decision makers are presumed to select output prices and input quantities to maximize an objective function that has quantity, quality, and profit as its arguments and is constrained by prevailing input and product market conditions and technology. Accordingly, the behavioral models typically include explanatory variables to reflect market demand conditions (e.g., ability to pay and need for hospital services), factor prices (e.g., wages), and the hospitals' fixed capital stock (e.g., beds). In addition, independent variables are entered to control for differences in case-mix (e.g., DRG Index or Resources Need Index), objectives (e.g., teaching orientation or ownership), and regulatory environment (e.g., hospital rate-setting or capital controls). Sloan and Steinwald (1980a) and Coelen and Sullivan (1981) used some of the most extensive sets of independent variables. At the other extreme of the cost function continuum are structural cost models that exploit the duality between production and cost functions. In these models, which are called technological or neoclassical cost functions, total cost is used as the dependent variable, and prices of inputs and quantities of outputs constitute the only independent variables (Brown, Caves, and Christensen 1979; Conrad and Strauss 1983). Recognizing the unique features of hospitals, a number of researchers have estimated quasi-technological cost functions by adding variables that depict hospital characteristics (e.g., teaching status or ownership) to the technological cost function (Pauly 1978; Salkever 1982; Cowing and Holtmann 1983; Grannemann, Brown, and Pauly 1986; Salkever, Steinwachs, and Rupp 1986).

Cowing, Holtmann and Powers (1983) discussed a number of problems associated with behavioral cost-function studies that limit their ability to estimate the structural aspects of production (i.e., economies of scale and scope) that affect hospital costs. The first problem noted was the absence of independent variables for input prices. This omission is equivalent to assuming zero input substitutability, which implies the existence of a technology that requires the use of resources in fixed proportions to produce hospital care. As suggested in the review of production functions in the previous chapter, this assumption is not valid. This problem is not likely to be resolved easily because of the unavailability of a complete set of valid data. Grannemann, Brown, and Pauly (1986,

p. 110), who argued that the absence of price variables is not likely to cause severe damage to the other parameter estimates, wrote: "Given the relatively poor quality of input price data, we did not judge the advantages of additional flexibility on this score to be worth the risk that poor price data would adversely affect measures of scale economies in a more flexible specification."

Second, many researchers used cross-section data to examine economies of scale in their behavioral cost functions. This method is inappropriate because hospitals are unlikely to be operating on their long-run cost function at any point in time (Salkever 1972). In a mathematical appendix to their literature review, Cowing, Holtmann, and Powers (1983) demonstrated that this problem can be avoided by using a short-run cost function as the basic model and then deriving long-run estimates from the envelope relationship between short-run cost curves and the long-run cost function. Salkever (1970) made a similar point with formal mathematical analysis as well as with cost function analysis of hospitals.

Third, many of the behavioral models did not incorporate correctly the multiple output dimensions of hospital services. The deficiency does not relate directly to the absence of suitable adjustments for case-mix variation (i.e., RNI or DRG index, etc.). Instead, Cowing et al. address an econometric estimation problem. Specifically, they imply that economies of scale in a multiproduct firm such as a hospital cannot be estimated by a single output model, even with adjustments for case-mix, because this type of model does not account for economies of scope. Therefore, if economies of scope are present, a specification error will occur.

In recognition of the recent increase in the use of quasi-technological, multiple-output cost functions for hospitals, we will provide a more detailed discussion of models in this genre. In addition to the technological cost function estimated by Conrad and Strauss (1983), at least five studies (see Table 8.1) that estimated quasi-technological cost functions for hospitals have been published (Pauly 1978; Salkever 1982; Cowing and Holtmann 1983; Grannemann, Brown, and Pauly 1986; Salkever, Steinwachs, and Rupp 1986). These analyses have relied on flexible functional forms that were first evaluated using data sets compiled from firms operating in the railroad industry (Brown, Caves, and Christensen 1979) and the electric power generation industry (Christensen and Greene 1976). A detailed technical discussion of flexible functional forms is provided in both articles.

Cowing, Holtmann, and Powers (1983) provided an extensive review of hospital cost-function studies. They argued that the quasi-technological or neoclassical joint cost function approach, which used flexible forms, was superior to the methods employed in the earlier behavioral cost function studies of hospitals because (1) this approach does not require any arbitrary a priori restrictions (e.g., fixed proportion technology) on the structure of the cost function, (2) estimates of economies of scope and economies of scale are available from the cost function, and (3) elasticities of input substitution can be derived from the parameter estimates of the joint cost function.

Table 8.1
Summary of Technological Cost Function Studies

Author, Year	Sample	Dependent Variables
Conrad and Strauss, 1983	Cross-section data of 114 North Carolina hospitals in 1978.	Total cost.
Cowing and Holtmann, 1983.	Cross-section of 138 New York hospitals in 1975.	Total operating costs.
Grannemann, Brown and Pauly, 1986	National cross-section of 867 hospitals, 1982 data.	Log(total cost)

Table 8.1 (continued)

Independent Variables	Primary Results

Vector of input prices for:
  nursing, ancillary service,
  administration and general
  services, and capital.
	Constant returns to scale;
	nursing and ancillary services
	are complementary to capital;
	general services and capital are
	substitutes.

Vector of outputs:
  child inpatient days,
  adult non-Medicare inpatient days,
  Medicare inpatient days.
 	
  (Translog function resulted in
  estimation of 36 parameters)	

Vector of outputs:
  Patient days in
  medical-surgical,
  maternity,
  pediatrics,
  other in-patient units, and.
  outpatient visits.
	Over capitalization
	Some diseconomies of scope
	Economies of scale
	Proprietary hospitals are 15%
	  less expensive
	Teaching coefficient not
	  significant (t = 0.92)
	73 of 107 coefficients were
	  not significant (p < 0.05)
	Economies of scope between
	  pediatrics and other services.

Vector of variable inputs:
  nursing, ancillary,
  professional, administrative,
  general, drugs and supplies.	

Two fixed inputs: capital, admitting physician.	
Ownership type, and teaching status.	
(Translog cost function resulted in estimation of 107 parameters).	

Vector of primary outputs:
  patient days in acute, intensive
  care, and other patient
  units; outpatient visits
  and emergency room visits.
	Economies of scale for
	  production of emergency service.
	Government hospitals 8.3% less
	  expensive.
	For-profit hospitals 14.7% more
	  expensive.
	COTH member hospitals 15.1% more
	  expensive.
	Costs directly related to age
	  of medical staff members.

Vector of inpatient discharges from:
  acute, intensive care, and other
  patient units.	

Vector of case-mix variables:
% admission and % outpatient
  visits classified as pediatric,
  surgical, psychiatric, OB/GYN,
  other.	

Vector of hourly input wages:
  maintenance, food service, lab
  tech, nursing.	

% Physicians under 45 years of age.	

Dummy variables for:
  government hospitals
  for-profit hospitals
  teaching hospitals
  region
  SMSA.	

Other variables included square and
  cubed output measures of interaction
  terms--63 coefficients were estimated.	

Table 8.1 (continued)

Author, Year	Sample	Dependent Variables
Pauly, 1978	Cross-section data for 50 California hospitals in 1975.	Total hospital costs.
Salkever, 1982	Cross-section data for 617 hospitals in MD, MA, NY, and PA in 1975.	Log(total costs minus direct expenses for non-reimbursable cost centers and physician compensation).
Salkever, Steinwachs and Rupp, 1986	Pooled cross-section and time-series data of 46 Maryland hospitals.	Log(inpatient costs). Log(routine cost). Log(ancillary cost).

Table 8.1 (continued)

Independent Variables	Primary Results

Admissions (adjusted for outpatient volume)
Vector of input prices for:
    nursing services, professional services, general services, administrative services.
 	
Vector of variables for proportion of primary attending physicians who are:
    board certified, pediatricians, internists, general surgeons, OB/GYN, otorhinologists, other surgical specialists, other specialists.
 	
Case-mix index based on mean charges.
Location in large urban area.
Output concentration index.
	Costs inversely related to physician concentration.
	
	Costs are lower if primary attending (PA) physician is a general surgeon and are higher if PA is a pediatrician or an internist.
	
	Mildly increasing returns to scale.
	
	Case-mix and teaching activities had a significant positive effect on total hospital costs.

Log (discharges)
Vector of 7 output mix variables including:
    emergency room visits per admission,
    outpatient visits per admission,
    births per admission,
    costliness index of facilities and services
 	
4 factor price variables:
    log (living costs)
    log (average service industry wages)
    log (union-adjusted compensation per hospital employee)
    log (unadjusted compensation per hospital employee)
 	
Dummy variables for:
    proprietary hospital
    government hospital
    teaching activities
    state location
    8 dimensions of union activities
	Unions increase total costs by 5.4 to 8.8 percent
	
	Non-wage impact of unions on total costs increases ranges from 3.3 to 6.7 percent.
	
	Higher total costs are associated with government-owned and teaching hospitals.
	
	Proprietary hospitals have lower costs.

Rate regulation variables. Proportion of beds which are special care. Available acute care bed days. Ratio of approved residents to beds. DRG case-mix index. Dummy variable for each hospital, except referent.	Weak and generally insignificant results were found for case-based payment program. Significant and negative coefficients were estimated for the more rigorous revenue cap program. Teaching activities had a much stronger positive impact on ancillary costs than on routine costs.

217

Our review of technological functions will be limited to those that used the multiple-output approach (Conrad and Strauss 1983; Cowing and Holtmann 1983; Grannemann, Brown and Pauly 1986) and, thus, are able to exploit the advantages of the joint cost function approach, which are very pertinent to multiproduct firms such as hospitals. As our review of quasi-technological cost function studies will show, however, the use of this type of model is not without substantial difficulties.

Conrad and Strauss (1983) used audited Medicare cost reports from 114 hospitals in North Carolina to estimate a translog cost function with total costs as the dependent variable. The independent variables consisted of prices for three inputs (nursing service, ancillary service, general service) and three outputs (child days, non-Medicare adult days, Medicare days) and interaction terms. A total of 36 parameters were estimated. Although the researchers attempted to reflect the multiproduct nature of the hospital in their model, the disaggregation of output by patient days in three age-related groups failed to capture the diversity of inpatient outputs. Further, Conrad and Strauss omitted other outputs, such as outpatient department and emergency room services, which have an important influence on the dependent variable, total costs.

Cowing and Holtmann (1983) obtained data from 340 hospitals in the State of New York. After removing specialty hospitals and all facilities with missing data, the sample on which the analysis was based consisted of only 138 hospitals. They estimated a short-run cost function because it is not likely that each hospital in the cross-section sample would be operating in a long-run equilibrium position. Accordingly, the dependent variable was defined as total operating costs, which included labor and supply expenses and excluded depreciation expenses. The independent variables, which were specified in translog form, consisted of a set of six output measures (i.e., number of emergency room visits, number of outpatient visits, and number of patient days in medical-surgical units, maternity units, pediatric units and other inpatient units), a set of five input prices (i.e., nursing labor, professional labor, administrative labor, general labor, and materials and supplies), a single measure of fixed capital stock (the book value of buildings and equipment), and the number of attending physicians. In addition to the interval scaled variables, two binary variables were used to represent proprietary hospitals and teaching hospitals. Although the inclusion of a more diverse set of output measures as well as two hospital characteristics variables represents an improvement over the Conrad-Strauss specification, this model is still deficient. Implicit in the use of patient days in the four inpatient service categories is the assumption that the output within each service is homogeneous. In light of the evidence summarized in Chapter 5, this assumption is not realistic.

Grannemann, Brown, and Pauly (1986) obtained data for a cross-section of 1689 short-term hospitals in 1981; however, complete data were available for only 867 hospitals, which were used in the analysis. In recognition of the unavailability of certain data as well as the unique cost-influencing features of hospitals, a translog functional form was not estimated. Instead, they selected a hybrid functional form that incorporated some of the desirable features of behavioral and structural cost functions.

The dependent variable of the cost function analysis was total annual hospital costs. The independent variables included measures pertaining to the hospital's primary outputs (expressed at their actual, squared, and cubed levels), miscellaneous outputs produced in some hospitals, input prices, sources of revenue, and case-mix. Although this model is a more realistic depiction of the heterogeneous nature of hospital output than the other quasi-technological cost functions, Grannemann et al. fail to overcome the previously discussed problems of quasi-technological models while introducing at least one new problem. Once again, output was defined in terms of broad categories (i.e., acute inpatient days, intensive care unit patient days, and subacute and other patient days). Unlike the previous quasi-technological cost-function studies, Grannemann et al. used multiple measures for the output of outpatient departments (i.e., outpatient visits and emergency room visits).

Recognizing the deficiencies in their output measures, the authors included what they called case-mix variables; however, these variables did not include standard case-mix measures such as the RNI or a DRG index. Instead inpatient case-mix was represented as the number of discharges in five broad service categories (i.e., pediatrics, surgery, psychiatry, OB/GYN, and other). These variables accounted for about 54 percent of total discharges. A rationale for the omission of other service category variables was not given. The use of these variables is troublesome for two reasons. First, given the observed heterogeneity of patients (Horn, Horn, and Sharkey 1984), these variables are too broad to represent adequately the multiproduct nature of the hospital, which was the intention of the research. Indeed, Grannemann et al. observed "that the variables included in the cost function do not fully capture the differences between large and small hospitals—unmeasured case-mix and service content differences may be responsible." Second, only 28 of 68 coefficients were significant at conventional levels ($p < 0.05$). Although a correlation matrix was not provided in the article, it is likely that strong inter-correlations among the variables reduced the reliability of the estimated regression coefficients.

In addition to the difficulties with output measures, Grannemann et al. reported difficulty in acquiring reliable price data for some inputs. Accordingly, rather than use poor quality data, they omitted variables for some input prices. This omission implies that the cost-minimizing mix of inputs is unaffected by the mix of outputs produced, an assumption that is contrary to the empirical results of Conrad and Strauss (1983).

In summary, our examination of the quasi-technological, multiple-output, hospital cost function studies suggests that, although this is a theoretically appealing model, and might provide new insights about hospital cost structures, the potential benefits described by Cowing et al. (1983) are unlikely to be achieved because of a number of data problems. First, an extremely large amount of detailed data, which is not routinely reported by all hospitals, is required.

Each of the three studies experienced large reductions in its sample size due to incomplete or unusable data. Since this may be related to the sophistication of the hospital's management information system, which, in turn, is likely to be correlated with other hospital characteristics, it is unlikely that the results of any of these studies can be generalized to larger populations. Second, a complete specification of these models requires the estimation of an extremely large number of parameters. This, in turn, requires a large sample size to provide a sufficient number of degrees of freedom to estimate a regression equation reliably. Paradoxically, a large sample size may not be available because of the extensive data requirements.

Third, each of the studies attempted to incorporate measures that depict the multiproduct nature of the hospital into the analysis. Although each cost function included several outputs, they were so broad as to be at best an extremely naive representation of the heterogeneous nature of hospital production.

Fourth, in order to estimate economies of scope, variables pertaining to input prices and output for each department where a joint production relationship occurs must be included in the cost equation; otherwise, a specification bias will occur. An examination of quasi-technological, cost function studies of hospitals suggests that such a specification error has occurred. For example, none of the hospital studies included variables for the number of residents and physicians in each specialty department. Price variables for these inputs were also omitted. In light of recent findings that suggest the existence of economies of scope in radiological residency programs between their education and patient care outputs (Hosek and Palmer 1983), a specification error is likely. Although not studied empirically, it is plausible that economies of scope between the social work department (for which data has not been entered into cost regressions) and patient treatment departments exist if the former is used to reduce lengths of stay of patients treated in the latter departments.

In conclusion, flexible multiple-output cost functions were initially validated empirically in the railroad industry and the electrical power industry (Christensen and Greene 1976; Brown, Caves, and Christensen 1979); however, these industries are comprised of firms that produce only a small number of outputs. Although it may be possible to estimate reliable multiple-output cost functions in these types of industries, formidable data requirements limit the transportability of this technique to the hospital industry.

In addition to the problems that are unique to the estimation of quasi-technological cost functions, the technological cost studies shared a problem common to many of the behavioral cost studies. Specifically, total hospital costs, including physician compensation, has been used frequently as the dependent variable; however, reported hospital costs include only the compensation of physicians with a contractual relationship with the hospital. Thus, institutions such as teaching hospitals, which have a greater percentage of their medical staff on their payroll, will report higher levels of physician-related expenses than nonteaching hospitals, even in situations where the total level of compensation received by the physicians in these different types of hospitals is the same. Obviously, an upward bias is created in estimates of the effects of teaching activities on hospital costs and in the coefficients of other variables that may be correlated with hospital-physician compensation arrangements. Accordingly, it is preferable to standardize the dependent variable by subtracting physician compensation from total costs (Coelen and Sullivan 1981).

Level of Aggregation

In addition to type of specification, health care cost function models can be classified according to level of aggregation, which can be as broad as the entire organization or as narrow as a department or functional group. Different problems and advantages are associated with each level of aggregation. Access to more aggregative organizational data is easy because it is readily available from archival sources such as the American Hospital Association (1987). Further, analysis of organizational level data avoids the problems associated with the arbitrary methods of allocating costs among departments. A number of disadvantages offset these advantages. First, the level of aggregation may be too broad to be meaningful. For example, a study that finds that long-term average costs of hospitals are minimized at 300 beds does not provide any information regarding how the hospital should be configured. Should it have one 300-bed ward or ten 30-bed units? How large should its various departments be? It is clear that studies which use the department as the unit of analysis may provide more meaningful information. Furthermore, since this level of aggregation increases product homogeneity, it reduces the problems associated with the multiproduct nature of the hospital. On the other hand, cost functions of departments do not provide any information about economies of scope. This could be a serious weakness of less aggregative studies because declines in economies of scope may offset gains associated with increases in the scale of operations, a plausible scenario under regionalization of services.

DETERMINANTS OF HOSPITAL COSTS

The following sections will examine the determinants of hospital costs, including economies of scale, economies of scope, teaching activities, behavior and composition of the medical staff, and ownership and control of hospitals. We will not repeat our analysis of other important determinants of hospital costs that are presented in other chapters; these include input prices (see Chapter 1), demand (Chapter 3), case-mix (Chapters 5 and 6), market structure (Chapter 11), and regulatory environment (Chapter 12). In the following sections, we refer to three tables that summarize multivariate studies that examined the relationship between hospital costs and teaching, medical staff, and case-mix (Table 8.2); state rate-setting activities (Table 8.3); and other cost determinants (Table 8.4). In most studies, however, the inclusion of other explanatory vari-

Table 8.2
Summary of Behavioral Cost Function Studies that Examined Teaching, Medical Staff, and Case-Mix

Author, Year	Sample	Dependent Variables
Anderson and Lave, 1986	National cross-section data for 5,000 hospitals in 1981.	Log (Medicare operating cost per case)
Barer, 1982	Cross-section, time-series data for 87 British Columbia hospitals during 1966-1973.	Estimated inpatient operating expenses per admission (Note: costs of educational research and outpatient services were subtracted from total costs).
Hornbrook and Monheit, 1985	National cross-section of 380 hospitals in 1977.	Cost per admission

Table 8.2 (continued)

Independent Variables	Primary Results

Log (Intern-resident to bed ratio)
Log (wage index)
Log (Medicare case-mix index)
Log (beds)
% population Medicaid
% population urbanized
Binary variables for metropolitan
   statistical areas (MSAs) in 6
   size classes.
	Costs are positively
	and significantly
	associated with all indepen-
	dent variables except MSA
	dummies for smaller areas.
	
	Results suggest that Medicare
	DRGs do not control variations
	in case-mix severity very well.

Personnel-mix index.
Wage index
Vector of variables for proportion
   of expenses allocatable to:
   outpatient department and
   educational activities.
Case-mix index
Average length of stay.
	Information theory approach
	generated intertemporally
	stable case complexity
	measures.
	
	Teaching activities generate
	substantial indirect costs.

Admissions
Admissions-squared
Case-mix index,
Scope of services,
Cost of capital,
Cost of labor,
# of interns/residents 	
Dummy variables for:
   rate-setting,
   PSRO,
   proprietary hospital,
   government hospital.
	Inclusion of case-mix measures
	   removes an upward bias in
	estimates of cost-volume
	relationships which causes
	researchers to conclude that
	diseconomies of scale exist.
	
	Constant returns to scale.
	
	Lower costs are found in
	proprietary and government
	hospitals.
	
	Costs are directly related to
	the number of interns and
	residents, case-mix index, and
	scope of services.

Table 8.2 (continued)

Author, Year	Sample	Dependent Variables
Pettengill and Vertrees, 1982	National cross-section of 5,071 hospitals in 1977.	Log (Medicare operating, costs per case).
Sloan and Becker, 1981	National cross-section of 1,228 hospitals in 1974.	Total expense per adjusted admission, total expense per adjusted patient day.
Sloan, Feldman and Steinwald, 1983	National pooled cross-section, time series of 390 hospitals in 1974 and 1977.	Non-physician cost per adjusted patient day and non-physician cost per adjusted admission. Utilization and cost measures for pathology and radiology departments.

Table 8.2 (continued)

Independent Variables	Primary Results
Log (intern-residents to bed ratio), Log (wage index), Log (case-mix index), Log (beds), Urban dummy variables for large medium, and small areas.	All coefficients (except small urban area) are positive and significant.
5 variables for physician contract-compensation arrangements pertaining to salary contracts and incentive contracts, as well as, limitations on physician affiliations with other hospitals. 3 departmentalization variables, 7 governing board and executive, committee variables, 5 demand variables, 4 factor supply variables. Other dummy variables for: government hospitals, proprietary hospital, size classes, teaching affiliations. RNI	Increased costs are associated with: salary physician contracts, departmentalization, case-mix, increased size, teaching activities, government ownership, presence of a union. Decreased costs are associated with: incentive physician contracts, physician membership on governing board.
Binary variables for 3 types of teaching hospitals. RNI, Payer mix, Size class dummies.	Increased costs are associated with teaching activities, size. Higher total costs in ancillary departments are due primarily to case-mix and secondarily to graduate training demands.

225

Table 8.3
Summary of Behavioral Cost Function Studies that Examined Prospective Payment

Author, Year	Sample	Dependent Variables
Coelen and Sullivan, 1981	National pooled time-series cross-sectional data from 2,693 hospitals during 1970-1977.	%Δ (Cost per adjusted patient day) %Δ (Cost per adjusted admission) %Δ (Cost per capita) Log (Cost per adjusted patient day) Log (Cost per adjusted admission) Log (Cost per capita) (Note: physician costs are not included in dependent variable).
Rosko, 1982	Pooled, time-series cross-sectional data from 142 hospitals in NJ and PA during the period 1971-1978.	Total cost per admission Total cost per day Routine cost per admission Routine cost per day Ancillary cost per admission Ancillary cost per day
Rosko, 1984	See Rosko (1982)	Total cost per admission Total cost per patient day
Rosko and Broyles, 1986	Pooled, time-series cross-sectional data from 84 hospitals in NJ during 1979-1982.	Cost per admission Cost per day
Rosko and Broyles, 1987	Pooled, time-series, cross-sectional data for 160 hospitals in NJ and PA during 1975-1982.	Log (Cost per admission) Log (Cost per day)

Table 8.3 (continued)

Independent Variables	Primary Results
A vector of 20 supply and demand variables for the county in which the hospital is located.	For-profit hospitals are less expensive. Results for government hospitals vary with model specification.
Dummy variables for: government hospitals, for-profit hospitals, rate regulation, PSRO, CON, time.	Mature rate regulation programs tend to contain costs.
Beds, scope of services, Volume of service, Dummy variables for rate regulation, catchment area, state. (fixed effects specification was used to control time-invariant differences in case mix).	Mature rate regulation program contains costs. Substantial indirect costs are associated with teaching activities. Costs are directly related to size and scope of services.
Same as Rosko (1982) except residents per bed was substituted for teaching dummy variable.	Mature rate regulation contains costs. Costs directly related to teaching activities, and scope of services.
Vector of 5 market area supply and demand variables, including: per capita income, % physicians who are specialists, % population receiving Medicare benefits Teaching dummies (a fixed-effects model was used to control inter-hospital differences, which were time invariant)	Compared to a per diem based prospective payment system, which operated simultaneously, the New Jersey DRG system reduced cost per admission but not cost per day. Higher costs are associated with teaching programs.
Vector of 5 market area supply and demand variables entered in logarithmic form. (fixed-effects model was specified)	Relative to cost-based retrospective reimbursement, per case and per diem prospective payment system constrained cost per admission and cost per day. Increased costs are associated

Table 8.3 (continued)

Author, Year	Sample	Dependent Variables
Salkever, Steinwachs and Rupp, 1986	Pooled cross-section and time-series data of 46 Maryland hospitals.	Log (total inpatient cost). Log (inpatient cost per case).
Sloan and Steinwald, 1980b	National pooled time-series, cross-section data from 1,228 hospitals during 1969-1975.	Total cost per adjusted admission. Total cost per adjusted patient day.

Table 8.3 (continued)

Independent Variables	Primary Results
A vector of 9 supply and demand variables for the county in which the hospital is located. Rate regulation variables. Proportion of beds which are special care. Available acute care bed days in hospital. Ratio of approved residents to beds. DRG case-mix index. (fixed-effects model was specified).	Weak and generally insignificant results were found for the case-based payment program. Significant and negative coefficients were estimated for the more rigorous revenue cap program. Cost per case and total costs were directly related to size and the ratio of special care beds to total beds.

A vector of 11 variables for young and mature cost control programs including:
    capital controls
    utilization review, and
    rate regulation.
 	
A vector of 8 demand variables
 	
A vector of 4 factor supply variables.
 	
Dummy variables for:
    government hospitals
    for-profit hospitals
    teaching hospitals
    hospitals in 3 size categories
	Ownership is not associated with cost variations.
	
	Costs are positively associated with teaching and union activities and size.

Table 8.4
Summary of Other Behavioral Cost Function Studies of Hospitals

Author, Year	Primary Area of Inquiry	Sample	Dependent Variables
Friedman and Pauly, 1981	Stochastic demand	National pooled cross-section, time-series quarterly data from 1973 to 1978.	Total expense per admission.
Friedman and Pauly, 1983	Stochastic demand	Same as Friedman and Pauly (1981).	Same as Friedman and Pauly (1981).
Renn, Schramm, Watt and Derzon, 1985	System affiliation	National cross-section of 561 hospitals in 1980.	Cost per adjusted admission. Case-mix index.
Robinson and Luft, 1985	Market structure	National cross-section of 5,103 hospitals in 1972. A subset of 1,084 hospitals was used in the equation containing case-mix.	Log (cost per admission). Log (cost per day).
Salkever, 1984	Unions	Cross-sectional data for 617 hospitals in MA,MD,NY, and PA in 1971 and 1975.	Log (total costs minus direct expenses for non-reimbursable cost centers and physician compensation). Log (cost per discharge). Log (cost per day). Log% Δ(total costs). Log% Δ(cost per discharge). Log% Δ(cost per day).

Table 8.4 (continued)

Independent Variables	Primary Results
Inverse of occupancy rate, beds, wage rate, vector of 5 service-mix variables, teaching affiliation.	Marginal cost of an expected admission is 98% of average cost; but for an unexpected admission marginal cost is only 35% of average cost.

Higher costs are associated with size, service mix and teaching activities. |
| Same as Friedman and Pauly (1981) except teaching variable is deleted and length of stay is added. | The change in model specification had little impact on major results.

The marginal cost of an expected admission is 100% of average cost, but for an unexpected admission marginal cost is about 58%.

Cost of an empty bed ranges from $2,400 to $3,800. |
| Vector of binary variables for hospitals classified as: investor-owned chain not-for-profit chain investor-owned freestanding not-for-profit freestanding government-owned.

Other variables for patient and payer mix, input costs, region, capacity, utilization, and teaching. | Significant differences were not associated with type of hospital.

Investor-owned hospitals had a less costly case-mix and a higher proportion of charge-based patients than freestanding not-for-profit hospitals. |
| Binary variables for: number of competitors, size class, public hospital, for-profit hospital, teaching hospital.

Residents per bed, MD, per 100,000 population, income per capita, 17 case-mix variables for the proportion of patients with a specified diagnosis or procedure. | Increased cost per admission is associated with: number of competitors, length of stay, size, income, physician-population ratio and teaching activities.

Lower costs are found in for-profit hospitals. |
| Vector of 11 product demand variables, including measures for : competition, ability to pay, and physician supply.

Vector of 4 capital stock variables including: size and mix of services.

Vector of 4 factor price variables.

Dummy variables for: proprietary hospital government hospital teaching activities state location 8 dimensions of union activities | Increased costs per discharge are associated with union activities, teaching hospitals, public hospitals, and mix of services.

For-profit hospitals are less expensive. |

231

ables provides estimates relevant to other cost determinants discussed in this chapter. For example, virtually every table includes results germane to the relationship between size and costs or teaching and costs.

The reader should note that the examinations of hospital cost determinants other than economies of scale and scope usually employed behavioral cost functions. The exceptions are the quasi-technological cost functions estimated by Salkever (1982) and Salkever, Steinwachs, and Rupp (1986). In our discussion of cost determinants, it is important to keep in mind that the specification of the model affects the interpretation of the regression equations. For example, in quasitechnological cost functions, the coefficients of the variables reflecting hospital characteristics (e.g., teaching or ownership status) estimate the impact of the effects of these factors on efficiency, that is, on the cost of producing any given volume and mix of output. In the behavioral cost equations, because output volume and product-mix variables are excluded, the estimated coefficients of the hospital characteristics variables reflect the impact of these determinants on efficiency as well as the cost implications of these variables on volume and mix of output (Salkever, Steinwachs, and Rupp 1986).

Economies of Scale and Scope

Most of the early investigations of economies of scale in the hospital sector employed data for the entire hospital. The goal of these studies was to determine the optimal size (in terms of beds) of the hospital. These studies provided ambiguous results that can be attributed to a variety of methodological problems associated with the use of behavioral cost functions (Cowing, Holtmann, and Powers 1983), as well as other research design errors summarized by Berki (1972). Several studies could not confirm the existence of economies of scale (Ingbar and Taylor 1968; Francisco 1970; Lave and Lave 1970). Researchers whose studies detected economies of scale could not agree on the location of the minimum point on the hospital's long-run, average cost curve, which ranged from 150 beds (Cohen 1967) to 900 beds (Ro 1968). The early studies of hospital cost functions suggest that if economies of scale exist, they are probably not substantial. As reported in the previous chapter, similar results have been reported by those who used the production function approach. More recent studies of economies of scale have not changed this conclusion. Jenkins (1980) reported the existence of overall diseconomies of scale with the optimal size of a hospital ranging from 100 to 300 beds, while Bays (1980) found constant returns to scale.

Vitaliano (1987) found a U-shaped average cost curve with a minimum point at 107 beds when a quadratic cost function was estimated; however, the estimates from a logarithmic cost function suggest significant economies of scale throughout the entire range of observations.

Since 1980, most of the published studies that provided evidence pertinent to economies of scale in hospitals consisted of two types: (1) studies that examined the utility of quasi-technological multiple-output models in the health care sector, and (2) studies that had other primary objectives but that controlled for the effects of size or volume on hospital costs. Many of the studies in the latter category did not include a quadratic term for size or volume of output, and thus, could not examine the existence of scale economies, although they could control the effects of size/volume on hospital costs.

The technological cost function studies reported conflicting conclusions regarding the nature of scale economies in hospitals. Given the previously discussed problems of these studies, the results should be accepted very cautiously. Cowing and Holtmann (1983) found a U-shaped, short-run, average cost curve, which suggested the existence of ''economies of scale with respect to variable costs in the short-run'' (p. 647). In contrast, Conrad and Strauss (1983) found constant returns to scale. Grannemann et al. (1986) detected strong economies of scale in the production of emergency department services; however, these researchers reported that they could not make valid estimates of inpatient cost structures because of their inability to control case-mix variations between hospitals.

In a related policy issue, Cowing and Holtmann also discovered positive economies of scope between pediatrics and other hospital services, and negative economies of scope for emergency department services. The former result suggests that any cost savings due to economies of scale that are gained by consolidating pediatrics services might be offset by negative economies of scope. Their latter result was corroborated by Grannemann et al. (1986); however, an alternative explanation that is simple and intuitively appealing can be offered. The admission of emergency room patients increases the complexity, and hence, the costliness of the patient mix (Munoz, Regan, Margocis, and Wise 1985); thus, if the hospital closes its emergency room, costly trauma patients are taken elsewhere.

We will conclude this section with a brief review of recent behavioral cost function studies that included size or volume variables. Sloan and associates have included three binary variables representing hospitals in different size classes in studies that examined the relationship between average hospital costs and prospective payment (Sloan and Steinwald 1980b), internal organization of hospitals (Sloan and Becker 1981), teaching (Sloan, Feldman, and Steinwald 1983), and ownership (Becker and Sloan 1985). In each of the four studies, a general pattern emerged. The average cost per day had a monotonically decreasing relationship with size, which implies increasing returns to scale; however, an opposite relationship was observed in the average cost per admission equations. ''These results, taken together, imply that length of stay is largest in the 400 bed-plus size category of hospitals. Since the first days of hospitalization tend to be comparatively expensive, a longer length of stay means, *ceteris paribus*, a lower cost per adjusted patient day'' (Sloan and Steinwald 1980b, p. 146). Robinson and Luft (1985), who included length of stay as an explanatory variable, found a monotonically increasing relationship between four size-related dummy variables and cost per case and cost per day. Although not definitive, and subject to the limitations of behavioral cost functions, which we discussed earlier in this chapter, the results of the more recent studies suggest a positive relationship between size and the cost per case.

Teaching Activities

Cost levels in teaching hospitals have been much higher than in their non-teaching counterparts. Given a substantial heterogeneity in resources committed to education among hospitals classified as teaching institutions, comparisons between teaching and nonteaching hospitals may result in misleading conclusions. Recognizing the need for a taxonomy of teaching hospitals, Sloan and Valvona (1986) developed the following hierarchy of hospitals, in descending order of involvement in teaching, with the number of hospitals in each category in 1982 in parentheses: flagship Council of Teaching Hospitals (COTH) member (116), other COTH member (198), medical school affiliated (442), and approved residency program (107). COTH members must have at least four approved residency programs and a medical school affiliation. Flagship hospitals are institutions that are owned by medical schools or are separate nonprofit or public hospitals in which the medical school department chairs and hospital chiefs of service are typically the same person.

Sloan and Valvona's hierarchy of teaching hospitals suggests that costs are positively related to the degree of teaching activity. For example, in 1982 the average cost per admission was $4,157 in flagship COTH member hospitals, $3,327 in other COTH member hospitals, $2,781 in medical school affiliated hospitals, $2,558 in hospitals with an approved residency program, and $2,345 in nonteaching hospitals. These striking cost differentials have stimulated public policy deliberations about payment formulas for teaching hospitals, which, in turn, have motivated a substantial amount of research on the impact of medical education programs on hospital costs. Before reviewing these studies, it is appropriate to summarize the ways in which teaching activities contribute to hospital costs.

Intern and resident programs generate direct and indirect costs. Direct costs include salaries paid to instructors, salaries paid to interns and residents, expenditures for teaching materials, the cost of classroom space, and overhead costs. Besides these direct costs, medical education programs may generate additional indirect costs associated with: a more complex case-mix attracted to tertiary teaching facilities (Becker and Steinwald 1981); decreased productivity of other employees who must assist in orienting new residents (Anderson and Lave 1986); increased availability of state-of-the-art technology (Russell 1979); increased use of ancillary services and diagnostic tests to support training requirements (Schroeder and O'Leary 1977; Garg, Elkhatib, Kleinberg, and Mulligan 1982; Rueben 1984).

There are conflicting positions pertaining to the issue of reimbursement for expenses associated with medical education programs. Insurance companies and government authorities have argued that payments to hospitals should be restricted to legitimate patient care expenses and should exclude expenses accrued in training interns and residents. Those who oppose this position make several arguments. First, interns and residents are substitutes for private physicians who receive compensation for treating patients in nonteaching hospitals. Second, medical education has a number of externalities that benefit society at large. Third, teaching hospitals, which tend to attract a more expensive case-mix, would be unfairly penalized in a payment system that does not recognize the indirect expenses of medical education. Finally, some of the direct expenses of medical education programs may be offset by increases in the productivity of other hospital personnel. To resolve these assertions, it is necessary not only to determine whether teaching hospitals are more expensive but also to determine the contribution of the indirect cost of educational activities to variations in hospital costs.

As indicated in Table 8.2, which summarizes results of multivariate studies on the effects of teaching programs on hospital costs, a consistently positive and significant association between teaching activities and hospital costs has been found. Corroborating evidence is also found in Tables 8.1, 8.3 and 8.4. These results are consistent over a variety of specifications including interval-scaled and binary teaching variables. Since the intensity of medical education activities is likely to vary by institution, an interval-scaled variable such as residents per bed may be more appropriate. Sloan and Steinwald (1980b) argued, however, that the residents per bed may be endogenous because both the numerator and denominator are subject to manipulation by hospital managers. Thus, in order to avoid simultaneity bias, a binary teaching variable (teaching versus nonteaching) should be used because a hospital is not likely to change its teaching status in the short-run. Hence, it is more realistic to treat a binary teaching variable as exogenous. Rosko and Broyles (1986) followed this approach but argued that the inclusion of two binary variables, major teaching hospitals and minor teaching hospitals, would provide more information. They found that after accounting for the effects of other market supply and demand conditions, major teaching programs contributed more than twice as much to the cost per admission as did minor teaching programs.

In the remainder of this section, we will discuss in more detail studies that provide greater insights into the determinants of cost variations between teaching and nonteaching hospitals.

Sloan, Feldman, and Steinwald (1983) conducted one of the most comprehensive studies of the effects of teaching activities on hospital costs. They analyzed performance measures pertaining to specific departments, as well as to total nonphysician hospital costs per adjusted day and per adjusted admission. In addition to 21 independent variables that were included in the regression equations to control for other determinants of hospital cost variations, such as case-mix, size, input prices, and payer-mix, the explanatory variables included three binary variables representing hospitals with an approved residency program, a medical school affiliation and a membership in the COTH. Regression analysis revealed a monotonically increasing relationship between the teaching variables (in order of their inclusion above) and costs per unit of output. The estimated regression coefficients indicated that major teaching hospitals (i.e., COTH members) and hospitals with a medical school affiliation had nonphysician hospital costs per adjusted admission that were, respectively, 13 percent and 5 percent more than their nonteaching counterparts; however, teaching hospitals with only an approved residency program did not exhibit costs per admission that were significantly higher than their nonteaching counterparts.

The univariate analysis of Sloan, Feldman, and Steinwald (1983) revealed that teaching hospitals had costs that were 33.3 percent more per admission than nonteaching hospitals, a differential that is more than twice as large as that implied by the largest teaching coefficient estimated in their multivariate analysis. These results suggest that a substantial portion of the cost differences between teaching and nonteaching hospitals is due to other factors that systematically vary with teaching activities. Among the other independent variables employed in this study, the most noteworthy was case-mix, which was measured by the RNI (resource need index). In this sample of hospitals, teaching hospitals had an RNI-value that was 7 percent greater than that of nonteaching hospitals. Further, the estimated regression equations revealed a consistently positive and significant ($p < 0.01$) relationship between the RNI variable and hospital costs, irrespective of the unit of output used in the dependent variable (i.e., adjusted admissions or adjusted patient days), or the data set employed (i.e., teaching hospitals only, nonteaching hospitals only, or the entire sample). Thus, the authors concluded that once patient mix variations are controlled, the cost differences between teaching and nonteaching hospitals are much smaller than commonly assumed.

Contradictory evidence is found in a more recent study in which 37 independent variables were used in regression analysis to control case-mix and other determinants of hospital costs. Sloan and Valvona (1986) found that major teaching hospitals (i.e., COTH members) were 21 percent to 41 percent more expensive than nonteaching hospitals. When only teaching status was used in the regression equation, the estimated parameters indicated that the cost per adjusted admission in major teaching hospitals was 37 percent to 59 percent more than in nonteaching hospitals. Thus, unlike the earlier studies, these results suggest that, even after controlling for the effects of case-mix and a large number of other factors, major teaching hospitals are much more expensive than nonteaching hospitals.

Sloan, Feldman, and Steinwald (1983) also analyzed the effects of teaching activities on the performance of specific hospital departments. They estimated equations for services per admission and costs per unit of output for the pathology and radiology departments. In general, ambiguous and sometimes conflicting results were found. For example, major teaching programs were associated with a significant increase in pathology services per admission but with a negative (but insignificant) change in radiology services per admission. A statistically significant ($p < .05$) relationship between teaching activities and department costs per admission was not found for either department. Indeed the most consistent pattern that emerged was that between case-mix and departmental performance. The RNI had a positive and significant coefficient in seven of the eight equations estimated for these departments.

Sloan et al. also provided a summary table for regression equations, which estimated the teaching effects on the performance of seven other departments. Although most of the coefficients reflected a positive relationship between teaching activities and departmental costs, less than one third of the coefficients were statistically significant ($p < .10$).

In addition to Sloan et al., two other recent studies have reported that teaching hospitals attract a more complex case-mix. Employing a data set compiled from 397 hospitals in 1974, Becker and Steinwald (1981) regressed three binary teaching variables (i.e., AMA-approved residency, medical school affiliation, and COTH membership), as well as 27 other independent variables, on the RNI. They found a monotonically increasing and significant ($p < .01$) relationship between the teaching variables and the case-mix index. Ament, Kobrinski, and Wood (1981) performed univariate analysis on a sample of 200 hospitals and reported that the RNI value for large and medium-sized teaching hospitals was significantly greater than that for their nonteaching counterparts.

Goldfarb and Coffey (1987) present an analysis that challenges the conventional wisdom about the propensity of teaching hospitals for attracting more severely ill patients. In a study that used a variety of case-mix measures (including DRGs and staging), they reported that case-mix differences between teaching and nonteaching hospitals were found only when the case-mix measure was based upon resource use; however, when a clinically oriented patient classification system was used, case-mix differences between teaching hospitals (except for medical school–based hospitals in two instances) and nonteaching hospitals were not discernible at conventional levels of significance (p < .05). Accordingly, Goldfarb and Coffey argue that some of the observed cost differences between teaching and nonteaching hospitals may be due to variations in physician practices resulting in a bias toward resource-intensive patient management in teaching hospitals. They support their argument with evidence from their study, which indicates that, when compared to nonteaching programs, teaching activities increase the length of stay, the use of surgery, the number of procedures, and the relative resource intensity of procedures regardless of case-mix adjustments. However, the conclusion is at variance with an earlier study (Becker and Sloan 1983), which employed a resource-related variable, the RNI, to control case-mix in the multivariate analysis.

Goldfarb and Coffey cite a number of problems that limit the usefulness of their results for policy deliberations concerning the compensation of teaching hospitals. First, the data are old, and treatment patterns that existed when the data were collected in 1977 may have changed over time with the advent of prospective payment and changes in medical science. Second, the cell sizes for some categories of teaching hospitals were small, resulting in unreliable estimates. Third, consistent with our discussion in Chapter 5, discharge abstract data in the 1970s were often very unreliable. Thus, although the evidence presented by Goldfarb and Coffey has provoked some rethinking of the conventional wisdom about the patient-mix of teaching hospitals, it is obvious that more research, which would correct the weaknesses they outlined, is needed.

Concerns regarding equitable payments for teaching hospitals have stimulated research about the indirect costs of educational programs. The magnitude of these costs reflects the important policy implications of this issue. For example, the federal government's decision to fund hospitals for the indirect costs of medical education resulted in over \$2 billion of expenditures by the Medicare program in 1985 (Anderson and Lave 1986). Furthermore, in this period of a perceived physician surplus, funding policy for medical education has profound implications for the number and distribution of medical residency programs.

In recognition of the association between teaching activities and case-mix, the HCFA (Health Care Financing Administration) conducted a study to determine if teaching hospitals incurred greater inpatient operating costs per case than nonteaching hospitals after controlling for case-mix by using the DRG Index and other factors (i.e., wages, number of beds, and size of city). The ratio of interns to beds was used to measure teaching activities. The regression equations revealed that the expected inpatient operating costs per case would be increased by 0.574 percent for every additional unit increase in its intern to bed ratio. Significant and positive coefficients were also estimated for the DRG case-mix index, wages, beds and the dummy variable for location in an area with population greater than 1 million (Pettengill and Vertrees 1982). These results suggest that an adjustment for *indirect medical education expenses* equal to the coefficient of the teaching activity variable would be inadequate for large hospitals or hospitals located in major metropolitan areas, characteristics that are highly correlated with large graduate medical education programs (Anderson and Lave 1986). Accordingly, Congress authorized the indirect medical adjustment to be 11.59 times the intern/bed ratio, an amount twice as large as the teaching activity coefficient. Anderson and Lave (1986) suggest that this apparently generous adjustment is attributable to doubts about the ability of the DRG patient classification system to account fully for factors such as the severity of illness of patients requiring the specialized services of teaching hospitals.

Using the same data base as HCFA, but employing a variety of model specifications, Anderson and Lave also demonstrated a significant association between the cost per admission and the ratio of interns to beds. They also reported, however, that the teaching activity coefficient varied by as much as 72 percent, depending upon the specification of the model. Since some specifications of the model included proxies for case-mix severity (i.e., percentage of population that is indigent) that had significant coefficients, they concluded that the current Medicare prospective pricing mechanism does not adequately compensate hospitals that have a more severe case-mix.

Welch (1987) also used the HCFA data and built upon the regression equation formulated by Anderson and Lave by adding some variables (i.e., number of patients transferred to the hospital and presence of open-heart surgery, organ transplant, and burn unit), which he argues reflect the severity of a hospital's case mix. Welch reports a positive and significant coefficient for the variable reflecting the ratio of interns and residents to beds and for patient transfers; however, the service variables, which probably fail to measure severity with precision, were not significant. In the equation in which a variable reflecting major teaching status was added, the coefficient of the variable that measured the ratio of interns and residents to beds dropped from .48 to .38. Welch cited these findings as evidence that supports his argument that only hospitals with extensive teaching commitments should receive additional payments under the Medicare prospective payment system.

Three other studies (Barer 1982; Rosko 1982; Salkever, Steinwachs, and Rupp 1986) provide evidence pertaining to the indirect costs of medical education. Employing an information theory approach suggested by Evans and Walker (1972) to control case-mix differences, Barer (1982) removed direct educational costs from the left side of the regression equation and found that a 1 percent increase in the ratio of educational expense to total inpatient expenses increased inpatient cost per case by $11 to $20, estimates that were significant $(p < 0.05)$. Since the dependent variable did not include the direct expenses of medical education, Barer suggests that these coefficients can be interpreted as the impact of teaching programs on what are often considered indirect medical education costs. Salkever, Steinwachs, and Rupp (1986) estimated regression equations for a number of dependent variables. In the total routine costs equation, the estimated coefficient of residents per bed was 3.38 $(p > 0.05)$, but in the ancillary cost equation, the coefficient was 329.9 $(p < 0.05)$. Assuming that the case-mix variables that they employed were sufficient to isolate the impact of patient needs on ancillary costs, the value of the residents per bed coefficients suggest that teaching programs contribute to increases in ancillary costs beyond that which might be attributable to case-mix. These findings are corroborated by Rosko's (1982) study, which reported that the value of the coefficient of the binary variable for teaching programs was much higher in the ancillary cost per admission equation (174.4) than in the routine cost per admission equation (128.8).

In contrast to the conventional wisdom, Hosek and Palmer (1983) suggested that intern and residency programs can result in savings. They argued that interns and residents have been substituted for more expensive physicians and in the absence of substantial differences in the efficiency of these two types of inputs, the costs of intermediate products and services (e.g., X rays used in the treatment and diagnosis of patients) have been reduced. Hosek and Palmer tested this hypothesis by using a data set consisting of cost and case-mix information compiled from the radiology departments in 90 Veterans Administration (VA) hospitals to estimate the determinants of total noncapital costs. The authors reported that radiology residency programs reduced the marginal costs of four of six primary outputs; however, only in the case of special examinations that were performed at the bedside or in the operating room was there a positive and significant relationship between costs and the existence of a radiological residency program. Hosek and Palmer also found that adding one resident, while holding the departments output-mix constant, would reduce the costs in hospitals that were already operating teaching programs by $1,700; adding one radiological resident in what was previously a nonteaching hospital would increase costs by $474 if this change did not affect the hospital's output-mix. This *ceteris paribus* assumption, however, is not realistic (Ament et al. 1981; Becker and Steinwald 1981; Sloan et al. 1983). Indeed, Hosek and Palmer (1983, p. 46) concluded that even though teaching programs may reduce primary product costs, their expenses may still be higher than nonteaching hospitals because of "differences in case-mix, case difficulty, medical techniques, or perceived quality of care."

In summary, our review of recent evidence supports the conventional wisdom that teaching hospitals are more expensive than nonteaching hospitals; however, studies that have used the RNI case-mix index found that, once case-mix differences are controlled, the cost differences between teaching and nonteaching hospitals decline dramatically. Unfortunately, a large scale analysis of the impact of teaching programs on hospital costs has not been conducted while using one of the more refined case-severity measures (i.e., Horn, Sharkey, and Bertram 1983; Young 1984). Hosek and Palmer's contention that the use of medical interns and residents as lower-priced substitutes can reduce primary production costs received some corroboration by Sloan and associates (1983), who found a negative but insignificant relationship between residency programs and the expenditures of radiology departments. Results from the same study, however, found the expenses in pathology departments are higher in major teaching hospitals. Accordingly, the results of Hosek and Palmer may not be generalizable beyond radiology departments in VA hospitals. Certainly, their study raises some interesting questions that should be addressed in future research in other departments of a representative sample of U.S. hospitals.

Medical Staff Organization and Composition

The studies reviewed so far in this chapter have taken a "black box" approach that ignores the internal organization of production within the hospital. This approach is consistent with most studies conducted by economists in other industries. Analysts can ignore the inner workings of firms in competitive industries without causing harm to the study, because firms with inefficient operating characteristics are eventually eliminated by the forces of the marketplace. In contrast, the structure of the hospital industry is influenced by a number of factors (i.e., not-for-profit orientation, consumer ignorance, regulation, and reimbursement policies) that tend to reduce competitive pressures. Thus, unlike highly competitive industries, a sizable amount of variation in organizational structures might exist between hospitals. Accordingly, the impact of organizational structure on costs is an important area for policy analysts to understand so that more relevant public policies can be formulated. Methodologists should also find results from this area of inquiry to be helpful in developing more realistic models of hospital behavior. Despite appealing reasons to study organizational determinants of costs, only size, teaching status, and ownership measures have been routinely incorporated in empirical research. The absence of variables pertaining to more specific dimensions of organizational structure can be attributed to a lack of a conceptual framework as well as the difficulty of obtaining this type of data.

Most of the detailed analysis inside the hospital's "black box" has examined medical staff characteristics. Pauly (1978) and Sloan and Becker (1981) conducted the most comprehensive multivariate studies of the relationship between medical staff characteristics and hospital costs (see Table 8.2). Shortell, Morrisey, and Conrad (1985) did not study costs; nevertheless, their study of hospital-physician relationships provides useful supplementary information. The following dimensions of medical staff characteristics and organizational structure have been examined: (1) compensation arrangements, (2) departmentalization, (3) governance and policy formulation, (4) medical staff composition, and (5) concentration of admissions.

Regarding the first dimension, a great deal of speculation has been expressed about the incentives provided to physicians by compensation arrangements. Many proponents of health maintenance organizations have criticized fee-for-service payments as inflationary because they induce physicians to provide unnecessary services.

Sloan and Becker (1981) found no association between the proportion of salaried hospital-based physicians (i.e., anesthesiologists, pathologists, and radiologists) and nonphysician expenses per adjusted admission. Further, contrary to their expectations, they found that costs were directly related to the proportion of non–hospital-based physicians who were on a salaried contract. One is tempted to attribute this seemingly anomalous result to observed correlations between the proportion of medical staff paid on a salary basis and case-mix (Shortell, Morrisey, and Conrad 1985). However patient-mix was controlled by the inclusion of a direct case-mix variable (the RNI) and a set of indirect case-mix variables (i.e., three teaching variables). Sloan and Becker suggested that the counterintuitive results were observed because the potential cost savings from having salaried medical staff were offset by the costs of the added bureaucracy needed to support the salaried physicians.

The second dimension of the organization of the medical staff is the degree of departmentalization. Sloan and Becker (1981) hypothesized that by organizing physicians into smaller groups, costs are controlled because a departmental structure: (1) subdivides the medical staff into much smaller groups, in which individual actions are more easily observed; (2) facilitates monitoring, to the extent that medical technology is more homogeneous within disciplinary fields; and (3) provides a unit in which a control and authority system can be derived consistently with the physician's discipline. Contrary to their expectations, all of the variables measuring degree of departmentalization were significantly ($p < 0.05$) related to cost increases.

The third dimension of medical staff organization, governance and policy formulation, included physician membership on the governing board, as well as the number of medical staff committees. The percentage of hospitals having active staff physicians as voting members of the governing board increased from 38.4 percent in 1972 to 81.7 percent in 1981 (Shortell, Morrisey, and Conrad 1985). Sloan and Becker (1981) found that hospitals with physicians on the governing board tended to have lower costs. This may be due to the stimulation of physician cost consciousness associated with medical staff participation on the governing board.

Another aspect of governance is measured by the number and type of medical staff committees. Between 1972 and 1981, the average number of medical staff committees increased from 5.4 to 14.7. It is interesting to note that in 1981, 20 percent of hospitals in states with a high degree of restrictiveness in their certificate-of-need regulation had cost containment or cost awareness committees in which physicians participated, a percentage that is significantly higher than that in hospitals operating in other states ($F = 6.34$, $p \leq .002$). Similarly, 21 percent of hospitals in states that operated highly regulated rate review programs had cost containment and/or cost awareness committees with physician members, versus only 13 percent of hospitals operating in less regulated environments (Shortell, Morrisey, and Conrad 1985). Although no correlations with costs have been performed, there is a very plausible relationship between the existence of these committees and cost control.

The fourth dimension of medical staff characteristics is composition, which has been measured by specialty mix variables and by the age of admitting physicians. Staff composition can influence hospital costs in two ways. First, the specialty mix of the medical staff undoubtedly affects the case-mix of the hospital. Second, the composition of the medical staff may predispose physicians to be more (or less) cost conscious. We have already discussed the impact of case-mix on hospital costs. Further, the studies reviewed in this section include variables that are designed to isolate the effects of case-mix from those of medical staff on hospital costs. Accordingly, we will restrict our discussion in this section to the effects of style or cost-orientation that may be associated with the composition of the medical staff.

Pauly (1978) reported that, relative to general practitioners as primary attending physicians, total hospital costs and the costs per case are higher if the primary attending physician specializes in pediatrics or internal medicine. Costs are lower if the primary attending physician is a general surgeon or a specialist in an area other than surgery or medicine. Costs are unaffected if the attending physician is a specialist in OB-GYN, otorhinology, or a surgical discipline. Although these results may indicate that specialty variables are better proxies for case-mix than the output variables employed in this study, they may also indicate that the cost-influencing aspects of practice style vary by specialty. Indeed, Pauly speculated that surgeons are likely to be more hospital-oriented than internists, pediatricians, or general practitioners because hospital care is more important to their practices. Therefore, surgeons, if they are more hospital-oriented, may be more concerned about excessive hospital costs. Further, since they use the hospital more frequently, surgeons may be better monitors of hospital activity, a factor that may allow surgeons to control costs more effectively than other specialists. It is important to reiterate that Pauly's findings pertain to the relative number of physicians in each specialty and thus should not be confused with the results from studies discussed in the chapters on demand and inflation, which measured the effects of increasing the physician-population ratio.

The last dimension of medical staff organization that we will consider is output concentration among physicians. A number of economists have hypothesized that if output is divided among fewer doctors and some costs are common, there should be a greater motivation and more ability to minimize costs. This is the well-known "size principle" (Olson 1962; Pauly and Redisch 1973; Pauly 1978). As expected, concentration of admissions is inversely related to the size of the hospital. In 1981, the top five admitters, in hospitals with fewer than 100 beds, accounted for 67 percent of admissions, while for hospitals in the 300 to 400 bed category, the top five admitters accounted for 17.6 percent of all admissions (Shortell, Morrisey, and Conrad 1985). Pauly (1978), who used the Herfindahl index to measure output concentration, found the expected inverse relationship between costs and concentration of admissions. Corroborative evidence is provided by an earlier study by Shortell, Becker, and Neuhauser (1976).

Union Activities

The labor intensive character of hospitals has prompted concerns that the rise of union activity in hospitals may result in substantial cost increases. In this section, we will provide a brief historical sketch of organized labor activity in hospitals, followed by an assessment of the impact of unions on hospital costs.

The National Labor Relations Act (NLRA) of 1935, popularly known as the Wagner Act, is the major federal law governing labor relations in the United States. Although this law initially included all private hospitals, the Taft-Hartley Amendment of 1947 exempted private, nonprofit hospitals from NLRA coverage. Thus, collective bargaining in these hospitals remained under the purview of state governments; however, few states filled the vacuum created by the Taft-Hartley Amendment. In 1974, the year in which the enactment of Public Law 93–360 amended the NLRA to place private hospitals under the jurisdiction of the NLRA, only 12 states had enacted laws to regulate hospital union activity (Becker, Sloan, and Steinwald 1982). In contrast, federal jurisdiction over union activity in hospitals was strengthened in 1962 when President John F. Kennedy signed Executive Order 10988, which established procedures for collective bargaining in federal hospitals.

Table 8.5

Hospitals with One or More Collective Bargaining Contracts, by Hospital Ownership, Selected Years, 1961–1980

Year	Percentage of Hospitals With Contracts		
	Federal Hospitals	Non-Federal Hospitals	All Hospitals
1961	0.0	3.4	3.2
1967	22.6	7.3	8.2
1970	51.9	13.3	15.7
1973	67.7	16.7	19.9
1975	77.0	19.2	22.8
1977	77.2	20.6	23.5
1980	86.1	23.8	27.4

Source: Becker, E., F. Sloan and B. Steinwald. 1982. "Union activity in hospitals: past, present and future." Health Care Financing Review 3(4):1-13.

The data summarized in Table 8.5 indicate the percentage of hospitals with one or more collective bargaining agreements and suggests that the growth in union activity in federal hospitals was stimulated by Executive Order 10988. Contrary to the expectations of many labor experts, little union growth in private hospitals was associated with the passage of the NLRA Amendments in 1974. In fact, the annual growth rate of hospitals with one or more unions was actually greater in the period from 1970 to 1973 (7.9 percent) than during 1975 to 1980 (3.6 percent). However, since the data on hospital unions summarized by Becker et al. (1982) does not include the number of employees who are represented by unions, it is possible that the growth of hospital union membership may have been understated.

Although the growth of hospitals with collective bargaining agreements slowed during the 1970s, many analysts feel that union activity in hospitals will be vigorous through the 1980s. Feldman, Lee, and Hoffbeck (1980) developed a number of multivariate models and predicted that about 65 percent of all hospitals will have one or more union contracts by 1990. Becker et al. (1982) wrote that this figure should be revised downward to about 45 to 50 percent.

The expansion of union activity into hospitals is expected to be inflationary because unions tend to extract higher wages without an offsetting increase in productivity. As summarized in Table 8.6, most studies have estimated a positive effect of unions on the compensation of their membership in hospitals. Consistent with the belief that registered nurses are attracted to unions for professional reasons, the impact of unions on wages appears to be the strongest for non-professional employees.

Although unions increase average compensation rates, union activities could actually reduce total hospital costs if productivity increases exceed compensation increases. Studies in other industries have found that unionization has increased factor productivity by 6 to 20 percent (Mandelstamm 1965; Frantz 1976; Brown and Medoff 1978; Clark 1980a, 1980b). Analyses of hospitals, however, indicate that unionization has increased costs by as much as 10 percent (Miller, Becker, and Krinsky 1979; Adamache and Sloan 1982; Salkever 1982, 1984), results that suggest that unionization has not improved the productivity of hospital inputs.

Further, contrary to the experience of other industries, Salkever (1982) found that the nonwage impact comprised two-thirds of the total union influence on hospital costs. Also of interest is the finding that the unions representing registered nurses and service employees have a smaller impact on costs than other unions.

Another noteworthy result is that the effect of unions on wages goes beyond their own bargaining unit. Adamache and Sloan (1982) reported significant "internal spillover effects" in which the presence of unions in one bargaining unit of the hospital positively affected the wages of other workers in the hospital. They also reported the existence of "external spillover effects" in which wages in one hospital were positively affected by the presence of unions in other area hospitals. Both results are consistent with the commonly held opinion that employers attempt to prevent union activity in their organization by matching pay

Table 8.6
Estimated Impact of Unions on Wages in Selected Hospital Occupations

Study	Occupation	Union Impact On Wages (percent)
Sloan and Elnicki (1979)	registered nurses	0 to 4
Sloan and Steinwald (1980b)	registered nurses	8
Feldman and Scheffler (1982)	registered nurses	3
Adamache and Sloan (1982)	registered nurses	4 to 11
Fottler (1977)	non-professional workers	4.5 to 8.2
Feldman and Scheffler (1982)	secretaries and housekeepers	11 to 12
Sloan and Steinwald (1980b)	non-professional occupations	4.9 to 17.6
Adamache and Sloan (1982)	non-professional occupations	6 to 17

increases gained by unions elsewhere. Since unions tend to organize in large hospitals and urban hospitals (Becker, Sloan, and Steinwald 1982), spillover effects provide another explanation for the positive coefficients usually associated with variables representing these characteristics.

Competition with Other Hospitals

The debate about the relative roles of competition and regulation in the health care industry has raised a considerable amount of interest about the impact of market structure on the performance of health care providers. Standard economic theory suggests that increased competition may force hospitals to vie for patients by reducing costs. On the other hand, recognizing the peculiarities of health care, as well as the experience of other service industries (e.g., hospitality and banking), some health economists argue that hospitals are likely to engage in nonprice competition, which might result in higher costs (Robinson and Luft 1987). Nonprice competition might be based on the three nonpecuniary dimensions of the marketing mix: service development, distribution policy, and advertising (Hillestad and Berkowitz 1984).

Unfortunately, the debate over the impact of market structure on hospital performance has generated more essays than sound empirical studies. Robinson and Luft (1985) have filled capably some of this vacuum by initiating the most sophisticated stream of research in this area of inquiry. Unlike others who used geopolitical areas such as counties to define market areas, Robinson and Luft operationalized the degree of competition as the number of hospitals within 15 miles of the study hospital. This measure was entered into the regression equation as four dummy variables (i.e., one neighbor, two to four neighbors, five to ten neighbors, and more than ten neighbors within 15 miles). In addition, they controlled for physician supply, case-mix, institutional size, capacity utilization, input costs, and regional patterns of medical care.

Using a national sample of community hospitals ($n = 5,013$) that reported data to the AHA in 1972, Robinson and Luft estimated separate sets of regression equations. One set included only indirect measures of case-mix, i.e., medical school affiliation, ratio of interns and residents to beds, and for-profit status. The other set of equations included these indirect measures as well as 17 case-mix variables (i.e., percentage of patients in seven diagnostic categories or percentage of patients in ten procedure-related categories). When direct case-mix measures were added to the equation with indirect case-mix variables, the R^2 increased slightly from 0.67 to 0.75, suggesting a high degree of correlation between the two sets of variables.

In each set of equations, a monotonically increasing relationship was found between average costs and the number of neighboring hospitals. This relationship contradicts standard economic theory, which predicts that hospitals will produce services more efficiently as competition is increased. Robinson and Luft suggest that hospitals respond to an increased number of competitors by increasing the intensity of hospital technology resulting in a "medical arms race." Using a similar group of independent variables on a set of data collected from a national sample ($n = 5,732$) of hospitals in 1982, Robinson and Luft (1987) once again found that hospitals in markets with more competitors tend to incur higher costs per admission. Joskow (1980) provides results that do not address costs directly but which, nevertheless, support Robinson and Luft's position regarding nonprice competition. He suggests that the stochastic nature of demand induces hospitals to reserve excess capacity to serve as safety stock for unanticipated surges in demand. Joskow argues that in a heavily insured marketplace in which consumers are price-insensitive, hospitals use safety stock to compete with other hospitals for patients and their admitting physicians. This argument is plausible because, *ceteris paribus*, patients and physicians are likely to prefer hospitals that provide greater access. Thus, hospitals are hypothesized by Joskow to respond to an increase in the number of competitors by increasing their safety stock. As expected, Joskow's multivariate analysis found that safety stock or reserve margin was directly related to the intensity of competition. The conclusion was corroborated by Mulligan (1985), who tested an alternate specification of Joskow's model on the same data set. Joskow argues that reserve margins are a surrogate for quality and quantity. Therefore, policies designed to facilitate entry and promote competition among hospitals in a price-insensitive market may exert undesirable consequences on the costs of hospital care. Joskow's analysis is weakened by the absence of a variable reflecting the proportion of admissions that are elective or the proportion of patients with life-threatening problems, factors affecting safety stock requirements.

Luft, Robinson, Garnick, Maerki, and McPhee (1986) also report evidence that supports the nonprice competition hypothesis. Using data for 3,584 community hospitals responding to a survey in 1972, they found that for most of 29 specialized clinical services, the probability of a hospital possessing a service is positively related to the number of neighboring hospitals.

A few studies provide evidence that weakens the support for the nonprice competition hypothesis. Romeo, Wagner, and Lee (1984) used 1980 data for the presence of five technologies in 469 hospitals located in Indiana, Maryland, and New York. They reported that the coefficient of their Herfindahl index (a commonly used measure of the degree of competition) was insignificant ($p >$ .05) in two of three equations for cost-enhancing technologies; the Herfindahl index was positive and significant in one of two equations estimated for cost-reducing technologies. Similar results were found by Lee and Waldman (1985), who studied the same hospitals but employed a different estimation technique. Sloan, Valvona, and Perrin (1986) examined the diffusion of five surgical technologies in 521 hospitals during the period 1972 to 1981. They found that the adoption of three of the five technologies was negatively associated ($p < .01$) with the intensity of competition (i.e., beds in other hospitals divided by county population). The competition variable had an insignificant coefficient ($p > .10$) in the equations estimated for the other two surgical procedures. It is important to note that in these studies (unlike Robinson and Luft who developed competition in terms of small market areas), variables depicting the intensity of competition were constructed by using the county as the market area. Given the wide variation in the size of counties and the frequent presence of nearby competitors who are located across political boundaries, it is clear that Robinson and Luft used the most accurate measure of hospital competition.

The weight of the evidence indicates that in heavily insured markets, an increased number of competitors is associated with higher hospital costs. However, we are not sure what type of competitive strategies are responsible for the increased costs. For example, only mixed support is available for the commonly cited *medical arms race hypothesis*. Alternatively, one might argue that these studies have measured external spillover effects of unions in nearby hospitals rather than the effects of competitive behavior (Adamache and Sloan 1982).

It is clear that the relationship between market structure and hospital performance should be explored in more detail. Most of the evidence pertains to the period before 1983. It is reasonable to expect hospitals to engage in vigorous nonprice competition when confronted with an environment in the 1970s that was dominated by cost-based reimbursement and few alternative delivery systems. However, the increased dependence upon prospective payment and the proliferation of alternate delivery systems that characterize the 1980s clearly alters this expectation. For example, Salkever, Steinwachs, and Rupp (1986), who conducted a study of the performance of hospitals in the Maryland prospective payment system, reported that inpatient cost per case was not associated ($p > .10$) with the intensity of competition; and Vitaliano (1987) found an insignificant ($t = 1.16$) association between market share and the costs of hospitals that operated under the New York prospective payment system in 1981. Accordingly, we are anxious to see the results of more studies conducted in an environment characterized by extensive reliance on rate regulation and the proliferation of alternate delivery systems. To date, most research has focused on the impact of HMO growth, a subject we will discuss in Chapter 11.

Other Determinants of Hospital Costs

We conclude our discussion of the determinants of hospital costs with a review of studies that examined the effects of ownership, control, organizational structure, and location on costs. The growth of proprietary hospitals, which increased from 3.5 percent of all hospital beds in the United States in 1960 to 8.3 percent of all beds in 1986, has created considerable controversy (American Hospital Association 1987). Proponents of investor-owned hospitals argue that the profit-motive creates incentives for these hospitals to operate more efficiently. The lower average costs and a shorter average length of stay are often cited as examples of the efficiency of proprietary hospitals. Critics claim that the values of these performance measures have occurred more from a selection of preferred patients, often termed "cream-skimming," than from greater efficiency (Relman 1980). Since an in-depth analysis of these and other issues is provided in a recently published book (Institute of Medicine 1986), we will limit our review of the performance of proprietary hospitals to a few recently published studies.

If lower costs per admission or length of stay are due solely to differences in case-mix, then these differences should disappear when case-mix is controlled in a multivariate analysis. However, mixed results are found in regression equations in which the average cost per admission served as the dependent variable and case-mix measures were used as independent variables. Some studies (Coelen and Sullivan 1981; Cowing and Holtmann 1983; Salkever 1984; Robinson and Luft 1985) found that proprietary hospitals were less expensive than not-for-profit hospitals, while negative but insignificant ($p < 0.05$) coefficients for the proprietary hospital variable were estimated by others (Sloan and Steinwald 1980b; Sloan and Becker 1981; Hornbrook and Monheit 1985). Two studies (Grannemann, Brown, and Pauly 1986; Institute of Medicine 1986) found that for-profit hospitals are more expensive than not-for-profit hospitals.

Becker and Sloan (1985) found that investor-owned hospitals that had recently entered multihospital systems (MHS) were more expensive than independent not-for-profit hospitals; they found that insignificant coefficients, however, were estimated for investor-owned hospitals that were either independent or had been in a MHS for more than four years. Further, when only ownership variables were entered in the cost per admission equation, the R^2 equaled 0.03, which was much less than the explanatory power ($R^2 = 0.68$) of the fully specified behavioral cost function. These results suggest that ownership has little impact on costs.

Analysis of differences in the length of stay between proprietary and not-for-profit hospitals may shed some light on the ''cream-skimming'' hypothesis. Freund, Shachtman, Ruffin, and Quade (1985), using a national probability-based sample of hospitals, found that the average length of stay was shorter in investor-owned hospitals (8.3 days) than in not-for-profit hospitals (9.6 days); however, the coefficient of the dummy variable for proprietary hospitals was insignificant ($p < 0.05$) in each of ten alternate specifications of regression equations in which length of stay, adjusted for case-mix, was used as the dependent variable. This result suggests that the shorter length of stay in investor-owned hospitals is due to differences in case-mix rather than to differences in efficiency in patient management. The conclusions advanced by Freund et al. are contradicted by Robinson and Luft (1985), who found that, even after including indirect and direct case-mix measures, the average length of stay was 10.6 percent shorter in proprietary hospitals than in not-for-profit hospitals. Worthington and Piro (1982), who used only indirect measures of case-mix, estimated coefficients of a similar magnitude. Thus, the controversy about investor-owned hospitals remains unresolved. Although proprietary hospitals may be slightly less expensive than not-for-profit hospitals, it is unclear whether these differences are due to case-mix, efficiency, or other factors.

Another possible structural determinant of hospital costs is membership in a multihospital system. In light of a recent review of studies pertaining to multi-hospital systems (Ermann and Gabel 1985), we will provide only a brief discussion of this cost determinant. Ermann and Gabel cited three possible advantages that system-affiliated hospitals have over independent hospitals: (1) economic benefits such as easier access to capital, increased efficiency, and economies of scale; (2) human resource benefits such as improved recruiting and ability to develop and retain high-caliber staff; and (3) greater ability to control environmental factors. Unfortunately, there is little empirical evidence to support these claims. We expect that two trends will result in more future research in this area. First, multihospital systems have become an important organizational structure in the hospital industry, representing one-third of all hospitals in the United States in 1982 (Ermann and Gabel 1985). Second, with the advent of annual surveys by the AHA in 1979, an easily accessible source of archival data has become available.

Ermann and Gable reviewed eighteen empirical studies that examined the influence of system-affiliation on hospital costs and concluded that the bulk of the evidence suggests that system affiliation results in an increase in hospital costs (on a per diem, per admission, or per capita basis), particularly during the years following a merger. These higher costs have been associated with capital expenditures required to modernize or expand the facilities of hospitals that joined the system. A recent study (Renn, Schramm, Watt, and Derzon 1985) used a national probability-based sample and provided different results. Costs per admission in system-affiliated hospitals were not significantly different than those in freestanding, not-for-profit hospitals. This regression equation, however, did not control for case-mix, a variable that Renn et al. (1985) found in another analysis to be negatively associated ($p < 0.05$) with investor-owned chains.

Many cost studies have included a binary variable for public hospitals with mixed results. Positive and significant coefficients have been estimated by Sloan and Steinwald (1980b), Sloan and Becker (1981), Salkever (1984), and Robinson and Luft (1985). These results support the contention that public hospitals are the victims of "patient dumping" or have liberal admission policies regarding low-income/high-risk patients who tend to have more complex needs.

In contrast, Grannemann, Brown, and Pauly (1986) reported a negative and significant coefficient for the variable representing public hospitals. These results may be an artifact of the sample, the model specification (i.e., a quasi-technological, flexible cost function), or the possibility that public hospitals respond to tight budget constraints by operating more efficiently and providing services of a quality that is less than nonpublic hospitals. Corroborative evidence for this position is provided by Hornbrook and Monheit (1985).

The last determinant of hospital costs we shall consider is location, a variable that has been entered frequently in behavioral cost functions to reflect differences in costs between urban and rural hospitals. Controversies about the existence of a substantial urban/rural payment differential (i.e., an average of about 25 percent) in the Medicare prospective payment system stimulated research to determine if continuation of this practice is justified.

A number of studies found a positive association between cost per admission and location in an urban area (Pettengill and Vertrees 1982; Anderson and Lave 1986; Cromwell, Mitchell, Calore, and Iezzoni 1987). Similar results were found when variables (i.e., population density, total population) correlated with metropolitan locations were used instead of an urban binary variable (Sloan and Steinwald 1980b; Watts and Klastorin 1980; Melnick, Wheeler, and Feldstein 1981; Sloan, Feldman, and Steinwald 1983; Rosko and Broyles 1987). It is not clear, however, why urban hospitals are more expensive than their rural counterparts. Some possible explanations for this cost differential include: nonprice competition among hospitals in close proximity, external union spillover effects, differences in case-mix severity, differences in input prices, and differences in efficiency.

Summary of Hospital Cost Determinants

In spite of a substantial amount of research, conclusive statements about the determinants of hospital costs are not possible. The bulk of the evidence indicates that costs are higher in teaching hospitals and government hospitals; however, the extra costs incurred by these types of hospitals are due more to case-mix and teaching activities than to other factors such as inefficiency. Hospital costs tend to be inversely related to physician participation on the governing board and the concentration of discharges among physicians and directly related to the presence of unions. The relationship between costs and other factors such as economies of scale, economies of scope, ownership (i.e., proprietary vs. not-for-profit), and other medical staff characteristics (compensation arrangements, average age of physicians, and specialty mix) are unclear, being obscured by methodological problems. In addition, evidence from studies reviewed in other chapters suggests that hospital costs are directly related to case-mix and input prices. On the other hand, as we will see in Chapter 12, prospective payment systems have restrained cost increases, while capital controls and utilization review have not been successful cost-containment mechanisms.

Although we are encouraged by the increased sophistication and rigor of recent hospital cost studies, we are not optimistic about the resolution of all of the technical problems facing those who wish to estimate cost functions in this industry. In particular, the development of case-mix measures that can be used to reflect the multiproduct nature of hospitals with precision has been slow and uncertain.

NURSING HOME COST FUNCTIONS

In this section, we will discuss the determinants of nursing home costs. As our review will show, research in the area has been less extensive, less sophisticated and more recent than in the hospital industry. In contrast to analysis of hospitals, with one exception (Ullmann and Holtmann 1985) only behavioral cost functions have been estimated for nursing homes. Since the estimation of nursing home cost functions has paralleled the estimation of behavioral cost functions in hospitals, a detailed discussion of the technical issues is not needed. Accordingly, the focus of the following sections will be on empirical results pertaining to the factors that influence the costs of nursing homes. Results from recent nursing home cost function studies are summarized in Table 8.7. Comprehensive reviews of earlier studies are found in Bishop (1980) and Birnbaum, Bishop, Lee, and Jensen (1981).

Volume and Rate of Output

Production of nursing home services may be viewed as a two-dimensional process with volume and rate aspects. The *volume effect* pertains to the capacity for which the nursing home is designed and is a relevant consideration only if scale economies are present in the industry. The *rate effect* is related to the intensity with which a facility of a particular size is used. A nursing home with a low occupancy rate is likely to incur higher than average costs because fixed costs are spread over fewer patient days. Conversely, a nursing home with an extremely high occupancy rate may experience higher than normal costs because capital is used too intensely relative to other factor inputs.

As summarized in a review of early cost function studies (Birnbaum et al. 1981), most research findings suggest that scale economies are minimal in the nursing home industry and that there are no pronounced scale effects beyond 40 beds. Most studies reported an insignificant coefficient for beds in the cost per patient day equation; studies with significant ($p < 0.05$) coefficients reported per diem cost differentials ranging from $-\$0.03$ to $\$0.007$ per extra bed.

Findings from Birnbaum et al. (1981); Meiners (1982); Traxler (1982); Ullmann (1984); Holahan (1985); and Sulvetta and Holahan (1986) support the hypothesized relationship between occupancy rate and average costs. Meiners reported that a 1 percent increase in the occupancy rate reduced average cost by about 2.7 percent; however, these cost savings approach zero as the occupancy rate approaches 100 percent. Although the results by Birnbaum et al. differ by state, their results suggest that average costs tend to decrease as occupancy rate increases, up to 97 percent. Beyond this point, average costs tend to increase.

Product Mix

Although it is likely that differences in product-mix will cause nursing home costs to vary, it has been difficult to define and measure the output of nursing homes. Three general types of product descriptors have been used: (1) certified level of care, (2) measures of service availability and intensity, and (3) patient characteristics.

Certified Level of Care

The Medicaid program has established criteria to categorize nursing homes into facilities that are capable of providing different levels of care. It is reasonable to assume that skilled nursing facilities (SNFs), which must meet higher standards than intermediate care facilities (ICFs), will experience greater average costs. The price differential is probably due to case-mix variations as well as differences in input utilization associated with the different standards set for these two types of long-term care facilities. This is further complicated in that each state is free to set SNF/ICF standards as long as they are consistent with loosely defined federal conditions of participation for SNFs and standards for ICFs. A number of studies have reported that certified level of care affects costs per day by an amount ranging from $\$2.55$ to $\$11.20$ (Bishop 1980; Ruchlin and Levy 1972; and Meiners 1982). Comparison of rates, however, is only appropriate for intrastate study and loses validity when utilizing aggregated interstate data that does not control for the definition of SNFs, which varies across states.

Services

Birnbaum et al. (1981) report that services provided, including occupational therapy (OT), physical therapy (PT), and nursing hours per patient day had a

Table 8.7
Summary of Recent Nursing Home Behavioral Cost Function Studies

Author, Year	Sample	Dependent Variables
Frech and Ginsburg, 1981	National cross-section data for 600 nursing homes located in urban areas in 1974.	Total operating expenses.
Holahan, 1985	Cross-section of data from nursing homes in 10 states during 1978-1980.	Percentage change in cost per day from 1978 to 1980.
Meiners, 1982	National cross-section data for 1147 nursing homes in 1974.	Total cost per patient day.
Smith and Fottler, 1981	Cross-section of 43 nursing homes in Southern California during 1979.	Costs per patient day.

Table 8.7 (continued)

Independent Variables	Primary Results

Input prices for labor and capital
Patient days
Index of services provided
Index of patient debility
Dummy variables for:
  for-profit status,
  6 types of Medicaid
    reimbursement systems,
  ownership/reimbursement
    interactions.
	Government-owned homes are the most expensive. Private non-profit homes are more expensive than for-profit homes in states with flat rate reimbursement but not elsewhere.
	
	Pure cost reimbursement systems (without ceiling) are associated with the highest costs. Homes in this type of system cost 21% more than those in simple flat-rate systems.
	
	Patient mix did not vary by ownership status.

Occupancy rate
Percent Medicare patients
Beds
Admissions per bed
Dummy variables for:
  ownership,
  location,
  prospective reimbursement,
  flat rate reimbursement,
  retrospective reimbursement.
	Lower cost increases are associated with:
	  for-profit status,
	  chain membership,
	  rural location,
	  higher occupancy rate,
	  and prospective payment.
	
	Higher cost increases are associated with:
	  size, admissions per bed,
	  and retrospective
	  reimbursement.

5 output/capacity measures
6 input price/location measures
Ownership status
Type of Medicaid reimbursement
  system
Level of certification
Service level indicators
12 resident characteristics
  variables, derived from ADLs
  and types of services
  received.
	Weak returns to scale,
	  least cost size is
	  330 beds.
	For-profit hospitals are
	  least costly.
	Prospective payment contains
	  costs.
	Chain membership does not
	  affect costs.
	Patients who score very high
	  or low on ADL are less costly.
	Costs positively associated
	  with quality index.

Beds
Percentage Medicaid patients
Staffing ratio
Occupancy rate
Nursing hours per patient day
	Costs were inversely related with
	  beds, experience of CEO,
	  percentage Medicaid patients,
	  occupancy rate,
	  and administrative costs.
	
	Costs were directly related with:
	  staffing ratio and nursing
	  hours per patient day.

Table 8.7 (continued)

Author, Year	Sample	Dependent Variables
Tamura, Lauer and Sanborn, 1985	Cross-section data from 163 nursing homes in Washington State during 1977.	Total cost per patient day.
Traxler, 1982	Pooled time-series and cross-sectional data for 68 nursing homes in Florida during the period 1971-1976.	Cost per patient day.
Ullmann, 1985	Cross-section data for 368 SNF's in New York State for 1976.	Total cost per patient day.

Table 8.7 (continued)

Independent Variables	Primary Results

ADL Index
Number of floors
  in the nursing home
Binary variable for
  hospital-based nursing home
	ADL was highly correlated
	with cost per day (r=0.711)
	
	Costs were positively associated
	with dependence in activities
	of daily living as well as with
	the number of floors in the
	facility and hospital-based
	location.

Beds
Beds^2
Occupancy rate
Input prices
% Medicaid patient days
Dummy variables for:
  government-owned and
  for-profit homes.
	Weak returns to scale, optimal
	size is 356 beds.
	
	Higher costs were associated
	with government-ownership,
	input prices, and degree
	of unionization.
	
	Costs per day were inversely
	related to size, occupancy rate,
	and administrative expense.

Patient days (PD), PD^2, PD^3 Investor-owned dummy DMS-1 case mix index Quality ratings Insurance mix Occupancy rate Facility age Hospital-based dummy	Slight diseconomies of scale in the range of 1 to 113 beds, constant returns to scale thereafter. Lower costs were associated with for-profit status and higher occupancy rates. Higher costs were associated with hospital based SNF's, average dependence of patients, and building features quality. Coefficients of nursing quality and rehabilitation services quality ratings were positive but insignificant.

positive impact on nursing home costs. Nursing homes that offered OT and PT cost from $0.85 to $0.91 per day more than nursing homes that did not provide these services. An extra nursing hour was estimated to cost the nursing home $3.29, and the cost of $3.14 per PT visit per patient day was estimated. Meiners (1982) used variables that were constructed by counting the number of professional rehabilitation services and the number of other services (i.e., private duty nursing, physician services, medical supplies, and special diets). Both variables exerted a positive and significant influence on costs. The results suggest that incremental rehabilitation services and other services cost the nursing home $0.59 per patient day and $0.15 per patient day, respectively. These variables need to be refined, however, in order to provide greater weights to the more costly services (Watts and Klastorin 1980).

Patient Characteristics

A number of patient characteristics variables have been used in nursing home cost functions. The most commonly used patient-mix description has been the Activities of Daily Living (ADLs) (Katz, Ford, Moskowitz et al. 1963). Meiners (1982) found that nursing homes with patients in midlevel patient dependence categories of ADLs tended to cost the most. Skinner and Yett (1973), whose results support this conclusion, assert that the very dependent nursing home residents are not capable of rehabilitation and thus require a lower level of care. Shaughnessy, Schlenker, Harley et al. (1980) and Ullmann (1984) also provide corroborative evidence for Meiners' findings.

Birnbaum et al. used ADLs, diagnoses, mental status, age, and gender as independent variables. Only the ADLs had a consistently positive and statistically significant relationship with average operating cost. However, multicollinearity between facility characteristics and patient attributes is likely to reduce the reliability of the estimated coefficients of each variable when they are entered in the same equation. Support for this proposition is given by analysis of cost functions in which case-mix and facility characteristics were entered in separate equations and in the same equation (Schlenker and Shaughnessy 1984).

Environmental Factors

A number of environmental factors, such as input prices, location and rate-regulation are expected to affect nursing home costs. Several studies have demonstrated a positive and significant relationship ($p < 0.05$) between input prices, measured as an index of wage rates or as wage rates, and nursing home costs (Birnbaum et al. 1981; Meiners 1982; Sulvetta and Holahan 1986).

Although operational definitions differ, a consistent body of evidence suggests that location is a determinant of nursing home costs. Using a binary variable, several studies have found that nursing home costs are less in rural areas, even when variations in the county wage rate are controlled (Birnbaum et al. 1981; Holahan 1985; Sulvetta and Holahan 1986). In addition, Meiners found that nursing home costs are greater in larger SMSAs (Standard Metropolitan Statistical Areas). Binary variables representing either regions (Birnbaum et al. 1981; Meiners 1982) or individual states (Holahan 1985) have also had significant regression coefficients suggesting that patterns of care differ by region.

Other Cost Determinants

Several studies found that proprietary status and membership in a chain of facilities are associated with lower costs (Holahan 1985; Sulvetta and Holahan 1986). Although Birnbaum et al. (1981), Traxler (1982), Schlenker and Shaughnessy (1984), and Ullmann (1984) did not include a variable for nursing home chains, they reported that proprietary nursing homes were less expensive. Meiners' study supports the results for proprietary homes; however, the coefficient for nursing home chains was positive but insignificant ($t = 1.15$). An excellent review of the effect of ownership on nursing homes is provided by Schlesinger, Marmor, and Smithey (1987).

Ullmann and Holtmann (1985), who conducted the only quasi-technological cost function analysis of nursing homes, reported that these facilities exhibited no economies of scope associated with the joint production of skilled nursing care and intermediate care. They also reported that the estimated coefficient of the beds variable, a surrogate for capital, was positive. This result indicates that nursing homes may have overinvested in capital.

In addition to the factors already discussed, it is clear that hospital-based nursing homes are more expensive than freestanding nursing homes. Sulvetta and Holahan (1986) reported that in 1983, the average cost per day in hospital-based nursing homes was $105.31, while cost per day in freestanding nursing homes was $61.12. Results from their regression analysis indicate that while controlling for the effects of location, ownership, size, input prices, and other determinants of nursing home costs, costs per day were $27.62 more in hospital-based nursing homes than in freestanding facilities. An earlier multivariate study by Meiners (1982) found that the cost per day was 17 percent higher in hospital-based nursing homes. Similar results were reported by Ullmann (1984).

There are several possible explanations for these cost-differentials. By refusing to adjust payments to hospital-based providers, HCFA has implied that the higher costs associated with this locus of care are the result of inefficiency and should not be recognized by third-party payers. On the other hand, hospital-based providers argue that their higher costs are due to treatment of patients whose care is more resource intensive, as well as to the provision of high levels of quality. This is an important issue to resolve because if hospitals receive inadequate payment for providing nursing home services in an efficient manner, they will have little incentive to convert acute care beds into long-term care units, a strategy that might simultaneously reduce the shortage of nursing home beds and the surplus of acute care hospital beds (Vladeck 1980).

Analyses of the variation in the costs of freestanding and hospital-based nursing homes have employed indirect and direct measures of case-mix. Percentage of patient days in the nursing home provided to Medicare patients has been employed as an indirect measure of nursing home case-mix. Its use is based on the assumption that Medicare patients, who are more likely to be recovering from an acute illness, trauma, or surgery, require greater intensity of services than long-term chronic patients (Shaughnessy, Kramer, Schlenker, and Polesovsky 1985). This assumption has received support from the results of two multivariate studies that found the ratio of Medicare patient days to total patient days is directly associated with nursing home costs per day (Meiners 1982; Sulvetta and Holahan 1986).

Studies that used direct case-mix measures also support the contention that hospital-based nursing homes have a case-mix that is more resource-intensive than that of freestanding nursing homes (Schlenker and Shaughnessy 1984; Shaughnessy et al. 1985). Given the weaknesses of the commonly used measures of the nursing homes' case-mix, these results should be accepted with caution.

HOME HEALTH CARE COST FUNCTIONS

The delivery of home health services has not been the subject of much economic inquiry; however, the recent emphasis on home health services, as part of a coordinated care program to reduce patients' stays in acute care settings, is likely to stimulate more research in this area. Only three cost function studies (Kurowski, Schlenker, and Tricarico 1979; Hay and Mandes 1984; Kass 1987) have been published. As discussed by Kass, however, the first two studies were small, restricted to one or two geographic areas, and subject to a number of other methodological problems. Accordingly, we will restrict our discussion to the study by Kass.

Kass used a national data base that was assembled from the Medicare Cost Reports of 1,704 home health agencies' cost reports. These data were used to estimate the parameters of a quasi-technological cost function in which a quadratic form was specified. The major findings of this study were the following:

1. Substantial economies of scale or scope in the provision of home health services were not evident.

2. Holding input prices constant, urban agencies are less expensive than rural agencies, a result attributed to less travel time for agency personnel in urban areas.

3. Costs are negatively related to the percentage of patient revenue accounted for by Medicare, a result attributed to restrictions on Medicare reimbursement imposed by HCFA.

4. Visiting Nurses Agencies (VNAs) incurred expenses per patient visit that were about 12 percent less than those found in other types of home health care agencies, a result that might be due to the nonprofit status of VNAs.

Although Kass' effort compares favorably to the most sophisticated studies of hospital cost-functions, we are cautious about generalizing from one study.

Further, we would like to see this type of study repeated to determine if the results are stable for different samples and over time. Given the changes in health care delivery associated with the introduction of case-based payment and other cost-containment programs, home health agencies may be reacting currently to an environment different from that which existed in 1982, the year in which the Kass study is based.

SUMMARY

It is not surprising that the most important determinant of costs of hospitals or nursing homes is case-mix. If a hospital (or any firm) changes its product-mix so that each unit of the new output requires more inputs than before, *ceteris paribus*, the new product will cost more than the old one.

Case-mix is such an important determinant of the costs of health care organizations that estimates of other determinants that are correlated with case-mix are obscured. For example, univariate analysis suggests that the cost per admission in teaching hospitals is as much as 33 percent more than in their nonteaching counterparts. Once the effects of case-mix and other factors are controlled, however, the estimated cost differential is reduced by half.

Contrary to popular belief, investor-owned and multi-institutional health care organizations are not significantly less expensive than independent institutions. It also appears that hospitals and nursing homes have a very shallow, "U-shaped," long-run, average cost curve, suggesting very weak returns to scale. Very little is known about the nature of economies of scope in the joint production of health care services. Recent advances in the estimation of flexible cost functions, however, may permit fruitful exploration in this area. Regarding future research, it is our hope that more refined measures of case-mix severity will become available so that concerns about bias resulting from differences in associated product-mix will be allayed in future studies.

REFERENCES

Adamache, K., and F. Sloan. 1982. Unions and hospitals: Some unresolved issues. *Journal of Health Economics* 1(1):81–108.

Ament, R. P., E. J. Kobrinski, and W. R. Wood. 1981. Case mix complexity differences between teaching and nonteaching hospitals. *Journal of Medical Education* 56(11):894–903.

American Hospital Association. 1987. *Hospital Statistics*. Chicago, IL: AHA.

Anderson, G. F., and J. R. Lave. 1986. Financing graduate medical education using multiple regression to set payment rates. *Inquiry* 23(2):191–99.

Barer, M. L. 1982. Case mix adjustment in hospital cost analysis: Information theory revisited. *Journal of Health Economics* 1(1):53–80.

Bays, C. W. 1980. Specification error in the estimation of hospital cost functions. *The Review of Economics and Statistics* 62(2):302–5.

Becker, E. R., and B. Steinwald. 1981. Determinants of hospital case-mix complexity. *Health Services Research* 16(4):439–58.

Becker, E. R., and F. A. Sloan. 1983. Utilization of hospital services: The roles of teaching, case mix and reimbursement. *Inquiry* 20(3):248–57.

Becker, E. R., and F. A. Sloan. 1985. Hospital ownership and performance. *Economic Inquiry* 23(1):21–36.

Becker, E. R., F. A. Sloan, and B. Steinwald. 1982. Union activity in hospitals: Past, present, and future. *Health Care Financing Review* 3(4):1–13.

Berki, S. 1972. *Hospital Economics.* Lexington, MA: Lexington Books.

Birnbaum, H., C. Bishop, A. J. Lee, and G. Jensen. 1981. Why do nursing home costs vary? *Medical Care* 19(11):1095–1107.

Bishop, C. E. 1980. Nursing home cost studies and reimbursement issues. *Health Care Financing Review* 1(4):47–64.

Brown, C., and J. Medoff. 1978. Trade unions in the production process. *Journal of Political Economy* 86(3):355–78.

Brown, R. W., D. W. Caves, and L. R. Christensen. 1979. Modelling the structure of cost and production for multiproduct firms. *Southern Economic Journal* 46(2):256–73.

Christensen, L. R., and W. H. Greene. 1976. Economies of scale in U.S. electric power generation. *Journal of Political Economy* 84(4):655–76.

Clark, K. B. 1980a. The impact of unionization on productivity: A case study. *Industrial and Labor Relations Review* 33(4):451–69.

Clark, K. B. 1980b. Unionization and productivity: Micro-econometric evidence. *Quarterly Journal of Economics* 95(4):613–40.

Coelen, C., and D. Sullivan. 1981. An analysis of the effects of prospective reimbursement programs on hospital expenditures. *Health Care Financing Review* 2(1):1–40.

Cohen, H. A. 1967. Variations in cost among hospitals of different sizes. *Southern Economic Journal* 33 (3):355–66.

Conrad, R. F., and R. P. Strauss. 1983. A multiple-output, multiple-input model of the hospital industry in North Carolina. *Applied Economics* 15(3):341–52.

Cowing, T. G., and A. G. Holtmann. 1983. Multiproduct short-run hospital cost functions: Empirical evidence and policy implications from cross-section data. *Southern Economic Journal* 49(3):637–53.

Cowing, T. G., A. G. Holtmann, and S. Powers. 1983. Hospital cost analysis: A survey and evaluation of recent studies. *Advances in Health Economics and Health Services Research* 4:257–303.

Cromwell, J., J. Mitchell, K. Calore, and L. Iezzoni. 1987. Sources of hospital cost variation by urban-rural location. *Medical Care* 25(9):801–29.

Ermann, D., and J. Gabel. 1985. The changing face of American health care: Multihospital systems, emergency centers, and surgery centers. *Medical Care* 23(5):401–20.

Evans, R. G. 1971. "Behavioral" cost functions for hospitals. *Canadian Journal of Economics* 4(2):198–215.

Evans, R. G., and H. D. Walker. 1972. Information theory and the analysis of hospital cost structure. *Canadian Journal of Economics* 5(3):398–418.

Feldman, R., L. F. Lee, and R. Hoffbeck. 1980. Hospital Employees' Wages and Labor Union Organization. Final Report on Grant HS 03649 submitted to the National

Center for Health Services Research, U.S. Department of Health and Human Services. The University of Minnesota.

Feldman, R., and R. Scheffler. 1982. The union impact on hospital wages and fringe benefits. *Industrial and Labor Relations Review* 35(2):196–206.

Feldstein, M. S. 1974. Econometric studies of health economics. In M. Intrilligator and D. Kendrick, eds., *Frontiers of Quantitative Economics.* Amsterdam: North-Holland.

Fottler, M. 1977. The union impact on hospital wages. *Industrial and Labor Relations Review* 39(3):342–55.

Francisco, E. 1970. Analysis of cost variations among short-term general hospitals. In H. Klarman, ed., *Empirical Studies in Health Economics.* Baltimore, MD: Johns Hopkins University Press.

Frantz, J. 1976. The impact of trade unions on production in the wooden household furniture industry. Seniors Honors Thesis, Harvard College.

Frech, H. E., III, and P. B. Ginsburg. 1981. The cost of nursing home care in the United States: Government-financing, ownership, and efficiency. In J. van der Gaag and M. Perlman, eds. *Health, Economics, and Health Economics.* Amsterdam: North-Holland.

Freidman, B., and M. Pauly. 1981. Cost functions for a service firm with variable quality and stochastic demand: The case of hospitals. *The Review of Economics and Statistics* 63(4):620–4.

Freidman, B., and M. Pauly. 1983. A new approach to hospital cost functions and some issues in revenue regulation. *Health Care Financing Review* 4(3):105–14.

Freund, D., R. H. Shachtman, M. Ruffin, and D. Quade. 1985. Analysis of length-of-stay differences between investor-owned and voluntary hospitals. *Inquiry* 22(1):33–44.

Garg, M. L., M. Elkhatib, W. M. Kleinberg, and J. L. Mulligan. 1982. Reimbursing for residency training: How many times? *Medical Care* 20(7):719–26.

Goldfarb, M., and R. Coffey. 1987. Case-mix differences between teaching and non-teaching hospitals. *Inquiry* 24(1):68–84.

Grannemann, T. W., R. S. Brown, and M. V. Pauly. 1986. Estimating hospital costs: A multiple-output analysis. *Journal of health Economics* 5(2):107–27.

Hay, J. W., and G. Mandes. 1984. Home health care cost-function analysis. *Health Care Financing Review* 5(3):111–16.

Hefty, T. R. 1969. Returns to scale in hospitals: A critical review of recent research. *Health Services Research* 4(4):267–80.

Hillestad, S., and E. Berkowitz. 1984. *Health Care Marketing Plans: From Strategy to Action.* Homewood, IL: Dow Jones-Irwin.

Holahan, J. 1985. State rate-setting and its effects on the cost of nursing home care. *Journal of Health Politics, Policy and Law* 9(3):647–67.

Horn, S. D., R. A. Horn, and P. D. Sharkey. 1984. The Severity of Illness Index as a severity adjustment to diagnosis-related groups. *Health Care Financing Review* 5 (Supp.):33–46.

Horn, S. D., P. D. Sharkey, and D. Bertram. 1983. Measuring severity of illness: Homogeneous case-mix groups. *Medical Care* 21(1):14–31.

Hornbrook, M. D., and A. C. Monheit. 1985. The contribution of case-mix severity to the hospital cost-output relation. *Inquiry* 22(3):259–71.

Hosek, J. R., and A. R. Palmer. 1983. Teaching and hospital costs: The case of radiology. *Journal of Health Economics* 2(1):29–46.

Ingbar, M. L., and L. D. Taylor. 1968. *Hospital Costs in Massachusetts: An Econometric Study*. Cambridge, MA: Harvard University Press.

Institute of Medicine. 1986. *For-Profit Enterprise in Health Care*. Washington, D.C.: National Academy Press.

Jenkins, A. 1980. Multiproduct cost analysis: Service and case-type cost equations for Ontario hospitals. *Applied Economics* 12(1):103–13.

Joskow, P. L. 1980. The effects of competition and regulation on hospital bed supply and the reservation quality of the hospital. *Bell Journal of Economics* 11(2):421–47.

Kass, D. I. 1987. Economies of scale and scope in the provision of home health services. *Journal of Health Economics* 6(2):129–46.

Katz, S., A. B. Ford, R. W. Moskowitz et al. 1963. Studies of illness in the aged: The index of ADL. *Journal of the American Medical Association* 195:914.

Kurowski, B. T., R. E. Schlenker, and G. Tricarico. 1979. Applied research in home health services-Vol. II: Cost per episode. Boulder: University of Colorado Medical Center.

Lave, J. R. 1966. A review of the methods used to study hospital costs. *Inquiry* 3(2):57–81.

Lave, J. R., and L. B. Lave. 1970. Hospital cost functions. *American Economic Review* 60(3):379–95.

Lee, R. H., and D. M. Waldman. 1985. The diffusion of innovations in hospitals. *Journal of Health Economics* 4(4):373–80.

Luft, H., J. Robinson, D. Garnick, S. Maerki, and S. McPhee. 1986. The role of specialized clinical services in competition among hospitals. *Inquiry* 23(1):83–94.

Mandelstamm, A. 1965. The effects of unions on efficiency in the residential construction industry. *Industrial and Labor Relations Review* 18(4):503–21.

Mann, J. K., and D. E. Yett. 1968. The analysis of hospital costs: A review article. *Journal of Business* 41(2):191–202.

Meiners, M. R. 1982. An econometric analysis of the major determinants of nursing home costs in the United States. *Social Science and Medicine* 16:887–98.

Melnick, G. A., J. Wheeler, and P. J. Feldstein. 1981. Effects of rate regulation on selected components of hospital expenses. *Inquiry* 18(3):240–6.

Miller, R., B. Becker, and E. Krinsky. 1979. *The Impact of Collective Bargaining on Hospitals*. New York: Praeger.

Mulligan, J. G. 1985. The stochastic determinants of hospital-bed supply. *Journal of Health Economics* 4(2):177–81.

Munoz, E., D. Regan, I. Margocis, and L. Wise. 1985. Surgonomics: The identifier concept. *Annals of Surgery* 202:119–25.

Olson, M. 1962. *The Logic of Collective Action*. Cambridge, MA: Harvard University Press.

Pauly, M. V. 1973. The economics of group practice. *Journal of Human Resources* 8(1):37–56.

Pauly, M. V. 1978. Medical staff characteristics and hospital costs. *Journal of Human Resources* 13 (Supplement):77–111.

Pauly, M. V., and M. Redisch. 1973. The not-for-profit hospital as a physicians' co-operative. *American Economic Review* 63(1):87–100.

Pettengill, J., and J. Vertrees 1982. Reliability and validity in hospital case-mix measurement. *Health Care Financing Review* 4(2). HCFA Pub. No. 03149, Office of Research and Demonstrations, HCFA. Washington, DC: U.S. Government Printing Office.

Relman, A. S. 1980. The new medical-industrial complex. *New England Journal of Medicine* 303(17):963–70.

Renn, S. C., C. J. Schramm, J. M. Watt, and R. A. Derzon. 1985. The effects of ownership and system affiliation on the economic performance of hospitals. *Inquiry* 22(3):219–36.

Ro, K. 1968. Determinants of hospital costs. Yale Economic Essays 8(2):187–257.

Robinson, J. C., and H. S. Luft. 1985. The impact of hospital market structure on patient volume, average length of stay, and the cost of care. *Journal of Health Economics* 4(4):333–56.

Robinson, J., and H. Luft. 1987. Competition and the cost of hospital care, 1972–1982. *Journal of the American Medical Association* 257(23):3241–5.

Romeo, A., J. Wagner, and H. Lee. 1984. Prospective reimbursement and the diffusion of new technologies in hospitals. *Journal of Health Economics* 3(1):1–28.

Rosko, M. D. 1982. *Hospital Responses to Prospective Rate Setting*, Unpublished doctoral dissertation. Philadelphia, PA: Temple University.

Rosko, M. D. 1984. The impact of prospective payment: A multidimensional analysis of New Jersey's SHARE Program. *Journal of Health Politics, Policy and Law* 9(1):81–102.

Rosko, M. D., and R. W. Broyles. 1986. The impact of the New Jersey all-payer DRG system. *Inquiry* 23(1):67–75.

Rosko, M. D., and R. W. Broyles. 1987. Short-term responses of hospitals to the DRG prospective pricing mechanism in New Jersey. *Medical Care* 25(2):88–99.

Ruchlin, H. S., and S. Levy. 1972. Nursing home cost analysis: A case study. *Inquiry* 9(3):3–15.

Rueben, D. B. 1984. Learning diagnostic restraint. *New England Journal of Medicine* 310(9):591–3.

Russell, L. B. 1979. *Technology in Hospitals*. Washington, DC: The Brookings Institute.

Salkever, D. S. 1970. Hospital cost studies and planning under uncertainty: Analysis of a simple model. *Southern Economic Journal* 36(3):263–67.

Salkever, D. 1972. A microeconomic study of hospital cost inflation. *Journal of Political Economy* 80(6):1144–66.

Salkever, D. 1979. *Hospital Sector Inflation*. Lexington, MA: Lexington Books.

Salkever, D. S. 1982. Unionization and the cost of producing hospital services. *Journal of Labor Research* 3(3):311–33.

Salkever, D. S. 1984. Cost implications of hospital unionization: A behavioral analysis. *Health Services Research* 19(5):639–64.

Salkever, D. S., D. M. Steinwachs, and A. Rupp. 1986. Hospital cost and efficiency under per service and per case payment in Maryland: A tale of the carrot and the stick. *Inquiry* 23(1):56–66.

Schlenker, R. E., and P. W. Shaughnessy. 1984. Case-mix, quality, and cost relationships in Colorado nursing homes. *Health Care Financing Review* 6(2):61–71.

Schlesinger, M., T. Marmor, and R. Smithey. 1987. Nonprofit and for-profit medical care: Shifting roles and implications for health policy. *Journal of Health Politics, Policy and Law* 12(3):427–57.

Schroeder, S. A., and D. S. O'Leary. 1977. Differences in laboratory use and length of stay between university and community hospitals. *Journal of Medical Education* 52(5):418–20.

Shaughnessy, P. W., A. M. Kramer, R. E. Schlenker, and M. B. Polesovsky. 1985. Nursing home case-mix differences between Medicare and non-Medicare and between hospital-based and freestanding patients. *Inquiry* 23(2):162–77.

Shaughnessy, P., R. Schlenker, B. Harley et al. 1980. Long-term care reimbursement and regulation: A study of cost, case-mix and quality. Working paper #4, University of Colorado Center for Health Services Research. (Report prepared pursuant to HCFA no.18-P–97145/8–01.)

Shortell, S. M., M. A. Morrisey, and D. A. Conrad. 1985. Economic regulation and hospital behavior: The effects on medical staff organization and hospital-physician relationships. *Health Services Research* 20(5):597–628.

Shortell, S. M., S. W. Becker, and D. Neuhauser. 1976. The effects of management practices on hospital efficiency and quality of care. *Inquiry* 13(suppl.):90–107.

Skinner, D. E., and D. E. Yett, 1973. Debility index for long-term care patients. In R. L. Berg, ed., *Health Status Indexes*. Chicago, Educational Trust.

Sloan, F. A., and R. Elnicki. 1979. Professional nurse wage-setting in hospitals. In R. Scheffler ed., *Research in Health Economics*. Greenwich, CT: JAI Press.

Sloan, F. A., and B. Steinwald. 1980a. Effects of regulation on hospital costs and input use. *The Journal of Law and Economics* 23(1):81–109.

Sloan, F. A., and B. Steinwald. 1980b. *Insurance, Regulation and Hospital Costs*. Lexington, MA: D.C. Heath and Co.

Sloan, F. A., and E. R. Becker. 1981. Internal organization of hospitals and hospital costs. *Inquiry* 18(3):224–39.

Sloan, F. A., and J. Valvona. 1986. The high costs of teaching hospitals. *Health Affairs* 5(3):68–85.

Sloan, F. A., J. Valvona, and J. M. Perrin. 1986. Diffusion of surgical technology: An exploratory study. *Journal of Health Economics* 5(1):31–61.

Sloan, F. A., R. D. Feldman, and A. B. Steinwald. 1983. Effects of teaching on hospital costs. *Journal of Health Economics* 2(1):1–28.

Smith, H. L., and M. D. Fottler. 1981. Costs and cost containment in nursing homes. *Health Services Research* 16(1):17–41.

Sulvetta, M. B., and J. Holahan. 1986. Cost and case-mix differences between hospital-based and freestanding nursing homes. *Health Care Financing Review* 7(3):75–84.

Tamura, H., L. W. Lauer, and F. A. Sanborn. 1985. Estimating "reasonable cost" of Medicaid patient care using a patient-mix index. *Health Services Research* 20(1):27–42.

Traxler, H. G. 1982. Determinants of nursing home costs in Florida: Policy implications and support in national research findings. *Public Health Reports* 97(6):537–44.

Ullmann, S. G. 1984. Cost analysis and facility reimbursement in the long-term health care industry. *Health Services Research* 19(1):83–102.

Ullmann, S. G. 1985. The impact of quality on cost in the provision of long-term care. *Inquiry* 22(3):293–302.

Ullmann, S. G., and A. G. Holtmann. 1985. Economics of scope, ownership, and nursing home costs. *Quarterly Review of Economics and Business* 25(4):83–94.

Vitaliano, D. F. 1987. On the estimation of hospital cost functions. *Journal of Health Economics* 6(4):305–18.

Vladeck, B. 1980. *Unloving Care*. New York: Basic Books.

Watts, C. A., and T. D. Klastorin. 1980. The impact of case mix on hospital cost: A comparative analysis. *Inquiry* 17(4):357–67.

Welch, W. 1987. Do all teaching hospitals deserve an add-on payment under the prospective payment system? *Inquiry* 24(3):221–32.

Worthington, N. L., and K. A. Piro. 1982. The effects of hospital rate setting programs on volumes of hospital services: A preliminary analysis. *Health Care Financing Review* 4(2):47–67.

Young, W. W. 1984. Incorporating severity of illness and comorbidity in case-mix measurement. *Health Care Financing Review* 5(Supp.):23–32.

9

THE SUPPLY OF PHYSICIANS: A
FOCUS ON SPECIALTY CHOICE

An understanding of factors that influence the supply of health resources and physicians in particular is of importance to policy analysts, medical educators, academics and planners. Historically, the policies implemented by federal authorities with regard to the supply of physicians were designed to (1) increase the supply of medical graduates and thereby reduce a perceived shortage of physicians, (2) reduce imbalances in the geographic distribution of physicians, and (3) alter the specialty mix of physicians. These policy initiatives were generally justified by the results of empirical research that indicated a need to increase the number of physicians, which, in turn, might enhance access to medical care, increase competition in local markets, and reduce the prices of services provided by physicians.

Contrary to federal policy, the American Medical Association and other physician groups may have attempted to erect barriers restricting entry to the practice of medicine that would reduce the flow of new practitioners and preserve the monopoly power or returns that accrue to established physicians (Friedman 1962; Feldstein 1983). Among the most commonly cited barriers are state licensure requirements, which not only impose restrictions on the flow of persons who enter the practice of medicine, but also limit the number of institutions authorized to provide medical education. In addition, the established medical profession has restricted entry by prolonging the period of training. Although an extension of the time required to complete internship and residency programs improves the competence of graduates, the prolonged period of training increases the costs of medical education and reduces the net rate of return expected by potential practitioners. Both factors tend to preserve the economic rents accruing to established physicians by limiting the flow of new practitioners. When viewed from a policy perspective, these observations suggest that the policies of the medical society were in conflict with those of the federal government and that the effects of legislative initiatives to alter the supply of physicians may have been mitigated by licensure and educational requirements imposed by the medical profession.

In addition to policy considerations, an understanding of factors that influence the supply of physicians is of importance to medical educators and health planners. For example, an improvement in the precision of estimates concerning the supply and distribution of medical personnel enables health planners and educators to reduce the magnitude of periodic shortages or surpluses. Similarly, an understanding of factors influencing career choices enables educators to attract and retain medical students who are likely to specialize or locate in those areas in which the number of established physicians is inadequate.

Recognizing the importance of ensuring an adequate supply, geographic distribution, and specialty mix of providers, we focus this chapter on career decisions implemented by physicians, a subject to be developed in essentially three phases. The first phase describes various methods that are commonly used to assess the adequacy of the physician supply. The discussion suggests that, in contrast to the period from 1960 to 1980, many analysts now argue that a surplus of physicians is likely and that the major policy concerns involve the specialty and geographic distribution of medical practitioners. Accordingly, the remaining sections of this chapter are committed to an examination of factors that influence the specialty choices of physicians. In particular, the second area of discussion focuses on the development of a theoretical framework for examining the selection of specialty or subspecialty, and the final section considers previous results concerning these decisions.

BACKGROUND STATISTICS

Of particular importance to this and the next chapter are recent changes in the stock and distribution of physicians. The data summarized in Table 9.1 indicate that during the period from 1960 to 1983, the increase in the stock of physicians, which nearly doubled, outpaced the growth in population. As a result, the number of physicians per 100,000 population rose from 151 in 1960 to 228 in 1983, a 50 percent increase.

The growth in the stock of physicians has shifted the focus of policy analysts from the effects of a shortage to those that are attributable to an impending surplus of physicians. Projections developed by the Department of Health and Human Services suggest that, by 1990 the stock of physicians will exceed the required number by approximately 50,000. Further, federal analysts project a surplus of approximately 80,000 physicians by the year 2000 (Iglehart 1986).

The growth in the stock of physicians has been accompanied by an expansion in the capacity of osteopathic medical schools, which, in turn, contributed to the increase in the number of students, from 32,000 in 1960 to 73,500 in 1983. Further, the number of graduates increased from 7,500 in 1960 to 17,600 in

Table 9.1
Physicians: Total, Per Capita, Total Newly Licensed, and Newly Licensed Foreign Medical School Graduates, 1960–1983

ITEM	1960	1970	1975	1980	1983
Total physicians* (000's)	275	348	409	487	542
Physicians per 100,000 population	151	168	187	211	228
Newly licensed physicians (000's)	8.0	11.0	16.9	18.2	20.6
Newly licensed graduates of foreign medical schools (000's)	1.4	3.0	6.0	3.3	4.8

Source: U.S. Bureau of the Census. 1986. Statistical Abstract of the United States: 1987 (107th edition). Washington, D.C.

*As of July 1

1984. During the same period, the number of newly licensed graduates of foreign medical schools grew from 1,400 to 4,800.

In addition to this, recent changes in the distribution of U.S. medical graduates by gender are worthy of note. During the 1965–1966 academic year, only 6.9 percent of medical school graduates were female. By contrast, this percentage grew to 30.7 during the 1985–1986 academic year. As will be indicated later, gender is thought to influence not only the selection of specialty but also the amount of time physicians commit to medical practice.

The final aspect to be described in this section is the distribution of physicians by specialty. As indicated in Table 9.2, the percentage of physicians engaged in general practice continued to decline during the 1970s. That decline, however, has been accompanied by a growing percentage of physicians engaged in the fields of internal medicine, pediatrics, and general surgery, which are commonly identified as areas of primary care.

MEASURES OF SURPLUS AND SHORTAGE

The adequacy of the physician supply and unevenness in the geographic distribution of medical practitioners were major policy issues in the 1970s and remain so, to a lesser extent, in the 1980s. This section examines the methods commonly used to assess the number, geographic distribution, and specialty mix of physicians. It is possible to identify essentially four approaches to the problem of assessing the supply of medical providers. The first, which was used extensively in early studies, relies on traditional economic theory to derive indicators of shortages or surpluses. The second approach focuses on variation in the ratio of physicians to population as a measure of the relative availability of health personnel. The third is a normative approach that relies upon professional judgments of the number and composition of physicians required to treat health problems associated with different population groups. As employed by the Graduate Medical Education National Advisory Committee (GMENAC), the fourth approach involves a comparison of the current or predicted number of physicians with the supply required to satisfy the health needs of the population at risk. Each of these approaches is considered in this section.

The Economic Definition

The economic assessment of the supply of physicians requires a distinction between the market for the services provided by practitioners and the market for practitioners. Referring to Figure 9.1, assume that the initial demand and supply curves prevailing in the market for physician services are represented by D_0 and S_0 respectively. In competitive equilibrium, market price and quantity are P_0 and Q_0 respectively, an outcome that yields neither an economic profit nor net loss. Assume that demand is constant and that the supply of physicians increases, resulting in a shift from S_0 to S_1 in Figure 9.1. Other things remaining constant,

Table 9.2
Physicians by Specialty, 1970–1983 (in thousands, percent of total in parentheses)

Specialty	1970	1975	1980	1983
General practice	57.9 (17.3)	54.6 (13.9)	60.0 (12.8)	64.2 (12.4)
Internal medicine	41.9 (12.5)	54.3 (13.8)	71.5 (15.3)	82.5 (15.9)
Pediatrics	17.9 (5.4)	21.7 (5.5)	28.3 (6.0)	32.8 (6.3)
General surgery	29.8 (8.9)	31.6 (8.0)	34.0 (7.3)	36.3 (7.0)
Obstetrics, gynecology	18.9 (5.7)	21.7 (5.5)	26.3 (5.6)	29.3 (5.6)
Orthopedic surgery	9.6 (2.9)	11.4 (2.9)	14.0 (3.0)	16.2 (3.1)
Opthalmology	9.9 (3.0)	11.1 (2.8)	13.0 (2.8)	14.3 (2.8)
Psychiatry	21.1 (6.3)	23.9 (6.0)	27.5 (5.9)	30.8 (5.9)
Anesthesiology	10.1 (3.0)	12.9 (3.3)	16.0 (3.4)	20.0 (3.8)
Pathology	10.3 (3.1)	11.7 (3.0)	13.4 (2.9)	14.9 (2.9)
Radiology	10.5 (3.1)	11.5 (2.9)	11.7 (2.5)	10.4 (2.0)
All Others	96.1 (28.8)	127.3 (32.4)	152.0 (32.5)	168.3 (32.3)
Total*	334.0	393.7	467.7	520.0

Source: U.S. Bureau of the Census. 1986. Statistical Abstract of the United States: 1987
(107th edition). Washington, D.C.

* As of December 31

and assuming physicians fail to induce demand, an increase in supply is expected to reduce price from P_o to P_1. As shown in Figure 9.2, a reduction in price may induce established physicians to commit less time to market activity and provide a lower volume of care (i.e., $Q'_o - Q'_1$). Also observe that, *ceteris paribus*, an increase in the supply of practitioners is expected to result in a net loss. Hence, these observations suggest that a surplus of physicians is characterized by low

Figure 9.1
Market Demand and Supply: An Increase in the Supply of Physicians

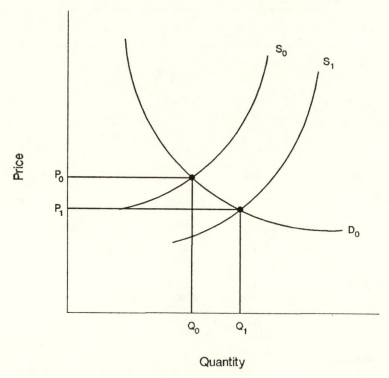

or negative returns and little or no exit of practitioners from the practice of medicine.

Referring to Figure 9.3, suppose next that rising disposable income results in an increase in demand, which, in the market for physician services, increases price from P_0 to P_1, and quantity from Q_0 to Q_1. In response to the higher price, the physician is induced to provide more care by committing additional hours to market activity or employing auxiliary personnel. As shown in Figure 9.4, these decisions not only increase volume from Q'_0 to Q'_1, but also enable the physician to earn economic profits. Suppose further that barriers to entry prevent the economic profits earned by established physicians from attracting new entrants to the practice of medicine. In such a situation, then, a shortage of physicians is characterized by high or rising returns and few new entrants to the practice of medicine.

The effects of barriers on the flow of entrants to the practice of medicine and the income of physicians were assessed recently by Noether (1986). As suggested by the discussion of Figures 9.1 to 9.4, a deterioration in the authority of the AMA and less restrictive barriers to entry are expected to result in not only an

Figure 9.2
The Physician Firm: The Case of Net Losses

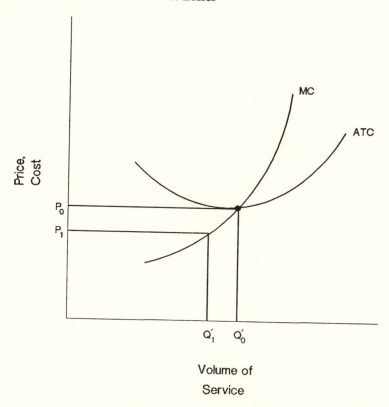

Volume of
Service

expansion in the stock of physicians, but also a decline in medical incomes. In an evaluation of these expectations, Noether examined the stock of physicians in relation to the supply that would prevail under perfect competition and the supply that would be produced by a perfect cartel. Focusing on the post–World War II period, estimates of a system of equations for the stock of physicians and medical incomes supported the conclusion that the "growth in physician competition has indeed been substantial" (Noether 1986, p. 529). After controlling for demand conditions and marginal cost, represented by the opportunity cost of becoming a physician, the results indicated that increased competition since 1965 has been accompanied by a 6 to 20 percent additional growth in the stock of physicians and a 19 to 45 percent decline in income. These conclusions are consistent with expectations and suggest that the effects of barriers to entry are less restrictive than assumed previously.

The discussion of Figures 9.1 to 9.4 also suggests that, in competitive markets, the long-run supply of physicians is in balance with demand when the returns in medicine are similar to those obtainable in occupations characterized by com-

SUPPLY-SIDE ANALYSIS

276

Figure 9.3
Market Demand and Supply: A Shift in Demand

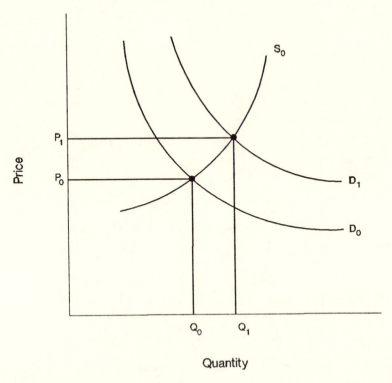

parable educational, skill, and job requirements. Conversely, after standardizing for differences in educational requirements, skills and nonpecuniary factors, the presence of relatively high returns or economic profits in a given occupation indicates a shortage; the obverse is also true.

Several early studies assessed the long-run supply of physicians in terms of differences in rates of return or lifetime earnings. For example, Fein and Weber (1971) used age-specific income to estimate the lifetime earnings of potential entrants to the practice of medicine in 1966. Employing earnings streams that were adjusted to reflect after-tax income, Fein and Weber calculated internal rates of return under different assumptions concerning the rate of inflation and growth in productivity. Compared to those with a Ph.D. in biological science, the internal rates of return accruing to the practice of medicine ranged from approximately 15 to 34 percent.

As indicated by Lindsay (1973), the high rates of return were attributable to a combination of several doubtful assumptions. In particular, it is likely that the internal rate of 34 percent is a product of assuming an inflation rate of 3 percent, of a high differential in the growth of productivity, and of employing the earnings

Figure 9.4
The Physician Firm: The Case of Economic Profits

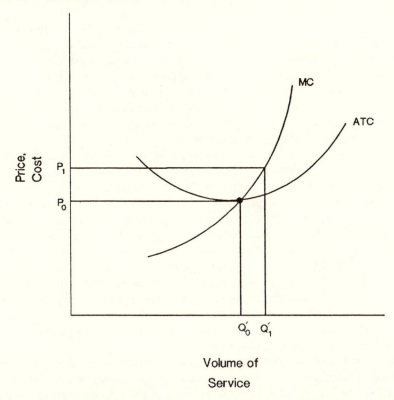

Volume of
Service

of a biological scientist as a measure of opportunity cost. Since the investment required to secure a Ph.D. in biological science was unprofitable during the study period, these assumptions combined to produce artificially high estimates of the returns to medical training.

In an attempt to determine if the decision to specialize is related to income differences, Sloan (1970) calculated the present values and internal rates of return that were based on differences in the lifetime earnings of those who practiced in one of several specialties and physicians who engaged in general practice. Present values and internal rates of return were based on differences in earnings during the years 1955, 1959, and 1965. Discount rates of 5 and 10 percent were used to calculate present values, while the internal rates of return reported in the study equated the present value of earnings in general practice with those in each of the specialties.

The results reported by Sloan indicated that returns were low or negative in several of the specialties (e.g., pediatrics and internal medicine). In addition, the measures of return to specialization were invariant with respect to time. Given the propensity of medical graduates to specialize at the time of the study, the results appeared to be inconsistent with expectations derived from normative theory (i.e., new entrants are attracted to a specialty area by high or rising returns).

In one of the earliest studies, Friedman and Kuznets (1945) estimated the proportion of the difference in the earnings of physicians and dentists that represented the rental values of the additional investment on medical education. The findings indicated that a difference of approximately 17 percent was required to ensure that the two careers were equally attractive; however, since relative income differed by approximately 32 percent during the period, an unexplained margin of 16.5 percent was reported, an outcome that was attributed to the relative difficulty of entering medical practice.

In an assessment of previous research, Lindsay contended that the results reported by Fein and Weber (1971), Friedman and Kuznets (1945), and by Sloan (1970) overstated differences in returns. The bias was attributed to the possibility that higher wages (returns) induce the individual to substitute hours of market for nonmarket activity. Hence, Lindsay suggested that differences in earnings were attributable more to longer hours of work than to barriers that prevent entry to the practice of medicine. After adjusting for differences in hours of work and employing a discount rate of 10 percent, revised estimates indicated that the net earnings reported previously were reduced or eliminated and that the returns to an investment in medicine were negative in several years during the post–World War II period. Lindsay concluded that the revised estimates fail to support the view that the limited capacity of medical schools creates a barrier to entry and inflates returns to practicing physicians.

In response to these observations, Sloan (1976) contended that, since occupational choices are based on nonpecuniary and financial factors, the internal rate of return is neither an adequate measure of the effect of barriers to entry nor an accurate indicator of surpluses or shortages. In addition, Sloan argued that the number of hours used by Lindsay to adjust earnings streams overstated the length of the work week of physicians, resulting in an understatement of the returns to medical practice. As a result, it is probable that variation in the number of hours committed to market activity did not represent a serious source of bias.

Revised estimates of the profitability calculated by Leffler (1975) indicated that in 1966 a career in medicine yielded an annual income that exceeded the yearly earnings of a college graduate by approximately $1,400. These estimates were based on life cycle, median incomes and adjusted for the higher mortality of physicians, a work week of 50 hours, and different probabilities of entering military service. Further, the adjustments failed to eliminate variation in the rate of return to specialists relative to general practice.

Although by no means conclusive or consistent, previous studies that employed differential returns to assess physician supply seem to suggest that, historically, a shortage existed in the health system. Among the methodological problems present in these studies are the questionable adjustments for differences in the amount of time committed to market activity and the appropriateness of the discount rate used to transform earnings into present value equivalents. In addition, the occupational alternative to which the returns of medical practice are compared also appears to be an unresolved issue. Finally, differences in the direct and opportunity costs of alternate educational programs were not considered in previous studies, another factor that contributes to the inconclusive nature of findings regarding the historical supply of physicians.

The Physician to Population Ratio

Perhaps the most commonly used measure of the availability of providers is the physician to population ratio. Appearing in the numerator is the actual or projected number of physicians, which serves as a surrogate for the supply of care, while the denominator of the ratio is the corresponding population, an indicator of demand for service. An imbalance in the supply of physicians is usually measured in terms of differences that are identified by comparing (1) current and projected ratios, (2) ratios of low and high income states or regions, and (3) existing and desired ratios that are based on normative judgments or evaluations. For example, the highest ratio prevailing in a state or region might be regarded as a standard that should be achieved in all areas during a future period.

The Reliability of the Physician to Population Ratio

The reliability of the physician to population ratio as an indicator of a shortage has been assessed previously. For example, Held and Reinhardt (1975) examined the relation of the physician-population ratio to indices of market tightness, such as waiting time for an appointment, number of visits per week, and willingness to accept new patients. Contrary to expectations, the results indicated that shortage areas, defined by a low physician-to-population ratio, were characterized by market indices that were comparable or less stringent than those prevailing in nonshortage areas. In a similar study, Wise and Zook (1983) examined differences in practice characteristics of general practitioners, internists, and pediatricians whose practices were located in shortage and nonshortage areas, as defined by the number of physicians per capita. The results indicated that, in general, measures of market tightness were similar in shortage and nonshortage areas, suggesting that the physician-to-population ratio is a poor indicator of an inadequate supply of practitioners.

Results reported by Kehrer and Wooldridge (1983) also suggest that the physician-to-population ratio fails to identify areas characterized by a shortage of physicians. The purpose of this study was to assess the reliability of the criteria used to designate health manpower shortage areas (HMSA). The first of these criteria specified that an HMSA must be a rational service area for the delivery of health services. The second criterion indicated that HMSAs were characterized by a population-to-physician ratio in excess of prescribed values. This criterion was satisfied by ratios of population-to-primary care physicians that exceed

3,500:1, or ratios of 3,000:1 when accompanied by evidence of either an insufficient capacity of providers or an unusually high health need of the population at risk. The final criterion specified that health manpower in contiguous areas must be overused, inaccessible, or excessively distant.

Applying these criteria to urban areas in Quebec, Kehrer and Wooldridge compared utilization and other measures of access in shortage relative to non-shortage areas. Among the dimensions examined (proportion with one visit, cost per service, number of visits per person, and number of examinations per capita), the utilization rates in HMSAs were virtually indistinguishable from those in nonshortage areas. These results were also consistent with those reported by Kleinman and Wilson (1977) and Berk, Bernstein, and Taylor (1983), who found few differences in the access of persons residing in underserved areas as compared with their counterparts in nondesignated areas.

Sources of Error in the Ratio

As suggested by the studies reviewed in the previous section, the use of the physician to population ratio as an indicator of market conditions and the adequacy of the number of providers is subject to criticisms that are related to the adequacy of the numerator to measure supply and the denominator to reflect demand. Regarding the latter, the discussion presented in Chapter 3 indicates that multiple factors influence the demand for health services, but these are not reflected by unadjusted measures of the population. For example, other things remaining constant, a change in the composition of the population may increase the demand (need) for health services per person, resulting in a shortage of physicians and an increase in the price of care. Hence, the adoption of policies designed to maintain a given ratio may result in a shortage of physicians and an increase in the price of care, an outcome that may prevent some from securing medical service.

Similarly, the unadjusted number of physicians appearing in the numerator of the ratio fails to measure the capacity of a given stock of physicians to provide service, a dimension that is a function of productivity and hours committed to market activity per period. Both determinants of productive capacity may be subject to systematic regional and temporal variation that is related to specialty mix, the rates of compensation or income earned by physicians, the demographic characteristics of providers, and the distribution of physicians with regard to mode of practice. Each of these factors is described in this section.

A major problem in using the unadjusted number of physicians as an indicator of supply involves not only the specialty mix in the numerator but also variation in the proportion of time devoted to direct patient care and the productivity of the physician population. Results presented by Werner, Langwell, and Budde (1979) indicate that primary care specialties differ in terms of hours committed to market activity (direct patient care), productivity and, hence, supply of patient care. These results suggest that, without adjustments for differences in specialty mix and productivity, the physician-to-population ratio is an unreliable indicator of the supply of services. For example, when accompanied by an increase in productivity resulting from a change in the mix of specialists, the maintenance of a constant ratio may result in a surplus of physicians.

In addition, the level of income earned by the physicians and the rate of compensation also influence the number of hours committed to medical practice. In a number of occupations, it is common for workers to substitute leisure time for income in response to an increase in the rate of compensation, resulting in a backward bending supply curve (Mansfield 1982). Similar responses by physicians have been documented by Feldstein (1970), Sloan (1975), Vahovich (1977) and Mitchell (1984). In addition, Sloan reported that the annual number of hours of work supplied per physician was inversely related to the income earned by the provider's spouse and other nonemployment sources. Hence, these findings indicate that the number of hours committed to market activity and, hence, the supply of services provided by a given stock of physicians, is influenced by earnings.

In addition to the influence of income, it is believed that preferences for market activity are influenced by marital status, sex, family size, age, specialty, and mode of practice. As suggested previously, it is common to argue that family responsibilities influence supply decisions and that, by virtue of their roles in family formation and caring for children, females are induced to substitute nonmarket for market activity. In the assessment of factors that influence the number of hours practiced per week and the annual number of weeks worked, however, Vahovich (1977) found that the sex of the physician failed to exert a significant influence on work effort.

Employing census data for 1960 and 1970, Sloan (1975) reported mixed findings concerning the influence of marital responsibilities on supply decisions. When the 1960 data were analyzed, the results indicated that being a parent significantly reduced the market activity of female physicians. These results were based on a small number of physicians, however, and were not replicated when census data for 1970 were analyzed.

The effects of marital status and responsibilities of child care on supply decisions of male and female physicians were also examined by Mitchell (1984). Relative to their single counterparts, married male and female physicians worked a fewer number of weeks per year, while female physicians who were married committed fewer hours to market activity than their single counterparts. The effects of marital status on the work effort of female physicians were attributed, in part, to the income earned by their spouses. As suggested by Kehrer (1976), the husbands of female physicians are probably also professionals who earn a high income. Conversely, the wives of male physicians are less likely to work and, among those who participate in the labor force, earn a lower average income. Accordingly, the relatively high family income of female physicians enables them to substitute nonmarket for market activity. That a rising income earned by the physician's spouse reduces the number of hours practiced per week was also suggested by results reported by Sloan (1975).

The general belief that women reduce the number of hours committed to market activity in order to care for children was not supported by findings reported by Mitchell (1984). Relative to their childless counterparts, female physicians with children worked the same number of hours per week and more weeks per year. Similarly, physicians who were fathers worked more hours per week and weeks per year than their childless colleagues. Although females who chose to work less than half-time were excluded from the sample, these results suggest that the need to support minor dependents induces male and female physicians to increase the number of hours devoted to market activity.

Age and years of medical practice are also expected to influence market activity. It is common to argue that, relative to their older counterparts, younger and less experienced physicians are likely to commit more time to market activity and the development of their practices. Further, the deleterious effects of age on health status and gradual retirement induce older physicians to reduce market activity. Hence, the age of the physician is usually expected to exhibit an inverted-U relation to market activity.

Relative to their older counterparts, Vahovich (1977) found that, in general, younger physicians worked more hours per week and weeks per year, a result that is also substantiated by Sloan (1975). Similar results are reported by Mitchell (1984), who found that, as expected, the number of hours devoted to market activity by male physicians exhibited an inverted-U relation to age; however, age failed to exert a significant effect on the number of hours per week or the annual number of weeks worked by female physicians. These results may reflect a peculiar career pattern of the female physicians included in the sample. For example, the age-specific work efforts of a subset of female physicians may have resembled those of their male counterparts. Conversely, a second group of the female physicians may have devoted more time to market activity during later stages in the life cycle when the responsibility for child care was reduced or eliminated.

That productivity and hours worked are related to mode of practice has been documented in a number of studies; however, since solo practitioners are typically compensated on a fee-for-service basis, while physicians who practice in health maintenance organizations (HMOs) are often paid on either a capitation or a salary basis, it is difficult to separate the effects of practice mode from compensation arrangements. Accordingly, we will discuss the effects of both of these factors on the supply of physician services in this section.

Our review of production-function studies in Chapter 7 suggested that physicians engaged in solo or small-group practices tended to enjoy increasing returns to scale and that large, multispecialty group practices exhibited decreasing returns to scale (Kimbell and Lorant 1977). Further, small single-specialty groups may be more productive than solo practices (Reinhardt 1972).

A number of analysts have addressed the impact of practice mode and compensation arrangement on the market activity of physicians. In a comprehensive review of previous evaluations of the performance of HMOs, Luft (1981) concluded that physicians participating in prepaid group practices worked fewer hours per week than solo practitioners. A review of the literature by Sloan (1974) suggested that salaried physicians commit less time to market activity than their self-employed counterparts. These conclusions were also substantiated by Sloan (1974), who found that salaried physicians committed fewer hours per week to medical practice than self-employed practitioners. The analysis indicated, however, that the type of employment failed to exert a significant influence on the annual number of weeks devoted to medical practice. In an attempt to assess the influence of practice mode and the payment scheme, Dutton (1979) and Mechanic (1975) found that, relative to fee-for-service solo practice, physicians participating in prepaid groups earned lower incomes and devoted less time to market activity, a finding that was also substantiated by Goodman and Swartwout (1984). In addition, Held and Reinhardt (1979) found that physicians participating in prepaid group practices not only commit fewer hours to market activity but also devote 10 to 15 percent less time to patient care than those who practice in more traditional modes.

Although previous findings suggest that group practice and the method of compensation for physicians may detract from work effort, contradictory results have been reported. For example, results reported by Mitchell (1984) indicate that, relative to solo practices, physicians associated with group practices committed a significantly higher number of hours per week to market activity. Even though group physicians worked fewer weeks per year, the results indicated that the annual number of hours devoted to market activity by those participating in group practices was greater than the corresponding measure of work effort by physicians in solo practices. The unexpected results reported by Mitchell may be attributable more to the surrogate used to indicate participation in group practice and a failure to measure differences in methods of compensation than to the systematic effects of organizational structure.

As suggested by this section, the unadjusted number of physicians appearing in the numerator of the provider-population ratio is probably an inaccurate reflection of the supply of care available in a given area or during a specified time interval. Hence, the interpretation of a change or variation in the ratio requires an assessment of the distribution of physicians with regard to specialty and mode of practice, their demographic attributes, and market decisions in relation to levels or rates of compensation. These observations suggest that, in isolation, the ratio of physicians to population is an insensitive indicator of a physician surplus or shortage.

Recognizing the inadequacies of the unadjusted physician-to-population ratio, the Bureau of Health Manpower developed a more sophisticated approach to the problem of developing forecasts of surpluses or shortages (Office of Technology Assessment 1980). The model of demand for medical care consists of essentially three stages. The first stage estimates future demand from the anticipated growth in the population and shifts in demographic attributes, such as age, sex, and income. The second stage, called the baseline configuration, focuses on the effects of historical trends on the per capita use of 20 types of care. Two trends are distinguished in developing the baseline configuration. The first involves the portion of the change in per capita use that is expected to result from the influence of changes in price on the decision to seek care. The second trend that is used to predict per capita use reflects changes in the accessibility of care, the incidence of disease, medical technology, and demographic attributes of the population. The third stage consists of a contingency modeling capability and focuses on changes in demand that emanate from such factors as anticipated growth of HMOs and delegation of tasks to midlevel practitioners.

Projections of the supply of physicians are based on the current stock, adjusted for deaths and retirements. Additions to the supply of physicians are forecast from trends in medical school enrollment graduates of U.S. medical and osteopathic schools, the immigration of foreign medical graduates, and the flow of U.S. citizens educated in foreign medical schools. Projected stocks are also adjusted to reflect such factors as specialty selection, productivity and geographic distribution. When combined with projected demand, these estimates yield estimates of the physician surplus or shortage.

The Normative Approach

The economic approach to the definition of a physician shortage or surplus focuses on the demand rather than the need for care. As described previously, the demand for health services is influenced by health status, the price of service, the income of the consumers, and perceptions concerning the efficacy of treatment. On the other hand, the need for medical services is usually defined in terms of the mix of service that experts believe ought to be consumed during a specified period of time by members of a reference group in order to preserve or restore health status, given the constraints imposed by medical knowledge and technology (Jeffers, Bognanno, and Bartlett 1971). Since care-seeking behavior entails out-of-pocket expenditures, opportunity costs, defined as foregone wages, and time costs, it is possible to argue that the demand for care is less than normative measures of need (Lave, Lave, and Leinhardt 1975).

In an early study, Lee and Jones (1933) employed the normative approach to determine physician requirements. As summarized by Lave, Lave, and Leinhardt (1975) the approach consisted of (1) determining the frequency with which each illness occurs in a population; (2) obtaining expert opinion on the amount of services needed to diagnose and treat each category of illness; (3) estimating the mean number of services provided per hour by a physician; and (4) securing professional opinion on the average number of hours spent in medical practice. Lee and Jones estimated that the United States required 135 physicians per 100,000 population instead of the 126 per 100,000 that existed at the time of the study.

The GMENAC Study

Employing the normative approach and the physician-to-population ratio, the results reported by the Graduate Medical Education National Advisory Committee (GMENAC) ushered in an era in which the focus of policy deliberations shifted from mechanisms of alleviating a perceived shortage of physicians to those that address a surplus. As summarized by Harris (1986), the GMENAC methodology followed two sequential steps. First, similar to the Lee-Jones study, GMENAC obtained from experts a consensus on norms of care for each health condition and each medical procedure. Second, the judgments of experts were modified to reflect the effects of economic, social, and behavioral constraints (GMENAC 1980). Projections developed by the GMENAC were based on essentially four scenarios and indicated that the physician-to-population ratio is expected to increase from 1.77 per thousand to 2.45 per thousand in 1990. In addition, the normative evaluation suggested that, relative to the need for 466,000 physicians in 1990, the physician surplus will range from 40,000 to 75,000 providers. Relative to the projected need for 498,000 physicians, estimates of the surplus ranged from 75,000 to 186,000 providers in the year 2000. In addition, the study also projected a maldistribution of physicians with respect to specialty and predicted shortages in pediatrics, family practice, and internal medicine. Based on these estimates, the GMENAC recommended the development of policies that attenuate the growth in medical school admissions, limit the number of graduates of foreign medical schools who enter the United States annually, and increase the number of physicians specializing in areas in which a shortage is expected.

Several analysts developed alternate estimates and challenged the recommendations of the GMENAC. For example, Lanska, Lanska, and Rimm (1984); Steinwachs, Weiner, Shapiro, Batalden et al. (1986); Jacobsen and Rimm (1987); and Weiner, Steinwachs, Shapiro, Coltin et al. (1987) adjusted projections for recent changes in factors that influence the productivity of physicians and the aggregate time committed to the practice of medicine. Lanska et al. reported data adjusted for the increased proportion of females in the physician supply and concluded that the surplus in the year 2000 will be 41,000 less than the GMENAC projection. Similarly, adjusting for decreases in the proportion of physicians who enter active practice, increases in the proportion of female physicians, and declines in productivity, Jacobsen and Rimm estimate a surplus of 39,000 physicians in the year 2000. The validity of conclusions based on sex-adjusted measures is weakened by the availability of only mixed evidence on the impact of gender upon physician productivity. Comparing the staffing patterns in three large HMOs with projections reported by the GMENAC, Steinwachs et al. concluded that, because of the proliferation of HMOs, 50 percent fewer primary physicians will be needed for adults and 20 percent fewer for children in 1990 than projected by the GMENAC. Hence, alternate projections seem to suggest that the estimates derived by GMENAC understate the impending excess supply of physicians.

Schwartz, Williams, Newhouse, and Witsberger (1988) also examined the impending surplus of physicians and the reduction of Medicare funding of post-graduate education for residents who are more than one year beyond the requirement for board certification in internal medicine. The study focused on the distribution of subspecialists in internal medicine with respect to community size and the supply of board certified subspecialists in relation to demand for their services. Unlike the projections derived by GMENAC, estimates reported by Schwartz et al. indicate that, by the year 2000, residents of medium and large cities will be either unserved or underserved. These results were attributed to a shortage rather than a maldistribution of subspecialists and suggest a need to expand the pool of these practitioners.

The recommendations to curtail the flow of foreign medical graduates have also been evaluated. For example, Way, Jensen, and Goodman (1978); Goodman and Wunderman (1981); Stimmel and Graettinger (1984); and Mick and Worobey (1984, 1986) argue that physicians trained in foreign medical schools tend to select specialties for which a shortage is forecast and locate in "underserved" areas. Hence, it is possible that a curtailment of the flow of foreign medical graduates may exacerbate the maldistribution of physicians with respect to specialty and geographic location.

Although federal policies supporting medical education appear to have eliminated the shortage of physicians and may have contributed to the projected surplus, several issues concerning the supply of physicians are unresolved. Among the more prominent of these is the distribution of physicians with regard to specialty. As indicated in the next chapter, the geographic distribution of physicians also constitutes a policy issue of concern to health planners and governmental authorities. Accordingly, the remainder of this chapter is committed to a discussion of factors that influence the selection of specialty, and the next chapter focuses on the location decisions of physicians.

THEORETICAL FRAMEWORK: DETERMINANTS OF SPECIALTY CHOICE

In any labor market, long-run adjustments in the supply and distribution of manpower are the product of a complex interaction among multiple factors. This section considers a theoretical approach for examining factors that influence the career choices and specialty decisions of physicians.

The framework proposed by Freeman (1971), as modified by Ernst and Yett (1985), assumes that an individual is confronted by a limited number of specialty alternatives represented by the set $O_i \ldots, O_k \ldots, O_n$. Consistent with normative theory, the model posits that the individual evaluates the alternatives and implements career decisions so as to maximize the utility function:

$$U[x_k R_k + WL + x_k P_k], \ k=1,\ldots,n \qquad\qquad (9.1)$$

where x_k is 1 if specialty k is selected, and 0 otherwise; R_k is the monetary returns or income derived from committing market activity to specialty k; W is non-professional income; L is the nonpecuniary value of nonmarket or leisure activity; and P_k is the psychic value or prestige derived from selecting specialty k.

Further, the monetary returns, R_k, may be expressed in the form:

$$R_k = f\ (w_k, \ s_k, \ H) \qquad\qquad (9.2)$$

where w_k is the expected pecuniary rate of compensation derived from market activity committed to specialty k; s_k is the anticipated proportion of time devoted to market activity (e.g., direct patient care); and H is the maximum amount of time available.

Similarly, let p represent the rate of nonpecuniary income derived from leisure activity and m_k correspond to the rate of psychic income derived from selecting specialty k. The nonpecuniary income derived from leisure activity may be expressed in the form:

$$L = g\ (p, \ 1\text{-}\ s_k, \ H) \qquad\qquad (9.3)$$

while:

$$P_k = h\ (m_k, \ s_k, \ H) \qquad\qquad (9.4)$$

identifies the arguments that influence the psychic or nonpecuniary income derived from selecting specialty k. The model proposed by Freeman assumes that the individual evaluates career alternatives in terms of the monetary returns, $x_k R_k + W$, and the nonpecuniary or psychic income, represented by $L + x_k P_k$.

As suggested above, it is reasonable to expect the individual to select the alternative that maximizes the utility function for which the arguments are pecuniary compensation, $x_k R_k + W$, and nonmonetary or psychic income, represented by $L + x_k P_k$. The evaluation process may involve an assessment of the tradeoff between monetary and nonpecuniary income. For example, if the increment in utility derived from additional monetary compensation is zero, the physician focuses on nonpecuniary returns, suggesting that noneconomic factors dominate the evaluation process. Conversely, if the increment in utility derived from a change in nonpecuniary income is zero, the physician focuses on monetary factors and is induced to select the alternative that is expected to maximize wealth. Hence, the individual will choose to invest in medical education if and only if pecuniary returns are expected to exceed monetary costs.

The model is of value when considering the effects of changes in monetary aspects on the occupational choices of the individual. For example, a reduction in the availability or the funding of low interest loans to medical students and an extension in the length of time required to complete training raise the costs of selecting medicine as a career. *Ceteris paribus*, an increase in these costs reduces the net increase in wealth expected by potential entrants to the practice of medicine and, as a result, it is reasonable to expect these changes to precipitate a decline in the relative attractiveness of a medical career.

Suppose the investment in medical education decreases as evidenced by fewer medical graduates or practitioners who select a given area of specialization. *Ceteris paribus*, fewer physicians may result in excess demand, resulting in higher fees, earnings and rate of return. The higher rate of return, represented by a shift in the demand for medical education, will induce a growing number of students to choose medicine or the specialty area as a career. The eventual increase in the stock of physicians not only reduces the inflationary pressure on fees and earnings but also lowers the rate of return and, hence, the demand for medical training.

In addition to the market forces that lead to an adjustment in the stock of physicians, public policy might be implemented to "control" the price of medical services. For example, low-interest loans might be offered to medical students, thus reducing the costs of investment and inducing more to select medicine as a career. Alternatively, public funding of medical education might be adopted to induce a greater flow of graduates and thereby reduce fees or the rate of increase in the price of service provided by physicians.

It is important to observe, however, that several factors reduce the precision with which the model explains or predicts career choices. First, the evaluation of alternatives usually occurs prior to entry into practice, suggesting that the expectations on which the assessment is based may be derived from imprecise or unreliable information. In addition, the monetary returns derived from market activity are influenced by discretionary and nondiscretionary factors. Consider, for example, expectations concerning the value of w_k, the pecuniary rate of compensation. Income expectations clearly depend on the pricing policies the potential physician might implement and the mix of care that will be provided. The latter consideration is influenced by the proportion of the capacity, s_k, that is committed to productive effort and the efficiency with which services are provided. Perceptions of the proportion of capacity used to provide service are related to a number of factors, such as location, mix of patients, and type of practice, while the efficiency of providing services is influenced by the scale of the practice and the use of physician extenders such as physician assistants or nurse practitioners. As a consequence, perceptions of professional income are likely to vary from physician to physician, and projections based on current or previous earnings are unlikely to reflect the expectations of potential entrants with precision.

Consider next the psychic or nonpecuniary returns to an investment in medical education. It is possible to argue that preferences for specialization and psychic returns are influenced by personal attributes such as age, sex, marital status, and ability. Similarly, several analysts contend that the prestige, relative attractiveness assigned to alternative specialties and, hence, career decisions implemented by potential entrants are influenced by the educational experience and attributes of the medical school. The next section considers empirical findings concerning the effects of pecuniary and psychic returns on the specialty choice of physicians.

EMPIRICAL RESULTS

As is well recognized, the flow of practitioners who select specialty k, F_k, is the culmination of multiple career choices, each of which is influenced by multiple factors. The discussion presented in this section is organized in accordance with:

$$F_k = f(r,z, m) \tag{9.5}$$

where it is assumed that the flow of new entrants to specialty k is influenced by the relative rate of return, r, a set of personal attributes, z, and a set of medical school attributes, m, that are thought to influence the relative prestige assigned to each specialty area. The following employs the general approach to assess the influence of economic factors, personal characteristics, and attributes of the educational experience on career choices that culminate in medical specialization.

Relative Returns

Several studies have attempted to evaluate the sensitivity of occupational choice to the rate of return of an investment in medical education and income differences among multiple specialties. For example, Sloan (1970) focused on nine fields of specialization and used two dependent variables in an examination of the demand for residency training. The first indicated the number of residents in each of the specialties during 1956, 1960, and 1966. The second measured the proportion of available residencies in each field that were occupied during each year of the study period. The independent variables used in the analysis of the number of residents in each field were (1) the present value of lifetime earnings in the specialty, lagged by one year, (2) the number of residencies available in the field, and (3) the number of foreign medical graduates occupying domestic residency positions. When the ratio of residents to available positions was examined, the number of positions in the field was eliminated from the set of independent variables.

Consistent with normative theory, Sloan examined the contention that career choice is influenced by income differences, and that higher lifetime earnings not only attract a larger number of residents but also increase the proportion of occupied positions. In each of the specifications, the results indicated that the present value of lifetime earnings exerted a positive and significant effect ($p < .05$) on the number of residents and the proportion of residencies that were filled. Even though the results were consistent with the expectations derived from normative economic theory, however, the elasticity coefficients were relatively low. As a consequence, Sloan concluded that dramatic changes in relative earnings are required to induce noticeable adjustments in the pattern of specialization.

Several comments concerning the design of Sloan's study are worthy of note. First, as suggested by Ernst and Yett (1985), the inclusion of the number of positions available (a surrogate for supply) in an examination of demand for medical education is questionable. Similarly, the number of residents in a given specialty relative to the number of positions available might be regarded as a ratio of "demand" for medical training relative to supply. Since medical schools may maintain or increase available positions even though the number of applicants is low or declining, reported coefficients probably fail to capture with precision the responsiveness of demand for specialty training to differences in monetary returns.

In addition, nonpecuniary considerations and preferences for various dimensions of medical training or specialization were excluded from the study. Hence, the study implicitly assumed that the incremental utility derived from a change in nonpecuniary factors is zero, and that career choice is based solely on income differences. Since subsequent research demonstrates that tastes and preferences exert a significant influence on career choice, however, the exclusion of surrogates for these factors probably represents an additional source of bias in the estimates of the relation between the demand for specialty training and differences in earnings.

Hadley (1977, 1979) employed a slightly different approach to the problem of assessing the influence of economic factors on career choice. Rather than focus on decisions implemented by a collectivity, the model proposed by Hadley used the individual as the unit of analysis and examined the effects of monetary, nonpecuniary and institutional factors on career choice. The model was predicated on the contention that career decisions are based, in part, on the expected monetary and psychic returns and costs assigned to each of the alternatives considered by potential entrants to specialty practice.

In the first of these studies (Hadley 1977), occupational choices among five specialty groups were examined, and in the second, Hadley (1979) assessed selections from nine categories. A set of binary dependent variables was used to indicate the actual specialty of 2,524 physicians engaged in direct patient care during 1972. Attributes that were specific to specialty choice were measured as ratios that compared pairs of values for specialty alternatives. For example, expected earnings were approximated by the mean net incomes of various specialties in each state during 1965. The independent variable incorporated in the regression analysis of the choice probabilities for the kth specialty was defined as a ratio of the form y_k/y_j, where y_k corresponds to the income proxy for the specialty. The denominator, y_j, was defined as the mean net income of (1) the actual specialty selected by the physician, if a field other than k was chosen, (2) the previous field preferred by the physician, if the individual selected k but had expressed a preference for j during the physician's longitudinal history, or (3) the physician's medical school class, if the individual selected k and did not express a preference for a different field. A similar approach was employed to construct explanatory variables that depicted prestige and length of postgraduate training. In addition to variables that were specific to specialty choices, Hadley examined the influence on choice probabilities exerted by personal attributes such as age, sex, marital status, socioeconomic origins, ability, and measures of the educational environment.

Ordinary-least-squares regression analysis was used to estimate the parameters of the linear probability functions. Unfortunately, such an approach may result in heteroscedastic error terms and the possibility that predicted values are not limited to the range (0,1). As a result, findings reported in the study must be interpreted with caution.

After controlling for other factors included in the model, the results of the 1977 study indicated that the relative income variable was significant and positive in only one equation. Further, in two of the three equations, coefficients relating relative income to occupational choice were negative, and one of the coefficients was found to be significantly less than zero ($p < .05$). The results of the 1979 study also failed to support the contention that variation in fiscal returns exerts a consistent, significant and positive effect on choice probabilities.

The failure of these studies to demonstrate that differences in relative earnings exert a significant and positive effect on choice probabilities may be attributable to the operational definition of the income variables. For those physicians who selected specialty k without expressing a prior preference for an alternative, the denominator of the relative income variable was assigned a quasi-arbitrary value. For those who selected a specialty and expressed a prior preference for an alternate field, the denominator presumably reflected the mean net income of a specialty that was actively considered. Similarly, it is doubtful that the income variable included in the regression analysis of the choice probabilities for specialty k measures the difference in earnings considered by those who selected j and did not express a preference for k. These observations suggest that the measure of the relative income was inconsistent across those included in the study group.

A second factor that may have contributed to the failure of these studies to verify expectations concerning the influence of differences in earnings on choice probabilities involves the implicit assumption that the relative length of training required for a given specialty is independent of the corresponding returns. When interpreting the coefficient that relates the relative length of training to choice probabilities, one assumes that all other factors, to include relative income, are constant. If a change in the relative length of training is not accompanied by an increase (or decrease) in relative earnings, physicians would presumably avoid specialties requiring long residency programs. Other factors remaining constant, however, a decline in the number of physicians would precipitate an increase in the net income of these specialty fields, suggesting that relative earnings, length of training, and specialty selection are interdependent.

As argued by Hay (1980, 1981), the joint dependence of specialty selection and income creates a bias in coefficients that relate choice probabilities to differences in relative earnings. Suppose individuals are confronted with a set of alternatives represented by A, B, C, and D. Presumably, those selecting specialty A anticipated greater financial returns in that field of specialization than in the other alternatives. Suppose further, that those who selected B, C, and D responded to similar expectations. Economic theory suggests that, if the first group of physicians selected alternatives B, C, and D, rather than A, earnings in these fields would be lower than actual or observed returns. Accordingly, the actual income of those engaged in alternatives B, C, and D overstates the returns physicians who selected A might have earned by selecting one of the other alternatives.

The simultaneous equation bias described above may produce spuriously low regression estimates, thus understating the sensitivity of specialty selection to differences in monetary returns. In an assessment of these effects, Hay (1980, 1981) developed a simultaneous-equation model of specialty choice in which selection probabilities and earnings were jointly endogenous. The study also focused on a single equation model of choice probabilities in which the set of independent variables were exogenous and represented the personal attributes of the physician, environmental factors depicting the educational process, and specialty earnings, measured by annual net income.

Parameter estimates of the two models supported the contention that specialty choices and earnings are jointly dependent. In the single equation model, the coefficients relating choice probabilities to net income were negative and not significant at conventional levels. Employing the same data and set of independent variables, the results obtained from the simultaneous equation model indicated that the relationship between the choice probabilities and net income was significant and positive.

The findings reported by Hay are of importance for several reasons. First, as suggested by Ernst and Yett (1985), the estimates of the simultaneous-equation model indicate that previous studies in which earnings were exogenous to the relationship understate the sensitivity of specialty selection to differences in monetary returns. In addition, the study provides evidence, based on a rigorous analysis, that supports the contention that specialty choice is motivated by income differences.

Several comments concerning previous evaluations of the influence of economic factors on career choice are appropriate. Implicit in each of these studies is the assumption that current or previous differences in earnings are congruent with the expectations of potential applicants or that current earnings are used to estimate life cycle returns, which form the basis for a career choice. For example, even though estimates of returns based on current earnings are low or negative, it is possible that anticipated changes in the pattern of demand may stimulate a growing number of applicants. It is also possible that medical graduates or potential applicants focus less on current or previous earnings and more on subjective estimates of market demand, prices, and net earnings for each of the future periods when evaluating specialty alternatives. In a similar fashion, the current number of hours committed to market activity may not be congruent with the expectations of potential applicants, suggesting that discounted returns, based on adjusted earnings, represent an imprecise indicator of the economic factors on which career choices are based.

Personal Attributes

As indicated previously, the change in the stock of physicians and the distribution of practitioners with respect to specialty are related to a set of noneconomic factors, represented by the vectors z and m in equation 9.5. Unlike differential earnings and returns to an investment in medical education, the effects of these factors on career choice have been examined extensively. For purposes of presentation, it is convenient to partition the discussion into an assessment of the effects of personal attributes and institutional characteristics that define the educational environment on career choice. The following relies on the reviews by Zuckerman (1977), who focused on the effects of institutional factors, and the review by Ernst and Yett (1985), who assessed previous findings concerning the influence of personal attributes on career choice.

Among the personal characteristics that have been related to career choice are age, sex, marital status, ability, and socioeconomic origins. These factors might be regarded as surrogates for preferences assigned to various career paths or as constraints that limit the set of feasible alternatives available to the individual.

Age

The commonly cited reason for using age as a proxy for preferences assigned to general versus specialty practice involves the anticipated effect of prolonged training on lifetime earnings. At the end of the first year of the residency program, the physician must choose between entering practice as a general practitioner or extending the length of training for a specialty career. Employing the analysis of the previous section, it is possible that those who elect to prolong the training period expect their annual net income to exceed the earnings of general practitioners and to compensate for the opportunity cost (i.e., net foregone income) of specialization. Accordingly, those who specialize expect a long work life, which is required to ensure that the present value of their lifetime earnings will exceed not only the present value of the earnings stream of the general practitioner, but also compensate for the net opportunity costs of prolonged training. Hence, physicians who are older at the end of the first year of residency training may expect a comparatively short working life and lower lifetime earnings, both of which increase the attractiveness of immediate entry into medical practice. Conversely, younger physicians might reasonably expect a longer working life and greater lifetime earnings, both of which increase the attractiveness of specialty training.

In general, previous findings are consistent with these observations. As summarized by Ernst and Yett, studies in which age is related to career choice indicate that general practitioners are older than others when they graduate from medical school. Similarly, findings reported by Hadley (1979) indicate that surgeons were younger than other medical graduates, an outcome that may be attributable to the prolonged period of residency training required for certification. Additional support for these expectations is cited by Weil, Schleiter, and Tarlov (1981) who found that residents who planned to specialize in internal medicine were older than those who planned a subspecialty career in the same field.

Sex

Previous studies also suggest that sex differences influence career choice. Perhaps the most consistent finding is that females exhibit a propensity to specialize in pediatrics, psychiatry and obstetrics-gynecology while avoiding those specialties, such as surgery, that traditionally are dominated by males.

The preferences of females for these specialty fields have been attributed to several factors. First, as suggested by Lopate (1968), discrimination may have excluded women from the specialties that are male-dominated. In addition, it is possible that females are attracted to those areas of medical specialty, such as pediatrics and psychiatry, in which tenderness, warmth, and understanding are of importance. Finally, the career choice of females may be influenced by a need to resolve conflicts between marital, personal, and professional goals. Since medical schools rarely permit students to interrupt their education for childbearing and related responsibilities, women may be more likely than men to select specialties that require shorter training periods, offer regular working hours, and permit interrupted or part-time employment. *Ceteris paribus*, these comments suggest that females are more likely than males to pursue careers in general practice, psychiatry, and radiology or pathology, a decision that might enhance the probability of securing employment in a hospital, where working hours are regular.

Several studies report findings that are consistent with these expectations. As summarized by Ernst and Yett, preferences of females for family formation are manifest in shorter training periods, lower rates of participation in the labor force, and in the selection of practice settings. Women are less likely to complete graduate programs resulting in board certification and, in general, devote less time to graduate training than do men. Further, the career choices of males and single females exhibit a high degree of similarity while those of males and married females with children are least similar. Accordingly, previous findings indicate that the preferences and roles of women in family formation exert a noticeable influence on career selection.

Socioeconomic Status

Closely related to the effects of age and sex on career choice are those exerted by the socioeconomic status of the individual, which is believed to exert two distinct and different influences on career choice. Concerning the first, various researchers contend that specialty selection is motivated by a desire to improve the socioeconomic status of the physician or the physician's family. If an improvement in socioeconomic status is a motive in specialty choice, it is reasonable to expect that, other things remaining constant, those of lower socioeconomic origins will select the most prestigious specialties.

Support for these expectations is found in the findings reported by Kritzer and Zimet (1967). This study examined the relation between the socioeconomic status (SES) of the families of residents of the University of Colorado and the perceived status of alternate specialties. The results revealed an inverse correlation between SES and perceived status, suggesting that the less wealthy selected the most prestigious specialty. Although the findings are consistent with the notion that an improvement in status is a motive that influences specialty choice, physicians of high SES who preferred less prestigious specialties appeared to exhibit perverse behavior in the selection of specialty. Hadley (1977, 1979) also found that career choice was significantly related to perceived prestige but unrelated to socioeconomic origins as measured by the occupation of the physician's father. These results indicate that the motive to improve economic status is a factor that influences career selection but conventional measures of SES fail to capture these incentives with precision.

Rather than using economic background as a proxy for the motive to improve status, it is possible to regard the origins of the physician as a surrogate for family wealth and the fiscal resources that are available to finance the costs of medical education. Unlike the status-related hypothesis, it is reasonable to argue that greater wealth enables the physician to finance the cost of education, suggesting that individuals of higher socioeconomic origins are more likely to select specialties requiring longer training periods than those of a lower status. Also supporting these expectations are perceived differences in the preferences of the poor and the wealthy for current and future consumption. Relative to their wealthier counterparts, those of poor origins are likely to exhibit a higher rate of time preference, suggesting that current consumption is preferred to future spending. Since a portion of the spending by wealthy families is discretionary, those of higher economic origins are more likely than their poor counterparts to forego current consumption in order to increase future consumption. Other things remaining constant, it is reasonable to expect that physicians from wealthier families are more likely to select specialties requiring extended training than the less affluent; however, the strength of the relation between family wealth and specialty choice is reduced by the possibility that the costs of prolonged training might be financed by debt sources.

Although contradictory results have been reported, most studies suggest that the socioeconomic status of the physician's family distinguishes general practitioners from other physicians. The weight of evidence indicates that those of poorer origins are likely to enter general practice; however, results reported by Oates and Feldman (1971), Otis and Weiss (1971), and Weil and Schleiter (1981) failed to support the expectation that SES significantly affects the types of careers preferred by physicians.

Marital Status

Similar to the use of SES in studies of factors that influence career choice, the marital status of the physician serves as a proxy for the marginal rate of time preference. Most analysts contend that preferences for current consumption are positively related to the number of dependents. Consequently, it is usually assumed that preferences for specialties requiring longer training periods diminish with the size of the physician's immediate family. *Ceteris paribus*, these observations suggest that married physicians with children are most likely to enter general practice after graduation from medical school, followed by married physicians with no children and single practitioners, a group that is expected to be least likely to select general practice as a career choice.

The weight of empirical evidence appears to support these expectations. Previous findings indicate that general practitioners are more likely than others to be married or to be married with children during medical school. In the assessment of career choices among internists, however, Weil, Schleiter, and Tarlov (1981) found that the number of dependents was not related to the decision to enter practice or to train for a subspecialty in internal medicine. As suggested by Ernst and Yett, differences in the training of a generalist or subspecialist in the field of internal medicine may be insufficient to induce the expected relationship.

Ability

An extension of normative theory suggests that the onset and effects of the principle of diminishing returns depends on the ability of the individual, and that those with a greater capacity will invest more in human capital than their less able counterparts. The most commonly used measures of ability are college grade point averages (GPAs), class rankings and performance on the Medical College Admission Test (MCAT), or the examination administered by the National Board of Medical Examiners (NBME). A number of studies have examined the relation between ability, as measured by these indicators, and the planned or actual choices of physicians.

Consistent with theoretical considerations, previous findings indicate that the measured abilities of academics are highest followed, in order, by internists, other specialties, and general practitioners. In particular, findings reported by Lyden, Geiger, and Peterson (1968) and Peterson, Lyden, Geiger, and Colton (1963) indicated that academics and internists were more likely to rank in the upper third of their class and MCAT group, while general practitioners were more likely to rank in the lowest third of their class and the lowest MCAT group. Similarly, a number of studies have indicated that graduates characterized by a relatively low class ranking and poor performance on the MCAT are the most likely to enter unspecialized internships. In addition to other variables, Fadem,

Nicolich, Simring, Dauber, and Bullock (1984) examined the congruence between performance on the NBME–Part II tests and specialty choice; the results indicated that high scores on the subtests pertaining to psychiatry, medicine, and surgery were associated with decisions to pursue postgraduate training in psychiatry, medicine, and surgery, respectively. These results suggest that specialty selection was closely related to performance on the NBME subtest; however, results reported by Rosevear, Tickman, and Gary (1985) failed to support the expectation that students pursue careers in those fields of specialization in which they excel academically.

Although several studies demonstrated that career choice is influenced by measured ability, it is also likely that those who perform well received more faculty attention than others. As indicated in the next section, measured ability may interact with the student-faculty relationship to influence career choice.

Institutional Factors

Although personal attributes or characteristics of the physician's background are of value when examining choices between general practice and specialization, these characteristics produce inconsistent results concerning secondary career decisions. As summarized by Zuckerman (1977), several studies suggest that the longer a medical student remains in the educational process, the more the components of the system become important determinants of behavior while the background characteristics become less influential. On the assumption that the process of training affects career choice, various researchers contend that decisions are influenced by (1) the relationship of the student to faculty members, (2) the values embraced by the medical school, and (3) the process of adult socialization that occurs during the educational process.

As indicated previously, the economic model of career choice emphasizes the individual and is predicated on the assumption that each physician forms expectations concerning the monetary and psychic attributes of available alternatives, evaluates each in terms of these dimensions, and selects the alternative that maximizes wealth. In contrast, Freidson (1970), Meyer (1977), Black (1972), and Mitchell (1975) among others contend that the characteristics and ambitions of the physician interact with the educational environment to form career choices. These analyses suggest that the educational process reinforces or alters the motives, knowledge, and values of the individual. Accordingly, it is possible that the educational environment modifies the career choices, suggesting that students respond more to the immediate influence of the training programs, the values of influential faculty, and peer group interactions than to personal attributes such as family origins or personality attributes.

Based on the assumption that career choices are developed during the educational process, the independent variables included in studies that focus on intraprofessional career choice include the medical school attended, type of internship, and the type of hospital in which the internship or residency is served.

The dependent variable focused on career choice, as measured by type of medical practice or specialty.

That the medical school and the values of faculty influence career choice has been documented by several studies. For example, Schumacher (1961) and Adler, Korsch, and Negrete (1985) report that intraprofessional choices occurred during medical school, suggesting that the environment created by the educational process modifies the career plans of physicians. As summarized by Zuckerman, disproportionate interest in general practice was induced by medical training at the University of Iowa. Conversely, those attending the University of Rochester expressed little interest in general practice, a preference that diminished during the educational process. Although the preferences of the two groups may be attributable to differences among students, these findings suggest that the educational process alters the career plans or choices.

Results reported by Becker, Hughes, and Strauss (1961), Marshall, Fulton and Wesser (1978), Zuckerman (1978), Weil and Schleiter (1981), and Adler, Korsch, and Negrete (1985) document the influence exerted on career choice by the educational environment represented by an exposure to faculty members as role models, differences between public and private medical schools, operating budgets, and the ratio of clinical to nonclinical staff. Additional support for the hypothesis that the educational environment influences career choice is found in the study by Paiva and Haley (1971), who concluded that those exposed to a research orientation during medical school were likely to select internships sponsored by university hospitals. Similarly, Peterson et al. (1963) concluded that graduates of private medical schools are more likely to pursue careers in specialty practice or academia, while those graduating from public schools are prone to enter general practice. Results reported by Weil, Schleiter, and Tarlov (1981) also confirm the notion that career choices are affected by the type of medical school and, to a lesser extent, by the type of residency programs. Wing and Blumberg (1971) also reported that the medical school's commitment to research, as evidenced by sponsored research spending, enhances the likelihood that graduates select academia as a career, while Fein and Weber (1971) reported that per capita and total school expenditures are positively associated with the likelihood that students select careers in teaching and research.

The type of internship has also been found to influence career choice. For example, findings reported by Caplovitz (1961) and Glaser (1959) indicate that straight internships were preferred by those who intended to pursue a career in academic or specialty practice. Early studies also suggest that straight internships were more likely to be (1) served in major affiliated hospitals, and (2) followed by residency training in teaching hospitals. Conversely, rotating internships were likely to lead directly to practice and less likely to lead to residency training; however, a rotating internship served in a hospital affiliated with a medical school increased the probability of residency training, suggesting that the type of hospital may offset the effects of the internship type.

In accordance with expectations concerning the effects of environmental factors on choices, studies have indicated that those who plan to pursue a career in academia are more likely to serve their internships in hospitals that are affiliated with medical schools. Conversely, those who prefer general practice are more likely to serve internships in private or municipal hospitals.

SUMMARY AND POLICY IMPLICATIONS

In the first part of the chapter, we examined various measures of the adequacy of the stock of physicians and found that none of the approaches are precise. Given unreliable forecasting measures, public officials must address the question—is a surplus of physicians or shortage of physicians more costly to society? Subscribers to the theory of supplier-induced demand and the target-income hypothesis argue that a surplus of physicians will be costly because it results in excessive physician-initiated demand as well as increased charges. As our review in Chapter 3 showed, however, the ability of physicians to induce demand may be much more limited than assumed in the past.

On the other hand, increases in the number of physicians might result in a better distribution of medical personnel resulting in a more equitable access to care. Further, it is commonly observed that the willingness of physicians to join alternate delivery systems or to offer office hours that are more convenient to patients has been a response by those who perceive a need to compete more vigorously for patients.

Most of the problems associated with a physician shortage are the converse of the benefits expected from a physician surplus; however, one aspect not considered in this brief analysis is that the quality of physician care tends to increase with the volume of care supplied. Thus, in a shortage, the volume of care per physician, and hence quality, may increase; unfortunately the increased quality is of little solace to those who are denied access to care. Thus, on balance, the weight of the evidence suggests that if errors in physician manpower policy are inevitable, public welfare will be better served by a bias towards a surplus.

In addition to our observations regarding the aggregate supply of physicians, the results summarized in this chapter suggest several policy implications concerning the projected shortage of pediatricians, family practitioners, and physicians who specialize in internal medicine. Perhaps the most striking finding of previous studies is the often inconsistent and rather small influence exerted by differences in monetary returns on specialty selection. These results seem to suggest that policies designed to alter the specialty mix by selectively increasing net returns are likely to yield uncertain effects. In addition, an increased dependence on economic incentives to influence the selection of specialty is likely to involve a substantial, if not prohibitive, financial commitment.

The distribution of physicians with regard to specialty might be influenced by implementing a mix of policies, however. For example, in addition to increasing the relative returns anticipated by those who might practice in a shortage area, the policies of medical schools ought to favor applicants who are likely to select pediatrics, family practice, and internal medicine. Among the attributes that might form the basis for such a policy are age, sex, and marital status. Although no single policy is likely to achieve desired results, a coordinated mix of public and private initiatives may reduce projected imbalances in the specialty distribution of physicians.

REFERENCES

Adler, R., B. M. Korsch, and V. F. Negrete. 1985. Timing and motivation in pediatric career choices. *Journal of Medical Education* 60(3):174–80.

Becker, H. S., E. C. Hughes, and H. L. Strauss. 1961. *Boys in White: Student Culture in Medical School*. Chicago, IL: University of Chicago Press.

Berk, M. L., A. B. Bernstein, and A. K. Taylor. 1983. Use and availability of medical care in federally designated health manpower shortage areas. Unpublished paper, Rockville, MD: National Center for Health Services Research, September.

Black, G. S. 1972. A theory of political ambition: Career choices and the role of structural incentives. *The American Political Science Review* 66:144–59.

Black, R. A., and K. F. Chui. 1981. Comparing schemes to rank areas according to degree of health manpower shortage. *Inquiry* 18(3):274–80.

Caplovitz, D. 1961. Reanalysis of 1958 institute data pertaining to the internship. *Journal of Medical Education* 36 (April, Part 2):68–81.

Dutton, D. 1979. Patterns of ambulatory health care in five different delivery systems. *Medical Care* 17(3):221–43.

Ernst, R. L., and D. E. Yett. 1984. Physicians' background characteristics and their career choices: A review of the literature. *Medical Care Review* 41(1):1–36.

Ernst, R. L., and D. E. Yett. 1985. *Physician Location and Specialty Choice*. Ann Arbor, MI: Health Administration Press.

Fadem, B. H., M. S. Nicolich, S. S. Simring, M. H. Dauber, and L. A. Bullock. 1984. Predicting medical specialty choice. *Journal of Medical Education* 59(5):407–15.

Fein, R., and G. Weber. 1971. *Financing Medical Education*. New York: McGraw-Hill.

Feldstein, M. S. 1970. The rising price of physicians' services. *The Review of Economics and Statistics* 52(2):121–33.

Feldstein, P. J. 1983. *Health Care Economics*, 2nd ed. New York: John Wiley & Sons.

Freeman, R. B. 1971. *The Market for College-Trained Manpower*. Cambridge, MA: Harvard University Press.

Freidson, E. 1970. *Professional Dominance: The Social Structure of Medical Care*. New York: Atherton Press.

Friedman, M. 1962. *Capitalism and Freedom*. Chicago, IL: University of Chicago Press.

Friedman, M., and S. Kuznets. 1945. *Income from Independent Professional Practice*. New York: National Bureau of Economic Research.

Glaser, W. 1959. Internship appointments of medical students. *Administrative Science Quarterly* 4(3):351–52.

Goodman, L. J., and J. E. Swartwout. 1984. Comparative aspects of medical practice: Organizational setting and financial arrangements in four delivery systems. *Medical Care* 22(3):255–67.

Goodman, L. J., and L. E. Wunderman. 1981. Foreign medical graduates and graduate medical education. *Journal of the American Medical Association* 246(8):854–58.

Graduate Medical Education National Advisory Committee (GMENAC). 1980. Summary Report of the Graduate Medical Education National Advisory Committee, Vol. I, DHHS Pub. No. [HRA] 81–651. Washington, DC: U.S. Department of Health and Human Services.

Hadley, J. 1977. An empirical model of medical specialty choice. *Inquiry* 14(4):384–401.

Hadley, J. 1979. A disaggregated model of medical specialty choice. In R. M. Scheffler, ed. *Research in Health Economics*. Greenwich, CT: JAI Press.

Harris, J. E. How many doctors are enough? *Journal of Health Affairs* 5(4):73–82.

Hay, J. 1980. Occupational choice and occupational earnings: Selectivity bias in a simultaneous logit-OLS model. Ph.D. dissertation, Yale University.

Hay, J. 1981. Selectivity bias in a simultaneous logit-OLS model: Physician specialty choice and specialty income. Farmington, CT: University of Connecticut Health Center.

Held, P. J., and U. E. Reinhardt. 1975. Health manpower policy in a market context. Paper presented to annual meetings of the American Economic Association, Dallas, TX, December.

Held, P. J., and U. E. Reinhardt. 1979. Analysis of economic performance in medical group practices. Princeton: Mathematica Policy Research.

Iglehart, J. K. 1986. Trends in health personnel. *Health Affairs* 5(4):128–37.

Jacobsen, S. J., and A. A. Rimm. 1987. The projected physician surplus reevaluated. *Health Affairs* 6(2):48–55.

Jeffers, J. R., M. F. Bognanno, and J. C. Bartlett. 1971. On the demand need for medical services and the concept of "shortage." *American Journal of Public Health* 61(1):46–63.

Kehrer, B. 1976. Factors affecting the incomes of men and women physicians: An exploratory analysis. *Journal of Human Resources* 11(4):526–45.

Kehrer, B. H., and J. Wooldridge. 1983. An evaluation of criteria to designate urban health manpower shortage areas. *Inquiry* 20(3):264–75.

Kimbell, L., and J. Lorant. 1977. Physician productivity and returns to scale. *Health Services Research* 12(4):367–79.

Kleinman, J. C., and R. W. Wilson. 1977. Are "medically underserved areas" medically underserved? *Health Services Research* 12(2):147–62.

Kritzer, H., and C. N. Zimet. 1967. A retrospective view of medical specialty choice. *Journal of Medical Education* 42(1):47–58.

Lanska, M. J., D. J. Lanska, and A. A. Rimm. 1984. Effect of rising percentage of female physicians on projections of physician supply. *Journal of Medical Education* 59(11):849–55.

Lave, J. R., L. B. Lave, and S. Leinhardt. 1975. Medical manpower models: Needs, demand and supply. *Inquiry* 12(2):97–125.

Lee, R. I., and L. W. Jones. 1933. *The Fundamentals of Good Medical Care*. Chicago, IL: University of Chicago Press.

Leffler, K. B., 1975. Quality, search and licensure. Ph.D. dissertation, University of California, Los Angeles.

Lindsay, C. M. 1973. Real returns to medical education. *Journal of Human Resources* 8(3):331–48.

Lopate, C. 1968. *Women in Medicine*. Baltimore, MD: Johns Hopkins Press.

Luft, H. S. 1981. *Health Maintenance Organizations: Dimensions of Performance*. New York: John Wiley & Sons.

Lyden, F. J., H. J. Geiger, and O. L. Peterson. 1968. *The Training of Good Physicians*. Cambridge, MA: Harvard University Press.

Mansfield, E. 1982. *Microeconomics: Theory and Applications, 4th Edition*. New York: W. W. Norton and Company.

Marshall, R. J., J. P. Fulton, and A. F. Wesser. 1978. Physician career outcomes and the process of medical education. *Journal of Health and Social Behavior* 19(2):124–38.

Mechanic, D. 1975. The organization of medical practice and practice orientations among physicians in prepaid and nonprepaid primary care settings. *Medical Care* 13(3):189–204.

Meyer, J. W. 1977. The effects of education as an institution. *American Journal of Sociology* 83(1):55–77.

Mick, S. S., and J. L. Worobey. 1984. Foreign and United States medical graduates in practice: A follow-up. *Medical Care* 22(11):1014–25.

Mick, S. S., and J. L. Worobey. 1986. The future role of foreign medical graduates in U.S. medical practice: Projections into the 1990s. *Health Services Research* 21(1):85–106.

Mitchell, J. B. 1984. Why do women physicians work fewer hours than men physicians? *Inquiry* 21(4):361–68.

Mitchell, W. D. 1975. Medical student career choice: A conceptualization. *Social Science and Medicine* 9(11/12):641–53.

Noether, M. 1986. The growing supply of physicians: Has the market become more competitive? *Journal of Labor Economics* 4(4):503–37.

Oates, R. P., and H. A. Feldman. 1971. Medical career patterns: Choices among several classes of medical students. *New York State Journal of Medicine* 71:2437–40.

Office of Technology Assessment. 1980. Forecasts of physician supply and requirements. NTIS no. PB80–181670, Washington, DC: Office of Technology Assessment.

Otis, G. D., and J. Weiss. 1971. Explorations in medical career choice. Report on contract No. (NIH) 71–4066, U.S. Department of Health, Education, and Welfare, May.

Paiva, R., and H. B. Haley. 1971. Intellectual, personality, and environmental factors in career specialty preferences. *Journal of Medical Education* 46(4):281–89.

Peterson, O. L., F. J. Lyden, H. J. Geiger, and T. Colton. 1963. Appraisal of medical students' abilities as related to training and careers after graduation. *New England Journal of Medicine* 269 (November 23):1174–82.

Reinhardt, U. 1972. A production function for physician services. *Review of Economics and Statistics* 54(1):55–66.

Rosevear, G. C., M. S. Tickman, and N. E. Gary. 1985. Relationship between specialty choice and academic performance. *Journal of Medical Education* 60(8):640–41.

Schumacher, C. F. 1961. The 1960 medical school graduate: His biographical history. *Journal of Medical Education* 36(5):401–2.

Schwartz, W. B., A. P. Williams, J. P. Newhouse, and C. Witsberger. 1988. Are we training too many medical subspecialists? *Journal of the American Medical Association* 259(2):233–39.

Sloan, F. A. 1970. Lifetime earnings and physician's choice of specialty. *Industrial and Labor Relations Review* 24(1):47–56.

Sloan, F. A. 1974. Effects of incentives on physician performance. In J. Rafferty, ed., *Health Manpower and Productivity*. Lexington, MA: D. C. Heath.

Sloan, F. A. 1975. Physician supply behavior in the short run. *Industrial and Labor Relations Review* 28:549–69.

Sloan, F. A. 1976. Real returns to medical education: A comment. *Journal of Human Resources* 11(1):118–26.

Steinwachs, D. M., J. P. Weiner, S. Shapiro, P. Batalden, K. Coltin, and F. Wasserman. 1986. A comparison of the requirements for primary care physicians in HMOs with projections made by the GMENAC. *New England Journal of Medicine* 314(4):217–22.

Stimmel, B., and J. S. Graettinger. 1984. Medical students trained abroad and medical manpower. *New England Journal of Medicine* 310(4):230–35.

Vahovich, S. G. 1977. Physicians' supply decisions by specialty: 2SLS model. *Industrial Relations* 16(1):51–60.

Way, P. O., L. E. Jensen, and L. J. Goodman. 1978. Foreign medical graduates and the issue of substantial disruption of medical services. *New England Journal of Medicine* 299(14):745–51.

Weil, P. A., and M. K. Schleiter. 1981. National study of internal medicine manpower: 6. Factors predicting preferences of residents for careers in primary care and in clinical practice or academic medicine. *Annals of Internal Medicine* 94(5):691–703.

Weil, P. A., M. K. Schleiter, and A. R. Tarlov. 1981. National study of internal medicine manpower: 5. Comparison of residents in internal medicine: Future generalists and subspecialists. *Annals of Internal Medicine* 94(5):678–90.

Weiner, J., D. Steinwachs, S. Shapiro, K. Coltin, D. Ershoff, and J. O'Connor. 1987. Assessing a methodology for physician requirement forecasting: Replication of GMENAC's need-based model for the pediatric specialty. *Medical Care* 25(5):426–36.

Werner, J. L., K. M. Langwell, and N. W. Budde. 1979. Designation of physician shortage areas: The problem of specialty mix variations. *Inquiry* 16(1):31–37.

Wing, P., and M. S. Blumberg. 1971. Operating expenditures and sponsored research at U.S. medical schools: An empirical study of cost patterns. *Journal of Human Resources* 6(1):75–102.

Wise, D. A., and C. J. Zook. 1983. Physician shortage areas and policies to influence practice location. *Health Services Research* 18(2):251–83.

Zuckerman, H. S. 1977. Evaluation of the literature on career choice within medicine. *Medical Care Review* 34(9):1079–1100.

Zuckerman, H. S. 1978. Structural factors as determinants of career patterns in medicine. *Journal of Medical Education* 53(6):453–63.

10

THE GEOGRAPHIC DISTRIBUTION OF PHYSICIANS: CHOICE OF LOCATION

With this chapter, the focus shifts from an assessment of factors that influence the selection of specialty choice to an examination of the economic variables and the attributes of the market area that affect the physician's selection of location. The manpower policies implemented during the 1970s were concerned with the geographic distribution, the specialty mix and the perceived shortage of physicians. As suggested by Schwartz, Newhouse, Bennett, and Williams (1983); Newhouse, Williams, Bennett, and Schwartz (1982); and Williams, Schwartz, Newhouse, and Bennett (1983) and Dionne, Langlois and Lemire (1987), the growing supply and diffusion of physicians into rural or underserved areas has reduced concern regarding the geographic distribution of medical practitioners; however, shortages of physicians in certain urban and rural areas are expected to persist into the 1990s (GMENAC 1980; Madison 1980; Fruen and Cantwell 1982; Hynes and Givner 1983; Leonardson, Lapierre, and Hollingsworth 1985). For example, a study of ten U.S. cities found that from 1963 to 1980, the ratio of physicians per 100,000 population in poverty areas increased by 21.8 percent; however, the number of office-based physicians per 100,000 population and the number of office-based physicians engaged in primary care per 100,000 declined in poverty areas by 6.5 percent and 45.1 percent, respectively (Kindig, Movassaghi, Dunham et al. 1987). Although many professions are characterized by a nonuniform distribution, unevenness in the location of physicians may create inequities in access and the use of care (Berk, Bernstein, and Taylor 1983). As a result, the geographic distribution of providers represents an issue that is not completely resolved and is of concern to governmental authorities.

As this chapter will indicate, most of the studies that examined factors that influence the geographic distribution of physicians employed regression analysis. The dependent variables usually measure the stock of physicians in a given location or the flow of practitioners entering the market area. The independent variables depict not only the income opportunities of different markets but also attributes of geographic areas that serve as proxies for nonpecuniary factors and tastes or preferences for practice conditions and living amenities.

The purpose of this chapter is twofold. The first is to consider a theoretical approach to explaining or predicting the pattern of the physician distribution and the results of studies that examined the influences of economic and noneconomic factors on location decisions. The second objective is to assess policy instruments that might be implemented to redress imbalances in the distribution of practitioners.

THEORETICAL FRAMEWORK

This section develops a theoretical framework that focuses on the flow rather than the stock of physicians. When evaluating empirical assessments of theoretical expectations, it is important to note that the monetary and psychic cost of relocating probably reduces the geographic mobility of physicians who enjoy an established practice. As a result, it is not likely that changes in the stock of physicians observed in cross-sectional analyses are sensitive to differences in net earnings or benefits among alternate market areas.

Similar to the discussion of specialty selection, economic theory suggests that the choice of location is influenced by differences in net earnings. Other factors held constant, it is reasonable to expect that physicians are attracted to markets in which net earnings are high and that the number of practitioners will decline in areas characterized by relatively low earnings. Further, an increase (or decrease) in the number of physicians is expected to reduce (or increase) net earnings, suggesting that adjustments in the location of physicians eliminate income differences among geographic areas in the long-run.

As is well recognized, however, geographic locations are not equally attractive, and each offers a different mix of nonpecuniary or psychic benefits to potential entrants into the market. For example, high earnings prevailing in an area characterized by an adverse climate and other undesirable factors may be insufficient to attract a flow of practitioners. As a result, differences in net earnings may persist indefinitely, suggesting that nonpecuniary and psychic factors play a role in adjusting the distribution of physicians among different markets.

Given that a physician selected specialty k, economic theory suggests that a practitioner implements location decisions so as to maximize a utility function in which the arguments are the present value of anticipated monetary earnings, net of the financial costs of locating or reestablishing a medical practice, and the present value of nonpecuniary returns, net of the psychic costs of relocating or establishing a medical practice in a given area. The second argument reflects the physician's preferences concerning climate, amenities and recreational opportunities that might be modified by prior contacts.

Differences in lifetime earnings derived from market activity are attributable to multiple factors. Perhaps the most important determinant of the income derived from professional activity is the density of market demand. The density of demand refers to the quantity and composition of care the physician expects to provide in a given location. Further, the density of demand depends on the size of the population, the incidence of demand (represented by the proportion of the population that demands care), and the intensity of demand, which is influenced by the amount of care or time consumed by those who seek service. For obvious reasons, then, the density of demand is affected not only by price, distance, and income but also by the type and severity of medical conditions prevailing in the population at risk.

A related factor that might influence expectations concerning lifetime income is the benefit of medical agglomeration. For example, the clustering of colleagues who serve as a source of referrals, not only affects income expectations but also is likely to be perceived differently by specialists and general practitioners. It is reasonable to argue that a source of referrals and the availability of hospital facilities, advanced medical technology, and support services are of greater importance to the specialist than to the general practitioner.

Consider next the monetary costs that might influence location decisions. In addition to the costs of moving from one location to another, the theory of regional economics indicates that transporting factor inputs to the producer results in transfer costs that might influence location decisions. Since physicians are producers *and* retailers of their services, it is unlikely that transfer costs, as traditionally defined, exert a dramatic influence on location decisions. Although the costs of transporting equipment and medical supplies may be incurred, especially by isolated practitioners, these items are not expected to represent a large portion of the expenses of operating a medical practice.

On the other hand, transportation costs are usually incurred by consumers and may exert an indirect influence on location decisions. For example, high travel and time costs may reduce the density of demand, thereby reducing the income opportunities in a given area. As a consequence, physicians may consider the distance to potential patients or the effects of transfer costs on the density of demand and potential earnings when selecting a site for their medical practices.

The monetary and nonpecuniary factors are likely to exert differential effects on the mobility of new entrants and established practitioners. For example, the earnings of a practitioner are closely related to the size of the practice and a system of referrals, both of which require a commitment of time in a given location; hence, the pecuniary earnings of established practitioners in a given location are greater than the income that would be earned if they recently entered the local market. All of these factors suggest that unusual income differences are required to motivate a decision to relocate. Further, in the absence of large income differences, the decision to relocate may depress lifetime earnings. The mobility of established physicians and their sensitivity to pecuniary factors are reduced further by the psychic costs of moving, represented by an aversion to

entering a new area or relinquishing established professional and personal relationships. These observations suggest that entrants to the practice of medicine
are more mobile than their established counterparts.

Among the commonly used measures of location decisions are the stock or
number of physicians in a given area, the physician-to-population ratio, the
number of physicians who initially located their practice in a given area, and
the change in either the stock of practitioners or the physician-to-population
ratio. The stock of physicians and changes in the number of practitioners capture
initial and subsequent location decisions, while the number of new entrants who
select a given site refers to initial location choices. Further, the physician-to-
population ratio, an indicator of access to patient care, is influenced by factors
that jointly influence the distribution of physicians and population. As such,
differences in the physician-to-population ratio describe the distribution of practitioners relative to the population, suggesting that the measure fails to capture
the responsiveness of location behavior to economic and nonpecuniary factors
with precision. As a consequence, the sensitivity of location decisions to the set
of pecuniary and "psychic" or nonpecuniary factors depends on the measure
used to depict behavior.

EMPIRICAL RESULTS

Studies of location decisions have usually employed regression analysis to
assess the relative influence of economic and nonpecuniary factors on the supply
of physicians in a given area. In addition to measures of income opportunities,
most studies have examined a set of area-specific factors thought to affect location
decisions. As described later in the chapter, however, simultaneous-equations
bias, the presence of multicollinearity and measurement error require a cautious
interpretation of reported results.

Economic Factors and the Location Decision

As indicated in the previous section, the economic factors that are believed
to influence the decision to establish or relocate a practice are differences in
potential earnings and the relative concentration of health resources that are
expected to complement or compete with the physician's practice. In this section,
the effects of differences in income on location decisions are considered first,
followed by an assessment of those exerted by medical agglomeration.

Differences in Income Opportunities

Previous findings concerning the influence exerted by differences in income
on decisions about location are mixed. Economic theory suggests that relatively
high earnings should attract a net flow of physicians into a given market. As
indicated previously, however, cross-sectional studies are likely to understate
the sensitivity of location decisions to income differences. In addition, the re-

lationship between the stock of providers or the physician to population ratio and income opportunities is difficult to estimate since the flow of physicians may be slow to adjust to differences in earnings.

Sloan (1968) used a single equation approach and a simultaneous-equations model to examine the stock of physicians practicing in a given state. The single regression analysis indicated that the stock of physicians was positively related to the net income of providers practicing in the state; however, estimates of the simultaneous-equations model suggested that the number of physicians was negatively associated with estimates of the net income earned by providers in the area. These results are supported by Yett and Sloan (1974) who reported a negative, but not significant, relation between the proportion of new entrants who initially selected a given state and the net income earned by physicians practicing in the state.

In addition, results reported by Hadley (1975) also fail to support expectations derived from economic theory. Limiting the analysis to medical graduates in 1960 and using the individual as the unit of analysis, this study indicated that the probability of selecting a given state as the site of medical practice was independent of the relative net income opportunities in the state. The state that served as the basis of comparison was not identified, however, and, as a consequence, it is difficult to believe that the surrogate for relative earnings adequately reflects differences in net income that were considered by graduates when reaching the initial location decision.

Conversely, findings reported by Wilensky (1979) are consistent with the expected relationship between income differences and location decisions. This study examined the probability of selecting Michigan as the site for establishing a medical practice and used a relative income variable to estimate differences in earnings. Unlike Hadley, however, Wilensky specified the income variable as the ratio of the net professional income prevailing in the state of practice and either the reported second choice of the subject or the state of most recent contact. The results indicated that the relation between the probability of locating in Michigan and the relative income proxy was significant and positive.

Similarly, Lee and Wallace (1970) and Fuchs and Kramer (1972) report a positive and significant relation between the ratio of physicians to population prevailing in a given state and surrogates for the physician's earnings in the state. Both studies examined the ratio as the dependent variable but defined the income surrogate differently. Lee and Wallace used the gross annual income of the physician group as the earnings surrogate, a procedure that failed to measure differences in the income potential of various specialties. Unfortunately, it is unlikely that gross annual earnings measure the income expectations of individuals with precision, while the failure to capture differences in the annual earnings of various specialties probably introduced an aggregation bias into reported results. Unlike the Lee and Wallace study, Fuchs and Kramer adjusted the income surrogate for specialty; however, the gross revenue per visit was used as an indicator of differences in earnings potential. For reasons cited previously, the average income earned by established practices may not correspond with precision to the revenue construction used by physicians to evaluate alternate locations.

In a related study, Cantwell (1979) developed a model of physician migration that focused on the influence of differences in Medicare compensation on the stock of physicians and the patient-practitioner ratio prevailing among standard metropolitan statistical areas, SMSAs, nonmetropolitan counties and states. Employing cross-sectional data, parameter estimates were derived for a single equation model in which the stock of practitioners and the physician-population ratio were dependent variables. Controlling for the quality of life, visits per capita, and the availability of hospital capital, the results indicated that the stock of physicians and the supply of practitioners per capita in an area are increased by higher fees.

Demand Density

Thus far, the review has focused on the responsiveness of location decisions to differences in potential earnings, a determinant that is influenced by the density of demand. Among the strongest and consistently positive correlates of the physician stock is the density of demand as measured by the size of the population at risk. That the number of physicians in an area increases with the size of the population has been confirmed by focusing on states, counties, and SMSAs as the geographic unit of analysis (Steele and Rimlinger 1965; Marden 1966; Benham, Maurizi, and Reder 1968; Fein and Weber 1971; Cantwell 1979).

Findings concerning the relation between the number of physicians per capita and the size of the population are less consistent; however, the major differences in reported results are attributable, in part, to the size of the geographic area selected as the unit of analysis. For example, several studies (Joroff and Navarro 1971; Blair 1975; Cantwell 1979) report findings that indicate a positive association between the number of physicians per capita and population. Also consistent with predictions derived from the theoretical model of regional economics are findings reported by Ball and Wilson (1968), Dougherty (1970), Blair (1975), and Coleman (1976). These studies employed the county as the unit of analysis and suggest that the supply of specialists exhibits a positive and significant relation with population size, population density, and degree of urbanization. Similarly, Yett and Sloan (1974), Coleman (1976), and Cantwell (1979) employed the state as the unit of analysis and concluded that the supply of specialists is more positively associated with the degree of urbanization than the supply of general practitioners. These results are consistent with the general view that a large population base is required to support specialty practice.

Conversely, Benham et al. (1968) employed the state as the geographic unit of analysis and reported a negative association ($p \leq .05$) between differences in the number of physicians per capita and population size. Similarly, Lee and Wallace (1970) and Benham et al. (1968) also found negative, but not significant, associations between state physician population ratios and population density;

hence, although contradictory results have been reported, the weight of the evidence confirms theoretical expectations and suggests that the supply of physicians becomes more abundant as population density increases.

In addition to the size of the population, theoretical considerations indicate that the density of demand is also influenced by the incidence of illness or injury. Further, it is reasonable to assume that the incidence of medical conditions increases as the population at risk ages, suggesting that physicians locate in areas characterized by disproportionately large proportions of elderly. Most studies define the age variable as the proportion of the population that is aged 65 or older. The overwhelming weight of evidence indicates that the number of general practitioners increases as the population at risk becomes more elderly (Marden 1966; Hambleton 1971; Joroff and Navarro 1971; Reskin and Campbell 1974; Blair 1975; Coleman 1976; Guzick and Jahiel 1976). Several studies also indicate that the stock of specialists increases significantly as the population ages; however, conflicting results are reported by Coleman (1976) and Evashwick (1976), who found negative or nonsignificant relationships between the number of physicians per capita and the proportion of elderly in the population at risk.

Although the incidence of need contributes to the density of demand, the discussion in Chapter 3 indicated that the decision to seek care is influenced by the ability of the individual to finance out-of-pocket expenses. As a result, it is reasonable to expect that perceptions of demand density and the attractiveness of a given area are positively associated with per capita or family income. Empirical findings that relate the stock of physicians or the number of physicians per capita to measures of consumer affluence confirm these expectations. Further, several studies report that those experiencing a prior contact are more likely to locate in a state where per capita income is high relative to other states (Fein and Weber 1971; Yett and Sloan 1974; Wilensky 1979). Similarly, Steele and Rimlinger (1965) reported a positive association between the ratio of growth in the county stock of physicians and the per capita income in the area.

Conversely, focusing on the county as the geographic unit of analysis, results reported by Benham et al. (1968), Coleman (1976) and Evashwick (1976) indicate that the flow of physicians is negatively associated with consumer affluence. Estimates derived by Wilensky (1979) also suggest that the likelihood of physicians trained in Michigan to locate in SMSAs declines as per capita income increases; hence, although the stock of physicians and the ratio of practitioners to population exhibit a positive association with per capita or family income, findings concerning the relation between the affluence of consumers and the flow of providers are somewhat inconclusive.

That specialists and general practitioners respond differentially to per capita or family income has also been examined. Most previous studies indicate that the stocks of specialists and general practitioners are positively related to per capita income and that the location decisions of specialists are more sensitive to consumer affluence than those of general practitioners (Benham et al. 1968; Hambleton 1971; Yett and Sloan 1974; Coleman 1976).

Medical Agglomeration

As indicated previously, the second major premise of the theory of regional economics is that the benefits of agglomeration influence the location decisions of physicians. Specifically, it is reasonable to argue that economies of scale in the production of medical services constitute the theoretical basis for expecting a relation between the supply of physicians and availability of hospital resources. In particular, many diagnostic and therapeutic services, which would include most surgical procedures, require the use of technology embodied in the capital equipment of the hospital. As a result, the provision of these services, and, hence, a component of the physician's income, is dependent on access to hospital resources that are usually unavailable in the physician's office. Further, given their relative dependence on these resources, it is reasonable to expect specialists to be more likely than general practitioners to locate their practices in areas characterized by an abundant supply of hospitals.

That the local supply of hospital resources might influence the location decisions of physicians was given explicit recognition in the majority of the studies reviewed in this chapter. Common measures of hospital supply in an area include the number of hospitals, the number of beds, and the number of beds per capita. Previous findings indicate that the stock of specialists and the number of specialists per capita exhibit a positive association with the availability of hospital resources. Among those practicing in urban areas, however, general practitioners are as likely as specialists to locate their practices near hospital resources.

The differential influence of hospital supply on the location decisions of specialists and general practitioners was explored by Rosett (1974). In this analysis, Rosett argued that hospitals complement specialists and compete with office-based practitioners in the provision of outpatient services. Further, the analysis suggested that hospital facilities are shared by those to whom privileges are extended and that an increase in capacity may yield only minimal benefits to office-based practitioners; hence, Rosett argued that the location decisions of office-based practitioners depend not only on the supply of hospital resources and the number of hospital-based physicians but also on the extent to which these facilities are regarded as competitors in the provision of outpatient services.

Empirical estimates were derived for four regression equations in which the dependent variables were the per capita number of general practitioners, surgeons, medical specialists, and other specialists practicing in 27 SMSAs. The independent variables that enabled an examination of these expectations were the number of beds per capita and the number of hospital-based physicians per person in the SMSA. Both of these variables represented variability in hospital resources while the number of hospital-based physicians was also thought to measure the degree of competition between hospitals and practitioners.

The results indicated that the per capita number of physicians in each of the four groups exhibited a negative relation with the per capita bed supply. Based on these findings, Rosett concluded that, when accompanied by few hospital-based physicians, an abundant supply of beds forces office-based practitioners either to accept a lower quality of care provided to their clientele or commit more time to the care of hospitalized patients.

Regarding the hospital as a source of competition, the coefficients relating the stock of physicians to hospital-based practitioners were positive while the number of general practitioners per person exhibited a negative correlation with hospital physicians. Accordingly, these results are consistent with the proposition that hospital-based physicians tend to increase the net income of specialists and that general practitioners regard the hospital as a competitor in the provision of outpatient care.

Feldman (1979) examined location decisions within the context of a simultaneous-equations model in which the supply function was similar to the one used by Rosett. Focusing on the same groups of physicians, the results indicated that, unlike Rosett's findings, the supply of office-based specialists was negatively associated with the number of hospital physicians per person. In addition, the supply of office-based general practitioners exhibited a positive and significant association with the number of beds per person, while the stock of practitioners in each of the specialty groups was unrelated to the ratio of beds to population. These results suggest that general practitioners, rather than specialists, are attracted by an abundance of hospital capacity and that office-based practitioners seem to perceive hospital physicians as competitors.

The tendency of specialists to establish their practices near hospitals has also been examined by Rushing (1975), who contended that these location decisions are responses to the growing importance of hospitals and a decline in the dependence on general practitioners as alternate sources of referrals. These expectations were examined by grouping U.S. counties in terms of the number of general practitioners per capita and degree of urbanization, a surrogate for hospital capacity. For each resulting subsample, regression analysis was used to establish the relationship between the number of specialists per person and the number of hospital beds per capita. Since the size of the coefficients relating the supply of specialists to hospital capacity varied inversely with the number of general practitioners per person, the results were consistent with expectations. Accordingly, Rushing concluded that specialists are more likely to establish practices in counties with a relatively low supply of general practitioners and that hospitals are a more important source of specialist referrals than general practitioners.

The diversity of theories and findings concerning the sensitivity of location decisions to differences in economies of scale or the benefits of agglomeration suggest that the interrelation of the distribution of physicians and the supply of hospital facilities is complex and not well understood. For example, among the unresolved issues is the causal effects exerted by the benefits of agglomeration on location decisions. Although previous studies seem to indicate that the availability of hospital capacity attracts specialists, it is possible that the stock of physicians located in an area is instrumental in stimulating growth in hospital capacity. Given the inconclusive and frequently contradictory evidence, it seems reasonable to conclude that the influence of economies of scale and the effects of the interrelationships among the components of the health market on location decisions are unresolved issues.

Methodological Concerns

The focus of empirical research on the effects of differences in earnings, demand density, and the benefits of agglomeration on location decisions suffers from several methodological difficulties that are well recognized and may have contributed to the diversity in the findings reported previously. Among the more important of these are the effects of multicollinearity, simultaneous-equations bias, and measurement error.

In regression analysis, *multicollinearity* is a term that refers to correlation among two or more independent variables. The presence of multicollinearity not only creates difficulties in estimating the separate effects of collinear variables on the dependent or response variable but also may produce regression estimates exhibiting a sign that differs from that of the corresponding parameter. In addition, multicollinearity inflates the standard errors of the coefficient assigned to collinear variables, thus reducing their statistical significance. The usual remedy for multicollinearity is to remove one or more of the offending variables, a practice that may result in the erroneous conclusion that the factors retained for analysis are significant, while those that were eliminated fail to exert an influence on the dependent variable. The presence of multicollinearity in location studies is well recognized. For example, the affluence of an area, the degree of urbanization and the supply of hospital facilities are interrelated, an outcome that mitigates the reliability of reported results derived from standard regression analysis.

The presence of simultaneous-equations bias also reduces the magnitude of reported coefficients. In terms of location studies, it is possible to argue that, in equilibrium, the number of physicians is determined by supply-and-demand decisions. Since both are influenced by the net income of the physician, the use of standard regression techniques to estimate a single supply equation erroneously assumes that net earnings are exogenous, rather than the product of a simultaneous system. As a consequence, previous results may understate the sensitivity of location decisions to differences in pecuniary factors.

The third major source of error that influences the results of location studies is measurement bias, which is attributable to the precision with which surrogates measure conceptual variables. For example, area differences in per capita income, population size, and the age distribution are probably imperfect measures of the physician's perception of demand density. Similarly, area differences in the net income of physicians may not correspond to the expectations or the revenue construction considered when evaluating alternate sites. Each of the surrogates approximates the expectations of physicians with an unknown precision. Accordingly, it is difficult, if not impossible, to measure either the direction or magnitude of the bias created by unavoidable measurement errors; however, the presence of these errors also reduces the reliability and complicates the interpretation of reported results.

Nonpecuniary Factors and the Location Decision

The discussion presented earlier suggested that nonpecuniary factors or psychic benefits, as measured by area attributes, and prior contact with the area might affect the decision to relocate or establish medical practice. Previous findings concerning the influence of these factors on location decisions are considered in this section.

Area Attributes

Available evidence indicates that area attributes such as climate and the availability of recreational facilities influence location decisions. For example, Yett and Sloan (1974), Coleman (1976), and Wilensky (1979) report findings that suggest that physicians are attracted by warm climates. Among the proxy variables for the quality of life are measures of availability of recreational facilities. Hambleton (1971), Fuchs and Kramer (1972), Held (1973), Rosett (1974), and Hadley (1975) report findings that indicate a positive association between the availability of recreational facilities and the stock and flow of physicians per capita.

Prior Contact

Thus far, the focus of the discussion has been on studies that are predicated on the assumption that location behavior is influenced predominantly by market forces. By contrast, a set of studies assumes that the physician's attachment to a given area is formed by past experiences that occurred during prior contacts and that the resulting attachment increases the probability of the physician establishing a practice in the location.

Among the personal events that are included in empirical examinations of the prior contact hypothesis are (1) the location of medical training, residency, and internship; (2) location of undergraduate education; (3) the size of the community in which the physician was raised; (4) the number of contacts with physicians in the area; and (5) the physician's birthplace. This section offers a brief overview of the influence of these factors on the location behavior of physicians.

Consistent with expectations, a number of studies have demonstrated that physicians are likely to locate in the area in which medical training occurred. The results of the discriminate analysis reported by Watson (1980) indicate that physicians established their practice in those states in which they were trained and reared. Similarly, Cooper, Heald, Samuels and Coleman (1975), and Yett and Sloan (1974) also found that physicians tend to practice in the area of their medical training and rearing. A positive association between location of training and practice setting was also reported by Burfield, Hough, and Marder (1986) and Leonardson, Lapierre, and Hollingsworth (1985). Burfield et al. also found that women and general practitioners were most likely to remain in the state where graduate medical education occurred.

In a related study, Aaron, Somes, Marx, and Cooper (1980) examined the relation among the sizes of the communities in which practices were located, medical education occurred, and physicians were reared. The results identified a congruence between the size of the communities in which physicians were reared, trained, and located their practices, a set of findings that were corroborated by Holmes and Miller (1986). In addition, Aaron et al. also identified similarities between the sizes of the communities in which physicians located their practices and received their undergraduate education, a set of results that are also consistent with the prior-contact hypothesis.

POLICY OPTIONS: A POTPOURRI

A number of policy options might be suggested to alter the geographic distribution of physicians. The potential effectiveness of each depends, in part, on the sensitivity of location decisions to prior contacts, economic incentives, and governmental controls that influence the flow of medical graduates, the number of residencies, the availability of hospital beds and the form of medical practice. Further, as suggested by Tierney, Waters, and Williams (1980), direct employment of physicians by the government and certificate of need for physician licensure might be adopted as methods of allocating physicians from surplus to shortage areas. Each of these policy options is described in this section.

The Distribution of Medical Schools and Residencies

Based on findings that suggest physicians locate in areas of their medical education, one solution to a maldistribution of physicians is to increase the capacity of medical schools in shortage areas and restrict capacity in surplus areas. For example, the distribution of medical school capacity might be altered selectively by reducing the level of support per capita in surplus areas and increasing governmental funding of medical schools located in shortage areas. Given the length of training and the probable intervention of educational facilities, however, control of medical school capacity and the flow of graduates is unlikely to alter either the geographic distribution or specialty mix in the short run.

The geographic distribution of residencies is probably subject to more direct control than medical school capacity. Similar to the discussion of policy options designed to alter specialty mix, national accrediting bodies might voluntarily alter the geographic distribution of residencies. Alternatively, governmental authorities and other third-party payers might deny compensation for care provided in association with "unapproved" residency programs, a policy that might precipitate legal action.

For reasons cited previously, selectively expanding and/or reducing medical school capacity or the availability of residencies is unlikely to exert a dramatic influence on the geographic distribution of physicians in the short run. In addition, the efficacy of these policy instruments depends on the association of location decisions and the site of medical education. Since a cause-effect relation has not been established by previous assessments of the prior-contact hypothesis, changes in the funding of medical education are not likely to result in noticeable adjustments in the geographic distribution of physicians unless these policies are accompanied by other initiatives.

Economic Incentives

Perhaps the most common approach to redressing imbalances in the geographic distribution of physicians is the imposition of economic incentives that induce providers to locate in shortage areas. Incentives to establish practices in underserved areas include (1) student loans with "forgiveness" provisions that apply to those who locate in shortage areas; (2) the provision of clinics or other facilities in underserved areas; and (3) direct placement of physicians who are government employees. Unfortunately, the current policies of third-party payers induce physicians to locate in urban or high-income areas. Perceived imbalances might be redressed by offering financial rewards to those who establish practice in underserved areas.

As suggested by the review of previous studies, however, empirical evidence indicates that location decisions are not sensitive to income differences. The effectiveness of the economic incentives appears to be limited to those who are subject to fiscal pressures and, in a review of the effectiveness of incentive mechanisms, Eisenberg and Cantwell (1978, p. 455) concluded that the reliance on these policies is not "justified by a consensus of empirical evidence."

Control by Hospitals

It is possible that adjustments in the distribution of hospital beds might redress imbalances in the allocation of physicians. For example, limiting the capacity of hospital facilities in surplus areas might reduce the flow of new entrants, while an expansion of capacity in shortage areas might increase the stock of physicians in underserved areas; however, the potential effectiveness of such a policy is mitigated by several considerations. First, although empirical evidence suggests that the stock of specialists is positively associated with the availability of hospital facilities, these studies failed to establish a causal relationship between these components of the health market. Further, increases in the proportion of medical and surgical procedures that are provided on an outpatient basis further reduce the potential effectiveness of altering the supply of physicians by adjustments in the hospital stock.

As a condition for continued fiscal support from public programs, governmental authorities might require hospitals to assess applications for privileges in terms of the health needs of the community or service area. Such a policy, however, might contravene the rights of physicians to engage in private practice, an outcome that would probably precipitate legal action. Further, the potential effectiveness of the approach is reduced by three additional factors. First, identifying the hospital as the locus of control ignores the ability of physicians to maintain viable practices in noninstitutional settings. Further, the effectiveness of such an approach is directly related to the dependence of hospitals on public programs as a source of funding. As a result, a hospital that receives little or no fiscal support from publicly funded programs would be unaffected by the policy. Finally, vesting hospitals with the responsibility of assessing community needs creates an environment in which the self-interests of the institution are in conflict with the process of defining community need, an outcome that may subvert the intended purpose of the policy. These observations suggest that the direct and indirect pressures exerted by hospitals are not likely to achieve a congruence between the health needs present in an area and the mix of physicians.

Certificate of Need

As recommended by Tierney et al. (1980), certificate of need might be employed to control the geographic distribution and specialty mix of physicians. The proposal requires an estimate of the health needs in the area and the maximum number of new entrants, distributed by specialty. These factors combine to determine the number of new licenses authorized for the area. In addition, unsuccessful applicants form a queue with their relative priorities established by board certification and other factors that contribute to the quality and accessibility of care.

Among the major impediments to the implementation of such an approach are the types or the volume of data required to establish limits on the mix of new entrants in a given area and the set of legal objections that might be posed by the medical society. Concerning the first, much of the information is currently assembled in the manpower survey component of the cooperative Health Statistics System. Further, with the passage of time, the licensing authority could develop a more comprehensive set of data to which an annual contribution of required information by practitioners should be mandatory; hence, although formidable, the problem of assembling required data is by no means insurmountable.

The legal objections of the AMA are expected to focus on essentially two issues. The first involves the potentially adverse effects the proposal might exert on the physician's right to due process. The inclusion of a ''grandfather'' clause that applies to established physicians and incorporating an appeal process in the certificate of need process address this legal objection. The second objection involves the possibility that such a policy may violate the fourteenth amendment, which guarantees equal protection. The AMA is likely to argue that, in order to improve quality, those to whom licenses are awarded should be identified only on the basis of qualifications; however, when the discrimination is not invidious and is rationally implemented to achieve a permissible state goal, the equal protection clause does not prevent unequal treatment of individuals. In this regard, an improvement in quality and a reduction in cost must be regarded as a permissible state objective, suggesting that such a proposal does not contravene rights guaranteed under the constitution. These observations indicate that neither the data requirements nor the legal objections of the medical society are insurmountable and that a certificate of need process is a potential vehicle for controlling not only the mix but also the geographic distribution of physicians.

Government Employment of Physicians

An extreme, but perhaps more effective approach to the problem of controlling the distribution of physicians is to implement a national health service in which providers are employees of the government. As proposed by the American Public Health Association, a national health service should entitle the entire population to a comprehensive range of health services provided through its own personnel and facilities. Such an approach not only contributes to an equitable distribution of health services but also creates an environment in which direct control is exerted over the number, mix, and geographic distribution of physicians.

In particular, a national health service centralizes funding responsibility and, thereby increases the extent to which direct control is exerted on the capacities of medical schools, the availability of internships and residencies, the number of medical graduates, and the mix of practitioners with respect to specialty. When combined with a certificate of need process described previously, a national health service also creates an environment in which the geographic distribution of physicians is controlled directly, an attribute that is not available in the other options described in this section.

REFERENCES

Aaron, P. R., G. W. Somes, M. B. Marx, and J. K. Cooper. 1980. Relationship between traits of Kentucky physicians and their practice areas. *Inquiry* 17(2):128–36.

Ball, D. S., and J. W. Wilson. 1968. Community health facilities and services: The manpower decisions. *American Journal of Agricultural Economics* 50 (5):1208–21.

Benham, L., A. Maurizi, and M. W. Reder. 1968. Migration, location and remuneration of medical personnel: Physicians and dentists. *Review of Economics and Statistics* 50(3):332–47.

Berk, M. L., A. B. Bernstein, and A. K. Taylor. 1983. The use and availability of medical care in health manpower shortage areas. *Inquiry* 20(4):369–80.

Blair, R. J. 1975. A multivariate analysis of factors influencing the location and distribution of physicians in the northeast U.S. Master's thesis, Pennsylvania State University.

Burfield, W. B., D. E. Hough, and W. D. Marder. 1986. Location of medical education and choice of location of practice. *Journal of Medical Education* 61(7):545–54.

Cantwell, J. R. 1979. Implication of reimbursement policies for the locations of physicians. *Agricultural Economics Research* 31(2):25–35.

Coleman, S. 1976. *Physician Distribution and Rural Access to Medical Services*. Publication no. R–1887–HEW. Santa Monica, CA: Rand Corporation.

Cooper, J. K., K. Heald, M. Samuels, and S. Coleman. 1975. Rural or urban practice: Factors influencing the location decision of primary care physicians. *Inquiry* 12(1):18–25.

Dionne, G., A. Langlois, and N. Lemire. 1987. More on the geographical distribution of physicians. *Journal of Health Economics* 6(4):365–74.

Dougherty, L. A. 1970. *The Supply of Physicians in the State of Arkansas*. Santa Monica, CA: Rand Corporation.

Eisenberg, B. S., and J. R. Cantwell. 1978. Policies to influence the spatial distribution of physicians: A conceptual review of selected programs and empirical evidence. *Medical Care* 14(6):455–68.

Evashwick, C. J. 1976. The role of group practice in the distribution of physicians in nonmetropolitan areas. *Medical Care* 14(10):808–23.

Fein, R., and G. I. Weber. 1971. *Financing Medical Education*. New York: McGraw-Hill.

Feldman, R. 1979. A model of physician location and pricing behavior. In R. M. Scheffler, ed., *Research in Health Economics*. Greenwich, CT: JAI Press.

Fruen, M. A., and J. R. Cantwell. 1982. Geographic distribution of physicians: Past trends and future influences. *Inquiry* 19(1):44–50.

Fuchs, V. R., and M. J. Kramer. 1972. *Determinants of Expenditures for Physicians' Services in the United States, 1948–1968*. DHEW Publication No. (HSM) 73–3013. Rockville, MD: U.S. Department of Health, Education, and Welfare.

Graduate Medical Education National Advisory Committee (GMENAC). 1980. Summary Report of the Graduate Medical Education National Advisory Committee, Vol. I, DHHS Pub. No. [HRA]81–651. Washington, DC: U.S. Department of Health and Human Services.

Guzick, D. S., and R. I. Jahiel. 1976. Distribution of private practice offices of physicians with specified characteristics among urban neighborhoods. *Medical Care* 14(6):469–88.

Hadley, J. 1975. Models of physicians' specialty and location choices. Ph.D. dissertation, Yale University.

Hambleton, J. W. 1971. Determinants of geographic differences in the supply of physicians' services. Ph.D. dissertation, University of Wisconsin, Madison.

Held, P. J. 1973. The migration of the 1955–1965 graduates of American medical schools. Berkeley, CA: Ford Foundation Program for Research in University Administration, University of California, January.

Holmes, J. E., and D. A. Miller. 1986. Factors affecting decisions on practice locations. *Journal of Medical Education* 61(9):721–6.

Hynes, K., and N. Givner. 1983. Physician distribution in a predominantly rural state: Predictors and trends. *Inquiry* 29(2):185–94.

Joroff, S., and V. Navarro. 1971. Medical manpower: A multivariate analysis of the distribution of physicians in urban United States. *Medical Care* 9(9):428–38.

Kindig, D. A., H. Movassaghi, M. C. Dunham, D. I. Zwick, and C. M. Taylor. 1987. Trends in physician availability in 10 urban areas from 1963 to 1980. *Inquiry* 24(2):136–47.

Lee, M. W., and R. L. Wallace. 1970. Demand, supply, and the distribution of physicians. Studies in Health Care, Report No. 5. Columbia, MO: Department of Community Health and Medical Practice, University of Missouri.

Leonardson, G., R. Lapierre, and D. Hollingsworth. 1985. Factors predictive of physician location. *Journal of Medical Education* 60(1):37–43.

Madison, D. C. 1980. Managing a chronic problem: The rural physician shortage. *Annals of Internal Medicine* 92:852–4.

Marden, P. G. 1966. Demographic and ecological analysis of the distribution of physicians in metropolitan America, 1960. *American Journal of Sociology* 72(3):290–300.

Newhouse, J. P., A. P. Williams, B. W. Bennett, and W. B. Schwartz. 1982. Where have all the doctors gone? *Journal of American Medical Association* 247(17):2392–6.

Reskin, B., and F. L. Campbell. 1974. Physician distribution across metropolitan areas. *American Journal of Sociology* 79(4):981–98.

Rosett, R. N. 1974. Proprietary hospitals in the United States. In M. Perlman, ed., *The Economics of Health and Medical Care*. New York: John Wiley and Sons.

Rushing, W. A. 1975. *Community, Physicians, and Inequality*. Lexington, MA: DC Heath and Company.

Schwartz, W. B., J. P. Newhouse, B. W. Bennett, and A. P. Williams. 1983. The changing geographic distribution of board-certified physicians: Facts, theory and implications. Santa Monica, CA: The Rand Corporation.

Sloan, F. A. 1968. Economic models of physician supply. Unpublished Ph.D. dissertation, Harvard University.

Steele, H. B., and G. V. Rimlinger. 1965. Income opportunities and physician location trends in the United States. *Western Economic Journal* 3(2):182–94.

Tierney, J. T., W. J. Waters, and D. C. Williams. 1980. Controlling physician oversupply through certificate of need. *American Journal of Law & Medicine* 6(3):335–60.

Watson, C. J. 1980. The relationship between physician practice location and medical school area: An empirical model. *Social Science and Medicine* 14D:63–9.

Wilensky, G. R. 1979. Retention of medical school graduates: A case study of Michigan. In R. M. Scheffler, ed., *Research in Health Economics*. Greenwich, CT: JAI Press.

Williams, A. P., W. B. Schwartz, J. P. Newhouse, and B. W. Bennett. 1983. How many miles to the doctor? *New England Journal of Medicine* 309(16):958–63.

Yett, D. E., and F. A. Sloan. 1974. Migration patterns of recent medical school graduates. *Inquiry* 11(2):125–42.

Part IV

Cost-Containment Strategies

11

COMPETITIVE APPROACHES TO
HEALTH CARE COST CONTROL

There has been considerable debate over the actions the government should take to control the rising costs of health care. The "proregulation" group has argued that the market system cannot assure efficient resource allocation or equitable distribution of health care services because of the special features of the market for health services (Arrow 1963). Advocates of "competitive" solutions argue that regulatory interventions have not constrained significant increases in health care costs and that centralized regulations provide incentives for health care providers to behave in socially undesirable ways (Pauly 1981; Arnold and Van Vorst 1985). Furthermore, they believe that there are many structural defects inherent in the regulatory process that cause regulators to favor industry interests rather than consumer interests (McClure 1981). Thus, they argue that increased reliance on market-like incentives is necessary to motivate producers to act in a more efficient manner and to encourage consumers to utilize health services more carefully or to seek out and use less costly alternatives. Although ideological differences have caused rancorous debate among members of the two camps, many observers believe that the health care industry will continue to have elements of competition and government regulations (Vladek 1981).

In Chapter 12, we will survey the empirical evidence pertaining to rate regulation and other forms of centralized controls. Although, like beauty, significant cost savings may lie in the eyes of the beholder, we concluded in our survey, in contrast to some competition advocates, that hospital rate regulation programs have contained significant increases in hospital costs. We do agree, however, with members of the procompetition group that unless structured carefully, hospital rate regulation can induce providers to behave in unintended ways.

In this chapter, our focus turns to an assessment of market-like approaches to health care cost containment. The market or competitive approach is not monolithic. The following policy approaches have been proposed:

1. Competition among alternative health delivery systems (Enthoven 1981);
2. Increased patient cost-sharing (Feldstein 1971; Pauly 1971; Seidman 1977);
3. Removal of bans on advertising (Greenberg 1985);
4. Vigorous application of antitrust laws (Havighurst 1983);
5. Competitive bidding for Medicaid contracts (Brecher 1984); and,
6. Managed care plans (Prottas and Handler 1987).

A paucity of empirical research precludes an assessment of all but the first two competitive approaches. Further, since we have already examined the evidence pertaining to patient cost-sharing in Chapter 3, The Demand for Health Services, we will restrict our attention in this chapter to competition among health systems.

Proponents of the growth of competition among health plans cite two general benefits of this approach. First, alternative delivery systems (ADS), such as Health Maintenance Organizations (HMOs) or Preferred Provider Organizations (PPOs), incorporate incentives that encourage providers to act more efficiently than those in the fee-for-service sector; hence, the growth of ADS should result in greater restraints on inflationary pressures. Second, as the enrollment in alternative delivery systems increases, price competition from these new providers would motivate traditional providers to participate in alternative systems or to make their existing operations more efficient.

A comprehensive examination of the impact of increased competition could easily fill an entire book. Thus, in order to limit our analysis to a manageable length, we will emphasize current findings pertinent to the ability of alternative delivery systems to control costs, without adverse consequences to health outcomes, over an extended period of time. Recognizing that the ability to constrain total expenditures for health care in the United States is influenced by unit cost savings as well as total number of units affected, we will limit our analysis to the following issues. First, are ADS really more efficient, or are their lower per capita expenditures due to other factors, such as biased enrollment or the provision of lower quality services? Second, what is the growth potential of ADS? Third, will growth of ADS stimulate price competition among traditional providers and insurers?

Recognizing that ADS is a generic concept pertaining to a variety of organizational forms, we describe the more common features of different types of ADS including HMOs, PPOs, and Managed Care Plans in the next section. Most of our attention, however, will be devoted to the HMO, which is not only the oldest type of ADS, but also is the dominant one.

CHARACTERISTICS OF ALTERNATIVE DELIVERY SYSTEMS

Health Maintenance Organizations

The ADS with which most Americans are familiar is the HMO. As of June, 1986, 23.7 million people, or about 10 percent of the U.S. population, were enrolled in HMOs (InterStudy 1986). Although HMOs follow a number of diverse structural patterns, Luft (1981) suggests they all possess the following attributes:

1. The HMO assumes a contractual responsibility to provide or assure the delivery of a stated range of health services. This includes at least ambulatory care and inpatient services;

2. The HMO services a population defined by enrollment in the plan;

3. Subscriber enrollment is voluntary;

4. The consumer pays a fixed annual or monthly payment that is independent of the use of services; and

5. The HMO assumes at least part of the financial risk in the provision of services.

Luft notes that the two major forms of HMOs, prepaid group practices (PGPs) and individual practice associations (IPAs), are distinguished by physician payment arrangements and location of services within the plan. Although there are some important exceptions, most IPAs are composed of physicians in private offices who are paid on a fee-for-service basis by the HMO, while physicians in PGPs provide services in the context of a single group and are compensated on a capitation or salary basis.

Managed Care Systems

Although there have been a number of demonstration projects in which Medicaid recipients were given the option of enrolling in HMOs, few states have relied extensively on this type of ADS to provide health services to the poor. A number of states, however, have recently implemented managed care systems for the poor. In some states, Medicaid recipients are not allowed to choose a particular health care system (Freund and Neuschler 1986). Since mandatory assignment violates a criterion used to define HMOs, we prefer to use the broader term *managed care system* to refer to a method of providing coordinated care to Medicaid recipients. Managed care systems may be operated by HMOs or by health insuring organizations (HIOs). Although enrollment of Medicaid recipients in HMOs and other prepaid plans has increased from .28 million in 1981 to .84 million in 1986 (Freund and Neuschler 1986), there is little empirical evidence pertaining to their cost and utilization experience. Case study analysis, however, suggests that managed care systems must overcome a number of political and bureaucratic obstacles if they are to succeed in controlling Medicaid expenditures (Prottas and Handler 1987). An analysis based on a case study in the state of Washington found that, contrary to expectations, the inpatient utilization experience of Medicaid recipients in an HMO was much higher than that of their counterparts in the fee-for-service sector. This result was attributed to adverse selection rather than provider behavior (Traska 1987a).

Preferred Provider Organizations

During the 1980s, PPOs experienced phenomenal growth rates with the number of individuals eligible to use them increasing from 1.8 million in December 1984, to 5.57 million in July 1985, to 16.5 million in June 1986 (de Lissovoy, Rice, Gabel, and Gelzer 1987). It is important to note, however, that the existence of a contract between an employer and a PPO does not mean that eligible persons will use the services of a PPO. Unfortunately, little is known about the use of PPO benefits or the actual cost savings achieved by PPOs. Accordingly our discussion of PPOs will be limited to a description of their key features and how they might affect costs. Given an absence of rigorous empirical analysis, we will resist the temptation to speculate as to their efficacy in controlling costs.

PPOs are generally defined as an arrangement in which a group of health providers agree to deliver care on a fee-for-services basis to a defined group of patients at an agreed upon set of charges. InterStudy (Ellwein and Gregg 1982) listed the following five components common to PPOs:

1. A provider panel limited to a specific group of physicians and hospitals;
2. Negotiated compensation arrangements;
3. Utilization controls;
4. Consumer choice of provider coupled with incentives to utilize PPO providers; and,
5. Rapid settlement of provider claims.

The last two components are used to stimulate consumer and physician participation in PPOs. As discussed by de Lissovoy et al. (1987), the first three features of PPOs can be used to contain costs. First, although providers may be selected to achieve geographic market coverage, many investor- or insurer-sponsored PPOs select physicians and hospitals on the basis of costs. Thus, PPOs may contain costs by diverting patients from high-cost providers toward cost-effective providers. If this occurs in substantial numbers, inefficient providers may be compelled to improve their performance.

Second, PPOs could encourage more cost-effective behavior by negotiating risk-sharing compensation arrangements with providers. Although charges and per diem rates are the typical basis of payments, a growing number of PPOs (27 percent) are using case-mix payment methods such as the diagnosis related group (Gabel, Ermann, Rice, and de Lissovoy 1986). It is unclear from this report, however, whether DRG rates are established prospectively and thus create incentives to contain costs. Physicians are reimbursed on the basis of a fee schedule by over 95 percent of PPOs, a feature lacking incentives to cut costs.

Finally, it appears that PPOs have relied on utilization controls as their most important cost-control instrument. PPOs require preadmission certification of patients (90 percent) and employ concurrent review of the necessity to continue the hospital stay (83 percent).

In summary, pressures on employers to contain costs will continue to stimulate the expansion of PPOs. Indeed, some Wall Street experts have speculated that by 1995, 40 percent of the United States population will be eligible to participate in PPOs (Abramowitz 1985). Although PPOs have some structural elements that might allow them to contain health care costs, Greaney and Sindelar (1987) suggest PPOs might engage in cartel-like collision resulting in price fixing, less aggressive utilization review, and restrictions on entry and innovation in the market. There is no rigorous empirical evidence to support this contention.

HMOs: PAST PERFORMANCE AND POTENTIAL GROWTH

In this section, our focus turns to an analysis of the past performance and future growth potential of HMOs. Rather than reinvent the wheel, we will refer extensively to Luft's (1981) comprehensive review of HMO studies. This will allow us to devote attention to more recent research. In this section, we will first examine the impact of HMOs on expenditures and utilization. We then examine biased enrollment and quality of care in HMOs to see if these factors have influenced cost and utilization. In the following section, we assess the growth potential of HMOs by examining attitudes toward HMOs. Next, recognizing the importance of HMO participation in the Medicare program, we assess the Medicare HMO capitation payment schemes. Finally, we examine the competitive effects of HMOs.

Methodological Perspective

Before turning to the analysis of HMO performance, it is appropriate to discuss the problems with the general methodology employed in the studies reviewed by Luft. First, most of the studies involved paired comparisons of HMO enrollee groups with groups of "similar" fee-for-service enrollees; however, since enrollees were allowed to choose and change their health plan on a voluntary basis, enrollment bias may threaten validity of the comparisons even though on a national level enrollment bias has been offset by counteracting experiences of different plans.

Second, it may not be appropriate to generalize results beyond the local area in which the paired comparisons were made. Further, the comparisons summarized by Luft were performed prior to the surge of HMO growth occurring during the current decade. Thus, his analysis is restricted primarily to California and other areas that were in the vanguard of the HMO movement. The applicability of the experience in these areas to that of new HMO markets is questionable.

Third, estimates of the differences between the performance of HMOs and conventional plans may have been confounded by the use of data that are uncomparable, lack sufficient detail to support the analysis, or were collected by inconsistent methods (Wolinsky 1980; Luft 1981; Cascardo 1982; Sauter and Hughes 1983; Mott 1986).

HMO COSTS

Unlike traditional fee-for-service practices in which the income of physicians is positively related to the number of services provided, the profitability of HMOs is related to reductions in the volume of services. Therefore, *ceteris paribus*, we would expect costs per subscriber in HMOs to be lower than those in traditional indemnity plans. As summarized by Luft (1981), evidence from six studies is consistent with expectations. Compared to HMOs, total expenditures (i.e., premiums plus out-of-pocket payments) per subscriber in traditional plans were 3 percent to 90 percent more. The distribution of cost differences were bunched from 15 percent to 30 percent; furthermore, differences may be increasing. Baker, McGee, and Shadle (1984) reported that the average HMO family premium rose by 13.7 percent in 1983, while average indemnity premiums increased by 25.0 percent. Although, as we will discuss later in this chapter, some apparent HMO cost savings may be due to biased enrollment, results from the Rand Health Insurance Experiment indicate the per capita cost of treating HMO enrollees is 25 percent lower than that of providing care to their counterparts in traditional fee-for-service plans, offering comparable benefits (Manning, Leibowitz, Goldberg, Rogers, and Newhouse 1984). The randomized procedures of selecting subjects in this experiment reduced the possibility that these results were due to biased selection; however, irrespective of the conceptual appeal and corroborating results from other studies, the generalizability of these results to other HMOs is questionable.

Most of the cost savings achieved by HMOs are due to lower utilization of hospitals. HMOs have up to 35 percent fewer hospital days per 1,000 population than their fee-for-service counterparts. Reductions in utilization in IPAs are not as great as those typically observed in PGPs; nevertheless, their use rates are 5 to 25 percent lower than those in indemnity plans (Luft 1981).

Differences in hospital use rates between HMO enrollees and subscribers to traditional plans are due more to reductions in the admission rate than to a reduction in the length of stay. HMOs were found to have lower rates of hospital admissions per 1,000 enrollees, ranging from 5 percent to 35 percent (Luft 1981) in 46 of 57 comparisons between group HMO enrollees and indemnity subscribers made during 1951 and 1975. In these comparisons, admission rates from IPAs were higher than those from PGPs; however, more recent evidence shows that IPAs reduced hospital utilization rates by almost 30 percent during the period 1980–1985 (Schlesinger 1985). This result has been attributed as a response of IPAs to increased competition (Ginsburg and Hackbarth 1986).

The results for the average length of stay are more ambiguous. In 30 out of 57 comparisons, HMO subscribers who were admitted to a hospital tended to have a lower length of stay than their counterparts in indemnity plans. Since

HMOs may avoid hospitalizing less severely ill patients who may have short stays, their performance in this dimension of utilization is not surprising.

Luft suggested a number of reasons for the lower rate of hospitalization experienced in HMOs. First, he expected that reductions in surgical admissions would account for a disproportionately greater amount of the differences in admission rates between HMOs and indemnity plans. This hypothesis is based on the assumption that fee-for-service surgeons have a greater financial incentive (caused by large surgical fees) to perform an operation in an ambiguous situation than internists or other nonsurgical medical specialists do to hospitalize a patient. Second, although the optimal surgical rate cannot be specified, it is reasonable to expect HMOs to achieve a greater reduction in the performance of those procedures for which there is a relatively high rate of surgery in the community. In an analysis of 25 pairs of HMOs and comparison groups, Luft concluded that HMOs appear to have equally lower rates of admission in both surgical and nonsurgical categories and that the rate of surgery in the community had no impact on the disparate admission rates between HMOs and their control groups.

It is difficult to specify, a priori, the impact of HMOs on use rates for ambulatory services. On one hand, ambulatory visits can be substituted for inpatient care and used to identify or treat problems before they become serious enough to require hospitalization. On the other hand, HMOs have financial incentives to reduce all but "necessary" care, including ambulatory visits. Luft reports that in 21 of 33 paired comparisons, HMO patients had higher rates of ambulatory care visits than those in the comparison group. Further analysis, however, suggests that these differences are attributable, in part, to the price-rationing function of cost-sharing by the comparison group. Indeed, ambulatory visit rates were lower among HMO enrollees than among their counterparts in the fee-for-service sector, who had indemnity plans without cost-sharing. The converse was found when HMO enrollees were compared with fee-for-service patients who paid some out-of-pocket costs for their ambulatory care visit.

In an attempt to find results that are more generalizable than the local paired comparison analysis reviewed by Luft (1981), Welch (1985a) used a national sample to determine if there are differences in utilization between HMO enrollees and subscribers to conventional insurance plans. Welch performed regression analysis on two randomly generated data bases: the National Medical Care Expenditure Study (NMCES) and the National Medical Care Expenditure and Utilization Survey (NMCEUS). We will not discuss any of the results from the analysis of the NMCEUS, however, because this data set had a number of consistency errors that were discussed in a critique written by Luft (1985). In addition to HMO enrollment status, Welch included a number of variables (e.g., health status, income, education, gender) commonly used to reflect differences in utilization. His results suggest that relative to subscribers in conventional insurance plans, HMO enrollees are 23 percent more likely to see a doctor and 26 percent more likely to be admitted to a hospital, but have 10 percent fewer physician visits and spend 25 percent fewer days in the hospital. Contrary to previous research, Welch estimated that HMO enrollees were 26 percent more likely to be admitted to a hospital; however, the low reliability ($p > 0.10$) of this estimate suggests that it should be accepted with caution. A rather heroic interpretation of these results suggests that, due to reduced financial barriers, HMO enrollees have greater access to physician care, resulting in more timely treatment of problems, which ultimately reduces the need for follow-up visits and lengthy hospital stays. Before rushing out and raising the procompetition banner, however, it is appropriate to mention a number of flaws of this study that were critiqued by Luft (1985). First, relatively weak measures of risk factors were used. Thus, it is not certain that Welch controlled for the possible existence of selection bias in HMOs. Second, the health insurance coverage variables were of questionable validity. Third, the NMCES data was collected in 1977 and may not reflect current conditions.

Analysis of differences between the performance of HMOs and fee-for-service providers may be distorted by enrollment or quality differences. We will discuss each of these in the next section, placing the greatest emphasis on enrollment bias.

Biased Enrollment in HMOs

The existence of biased enrollment in HMOs has been the subject of extensive inquiry. HMOs may suffer from adverse selection, a phenomena in which a disproportionate number of high-risk/high-use patients enroll in the HMO, thereby increasing utilization rates and per capita expenditures. Conversely, an HMO may benefit from favorable selection. It is difficult to predict, *a priori*, whether an HMO will experience a particular type of biased selection because there are plausible reasons for both to occur.

Proponents of the risk-vulnerability hypothesis (Bashur and Metzner 1970; Moustafa, Hopkins, and Klein 1971; Tessler and Mechanic 1975a; Bice 1975; Berki, Ashcraft, Penchansky, and Fortus 1977) suggest that individuals who consider themselves to be at high risk in terms of expected illness and who feel financially vulnerable because of potentially high out-of-pocket costs are more likely to enroll in an HMO.

Some analysts, who have observed the low utilization rates of HMO enrollees, speculate that these plans operated under a financial incentive to practice cream-skimming, resulting in a favorable selection; however, HMOs could experience favorable selection through less overt activities. For example, enrollment in new alternative delivery systems may be inversely related to the transition costs of leaving existing health care arrangements. Thus, the young (healthy) may be more predisposed to enroll in HMOs because they have experienced a shorter period of association (less contact) with a physician, which results in lower transition costs.

Appearing in Table 11.1 is Wilensky and Rossiter's (1986) summary of results from 21 patient self-selection studies that were conducted from 1975 to 1986.

Table 11.1
Summary of Patient Self-Selection Studies

Study	Population	Measurement	Findings
Bice (1975)	Low-income families	Preenrollment claims	HMO adverse selection
Hetherington, Hopkins, Roemer (1975)	Employment-based	Chronic health problems	HMO adverse selection
Tessler, Mechanic (1975a)	Employment-based	Chronic health problems	HMO adverse selection
Berki, Ashcraft, Penchansky, Fortas (1977)	Employment-based	Self-reported health status	No evidence for biased selection
Scitovsky, McCall, Benham (1978)	Employment-based	Self-reported health status	No evidence for biased selection
Eggers (1980)	Medicare	Preenrollment service use	HMO favorable selection
Juba, Lave, Shaddy (1980)	Employment-based	Chronic health problems	Not conclusive
McGuire (1981)	Employment-based	Years of age	Not conclusive
Eggers, Prihoda (1982)	Medicare	Prior service use	HMO favorable selection
Jackson-Beeck, Kleinman (1983)	Employment-based	Preenrollment claims	HMO favorable selection
Price, Mays, Trapnell (1983)	Employment-based	Premium changes	HMO favorable selection

Table 11.1 (continued)

Study	Population	Measurement	Findings
Welch, Frank, Diehr (1984)	Employment-based	Service use and imputed costs	Not conclusive
Dowd, Feldman (1985)	Employment-based	Chronic health problems	HMO favorable selection
Ellis (1985)	Employment-based	Prior year enrollment claims	Not conclusive
Farley, Monheit (1985)	Employment-based	Expenditures and premiums	No evidence for biased selection
Lubitz, Beebe, Riley (1985)	Medicare	Medicare claims, service use	Not conclusive
Luft, Trauner, Maerki (1985)	Retired employee	Age-sex distribution	HMO favorable selection
Price, Mays (1985)	Employment-based	Premium changes over time	HMO favorable selection
Welch (1985b)	Medicare	Preenrollment claims	HMO favorable selection but declines
Merrill, Jackson, Reuter (1985)	Employment-based	Prior year enrollment claims	HMO favorable selection
Buchanan, Cretin (1986)	Employment-based	Prior claims	HMO favorable selection

Source: Wilensky, G.R. and L.F. Rossiter. 1986. Patient self-selection in HMOs. Health Affairs 5(1):70.

As their summary indicates, mixed results have been reported. The early studies tended to report that HMOs suffered from adverse selection or that there was no evidence for biased selection. In contrast, the more recent studies reported that when conclusive evidence for biased selection was found, it suggested HMOs enjoyed favorable risk selection. Although a majority of the studies conducted since 1980 have concluded that HMOs experienced favorable selection, it is difficult to conclude unequivocally that analyses of HMO performance in terms of utilization and costs have been biased because these studies focused on selection bias and not on the total bias of the enrollee population. The latter is influenced by who enrolls (selection bias), who disenrolls, and how enrollees change in the interim (Welch 1985b). Although the first component has been examined extensively, the other two types of bias have received little attention.

Most of the studies of biased disenrollment have found that the utilization of "leavers," prior to disenrollment, has been lower than that of "stayers" (Wollstadt, Shapiro, and Bice 1978; Gold 1981; Wintringham 1982; Wersinger and Sorenson 1982; Mechanic, Weiss, and Cleary 1983; Hennelly and Boxerman 1983; Lewis 1984; and Stiefel, Gardelius, and Hayami 1984). These results are consistent with the risk-vulnerability hypothesis and our expectations that plan switching is inversely related to integration into the medical care system, which, in turn, is positively related to the amount of consumer interaction with the medical care system. Although consistent with theoretical expectations, the results from these studies are clouded by a number of methodological problems that were summarized by Welch (1985c). First, several studies did not include out-of-plan utilization, which may be related to dissatisfaction with the plans. Of those who included it, Mechanic et al. (1983) and Wollstadt et al. (1978) found out-of-plan visits of leavers to be greater than that of stayers, while Hennelly and Boxerman (1983) found out-of-plan visits to be about the same for the two groups. Second, most of the studies did not distinguish between mandatory and voluntary disenrollees. Hennelly and Boxerman found that the utilization patterns differed significantly between members of these two groups. Finally, Wintringham (1982), Wersinger and Sorenson (1982) and Lewis (1984) analyzed HMOs whose premiums had recently increased, a situation that limits generalizations to HMOs with stable premiums.

Little research has been conducted on the third component of the total bias of HMO enrollee population—temporal changes in enrollee utilization. A few researchers (Eggers and Prihoda 1982; Anderson and Knickman 1984; Blumberg 1984; Beebe 1985) report that the initial cost advantages gained by preferential selection of HMO enrollees are reduced by *regression-to-the-mean* of abnormally low users. For example, Eggers and Prihoda reported that Medicare enrollees had preenrollment expenditures below those of their counterparts who stayed with traditional providers. Following enrollment in 1980, however, enrollee utilization, measured in hospital days per 1,000 enrollees, increased to 1,667 in 1981; 1,607 in 1982; 1,976 in 1983; and 2,116 in 1984. Welch (1985b) reports that one-half of the utilization increase by the enrollees can be attributed to aging and that the residual increase is due to regression-to-the-mean and adverse dis-enrollment. Two studies, reporting that members of high- (or low-) use groups tend to remain high (or low) users (Eggers 1980; McCall and Wai 1981), con-tradict the regression-to-the-mean hypothesis.

In sum, a consensus of findings suggests that despite the existence of favorable selection into HMOs, the health status of HMO members is not significantly different from that of persons in fee-for-service plans (Freeborn and Pope 1982; Sorenson and Wersinger 1981; Diehr, Martin, Price et al. 1984; Welch 1985b; Welch and Frank 1986). A review of the literature suggests that the answer to this apparent paradox lies with adverse disenrollment from HMOs and regression-to-the-mean.

The only unequivocal conclusion previous research suggests is that the impact of biased enrollment on HMO performance makes analysis difficult. Conflicting reports suggest that HMOs either have more low-risk enrollees or that there is no difference between the pre-enrollment utilization patterns of HMO subscribers and members of conventional plans. Ironically, both conclusions may not be contradictory. For example, analysis of new and growing HMOs may be biased by favorable selection because insufficient time may have elapsed for the effects of regression-to-the-mean, aging, and adverse disenrollment to take effect. In contrast, comparisons of mature HMOs, in which the full effects of these phe-nomena have been experienced, may not be affected by enrollment bias. Con-sequently, it is clear that results of studies, which examined HMO performance (i.e., cost and utilization), should be accepted with caution only after a critical examination of the research methods of the study.

Quality of Care in HMOs

Although the prepaid features of HMO contracts provide desirable incentives for efficiency, some analysts are concerned that resource constraints will reduce the quality of care provided to HMO enrollees (Hornbrook and Berki 1985). The difficulties of measuring the quality of health care are legion and well known. Although quality of health care has been measured in a variety of ways, the tripartite classification of structure, process, and end results is common (Don-abedian 1966; Brook 1973). The structural approach, which is based on the assumption that outcomes are related to the types of inputs available to the provider, measures various characteristics of providers such as place and type of medical training, specialty certification, availability of equipment and accre-ditation status. Process evaluations consist of a review (e.g., medical audits) of actions taken by providers. End results examine the outcomes of health care and focus on measures such as mortality and morbidity rates or improvements in health status.

Luft's (1981) comprehensive review of the literature indicates that irrespective of which of the three dimensions of quality is evaluated, the level of quality provided in HMOs is not distinguishable from that provided in the fee-for-service sector. Cunningham and Williamson (1980) reported, in a literature review, that 19 of 27 studies conducted during the period 1958 to 1979 found quality of care in HMOs superior to that in fee-for-service settings. In the other 8 studies, the quality of care was similar in both settings. Hornbrook and Berki (1985) suggest that this result is reasonable since HMO physicians must provide the prevailing standard of care to limit their exposure to malpractice litigation. Indeed, since the corporate nature of HMOs makes them better targets for litigation than individual practitioners, they may be under more pressure to develop strong quality assurance mechanisms as part of their risk-management program.

Satisfaction and Growth of HMOs

In order to remain viable over a long period of time, HMOs must attract and retain members. Accordingly, consumer satisfaction should be viewed as one of the most important dimensions of HMO performance. Luft (1981) reports that analyses of patient or consumer satisfaction with health care began only recently. Consequently, there is no generally accepted theoretical framework for this concept, a situation resulting in the use of different measures and questions in each study. In general, the patient satisfaction studies have focused on two of the components of attitudes—feelings and behavior. Both approaches suffer from a number of problems that threaten the validity of results. Satisfaction studies, which measure feelings of consumers, must rely on interviews and self-reporting. Interviewers introduce the biases of selective memory and systematic response tendencies (Kinnear and Taylor 1979). On the other hand, behavioral measures such as disenrollment may reflect the availability of good substitutes rather than dissatisfaction with the current plan.

Although a number of individual factors that might affect satisfaction have been studied (Luft 1981), there is a paucity of rigorous empirical research on the determinants of enrollee satisfaction with HMOs (Francis 1986). Accordingly, our discussion of satisfaction with HMOs is limited to an examination of national enrollment trends and to results gained from national surveys conducted by Harris and Associates in 1980 and 1984 (Taylor and Kagay 1986). In recognition of the influence of corporate benefits managers and physicians on HMO growth, we also review results pertaining to their attitudes toward HMOs.

As indicated by the accelerated growth in enrollment shown in Table 11.2, HMOs are gaining acceptance as an alternative to traditional indemnity plans in the United States. Due to a smaller enrollment base, IPA-HMOs grew at a faster rate in the 1980s; however, PGP-HMOs have enjoyed larger increases in total enrollments than IPAs. HMO enrollment is not distributed uniformly across the country. Five states (with percentage of total HMO enrollment in parentheses) accounted for almost one-half of total enrollment: California (27.3 percent), New York (7.1 percent), Michigan (5.0 percent), Illinois (4.8 percent), and Minnesota (4.4 percent). HMO market penetration exceeded 20 percent in two states, California and Minnesota, and over 15 percent in five others (InterStudy 1986).

Table 11.2
Health Maintenance Organization Growth: Selected Years, 1970–1986

		All Plans			Plan Type			
					Staff, Group/Network Plans (combined)		IPA Plans	
		Number of Plans[a]	Enrollment (Millions)[a]	Enrollment (Percent of U.S. Population)	Number of Plans	Enrollment (Millions)	Number of Plans	Enrollment (Millions)
January	1970	26	2.9	1.4				
June	1975	178	5.7	2.6				
June	1980	236	9.1	4.0				
June	1981	243	10.2	4.4	153	8.7	90	1.6
June	1982	265	10.8	4.7	168	9.4	97	1.5
June	1983	280	12.5	5.3	181	10.6	99	1.9
June	1984	306	15.1	6.4	180	12.2	126	2.9
June	1985	393	18.8	7.9	212	14.2	181	4.6
June	1986	595[b]	23.7[b]	9.8	250	15.4	345	8.3

Sources: [a] National HMO Census – 1984 (Excelsior, MN: InterStudy, 1985).
[b] National HMO Census June Update (Excelsior, MN: InterStudy, 1986).

In 1980 and 1984, Harris and Associates conducted opinion polls in which representative samples of adult employees, corporate benefits managers and physicians were asked to respond to questions about HMOs (Taylor and Kagay 1986). The Harris Poll found that 90 percent and 76 percent of HMO subscribers were satisfied with the quality of their physicians and the quality of their hospital care, respectively. Satisfaction with HMO services is inversely related to disenrollment (Moustafa, Hopkins, and Klein 1971; Galiher and Costa 1975). Thus, it is not surprising that 93 percent of the HMO enrollees surveyed in 1980 and 1984 said they would probably renew their HMO contract when it expires (Taylor and Kagay 1986). The results from these "intention-to-behave" statements are consistent with previous behavior (i.e., disenrollment rates) summarized by Luft (1981).

Further analysis of the results from the Harris Poll suggests that HMO enrollees are more satisfied with most plan features than their counterparts in conventional plans. About 55 percent of HMO enrollees, in contrast to 38 percent of fee-for-service plan subscribers, responded that they were very satisfied with the overall level of health services. As expected, satisfaction with costs distinguished HMO enrollees from nonmembers. About 59 percent of HMO members were fully satisfied with the costs they and their families paid for health care. The corresponding figure for nonenrollees was only 27 percent. Finally, compared to nonenrollees, HMO members were more satisfied with access to health care services.

Although HMOs are granted access into many corporate benefits programs by the provisions of the HMO Act of 1973, employer cooperation is likely to facilitate HMO penetration into the marketplace. The results of the Harris Polls suggest that, among employees, HMOs have increased their name recognition and their image as efficient providers from 1980 to 1984. Both of these changes may stimulate enrollment in HMOs.

In order to grow, HMOs must obtain broader participation from physicians. Luft (1981) summarized a number of factors that might encourage (or discourage) physician participation in HMOs. The Harris Poll revealed that from 1981 to 1984, the percentage of physicians reporting at least a somewhat favorable attitude toward HMOs increased from 36 to 50. Unfortunately, this survey did not ask physicians to distinguish between IPA and PGP models of HMOs in their attitudes. It is likely that physicians object to a loss of autonomy in the latter type of HMO. Although a more favorable attitude is emerging, the 1984 survey revealed that most physicians (65 percent) believed that HMOs offer inferior care.

Taylor and Kagay (1986) reported that this attitude was influenced by the widely held perception that HMOs perform fewer laboratory and other diagnostic tests than may be necessary, employ less qualified doctors, or do not allow for an adequate doctor-patient relationship. Contrary to physician perceptions but consistent with earlier findings summarized by Luft (1981), the results of this survey suggest that there was not a significant difference between HMOs and fee-for-service physicians in terms of the proportion of board-certified physicians, a commonly used structural measure of quality.

In summary, the "proof of the pudding is in the tasting." An unprecedented number of individuals have tasted HMOs during the 1980s and reported that, in general, they liked what they experienced. Apparently, either from positive word-of-mouth advertising or through mere exposure, nonenrollees are developing a more positive attitude towards HMOs, a trend also experienced by physicians and corporate benefits managers. Accordingly, there is good reason to believe that HMO enrollment will continue to grow, albeit eventually at a slower rate, as the market matures.

MEDICARE HMOs

As part of a procompetitive cost containment strategy, the federal government has encouraged HMOs and Competitive Medical Plans (i.e., organizations that offer prepaid health services but are not federally qualified HMOs) to enter into risk contracts for Medicare beneficiaries under regulations published by the Health Care Financing Administration (HCFA) in 1985. HMOs, which sign risk contracts, are paid a capitation rate equal to 95 percent of the adjusted average per capita cost (AAPCC) of health services, a measure of the cost of treating Medicare beneficiaries in the fee-for-service sector in each county. In the following sections, we examine the previous growth of Medicare participation in HMOs and prospects for future increases in beneficiary enrollment. Next we consider the deficiencies in the current capitation arrangements and how they can be improved.

History of Medicare Capitation Payments

The Social Security Amendments of 1966 authorized the Medicare program to contract with HMOs for the payment of 80 percent of the reasonable costs of providing Part B services (medical and other professional services). In order to increase the participation of HMOs in the Medicare program, Congress passed Section 1876 of the Social Security Amendments of 1972, which allowed HMOs to enter into risk-based or cost-based contracts with Medicare for both Part A and Part B services. This law, however, limited risk-based contracts to HMOs with more than 25,000 enrollees and stipulated that HMOs could not keep more than 10 percent of the savings earned by providing services at levels less than the AAPCC. Given these restrictive covenants, it is not surprising that by the end of 1979, only two HMOs chose to enter into a risk-based contract with Medicare under the provisions of the Social Security Amendments of 1972. HMOs viewed Medicare cost contracts in a similar light. By December 31, 1979, only 31 HMOs with 42,766 Medicare beneficiaries enrolled signed cost contracts with HCFA (Adamache and Rossiter 1986).

In order to determine if other forms of risk-contracting would stimulate increased HMO participation in the Medicare program, HCFA developed a series of capitation demonstration projects. In the first of these experiments, the Medicare Capitation Demonstrations, eight plans began operations between 1980 and 1981. In 1982, HCFA initiated a second series of experiments, called the Medicare Competition Demonstrations. By 1984, 117,000 beneficiaries were enrolled in 26 operational plans under the demonstration. In this project, the HMOs received a monthly capitation payment from HCFA equal to 95 percent of the AAPCC. The HMOs were required to provide the current Medicare benefit package; however, they were allowed to provide additional benefits and to charge premiums to enrollees (Langwell and Hadley 1986).

The more attractive HMO participation provisions in the demonstration projects were included in the Tax Equity and Fiscal Responsibility Act of 1982 (TEFRA). Accordingly, as of June, 1985, 25 of the 26 HMOs were induced to convert to operational TEFRA HMOs. By April, 1986, 119 plans with 556,190 Medicare beneficiaries enrolled had signed TEFRA risk contracts. In addition, 64 applications for TEFRA risk contracts were awaiting federal approval.

In contrast to the early sluggish experience, HMO participation in the Medicare program grew dramatically during the 1980s. The enrollment of Medicare beneficiaries in HMOs with risk contracts increased by 300 percent from January 1, 1980, to March 31, 1986. Despite this trend, however, by the end of the first quarter of 1986, only a small proportion (4.6 percent) of the Medicare population had enrolled in some type of a prepaid health plan, with 2.2 percent enrolled in a prepaid plan with a risk contract (Langwell and Hadley 1986).

Although the recent growth of HMO participation in the Medicare program has encouraged those who favor a procompetition strategy, questions still remain about the long-term participation of HMOs in the market, as well as about their ability to achieve the goals established by federal health care officials. A recent article by Adamache and Rossiter (1986) reported findings that may help answer these questions about Medicare HMOs. Using data from the 1982 National HMO Census (InterStudy 1983), which contained information on 263 HMOs, 40 of which participated in the federal Medicare capitation experiments, the researchers used regression analysis to test a number of hypotheses regarding the factors influencing an HMO's decision to enter into a Medicare risk contract.

Adamache and Rossiter reported that the single most important predictor of market entry is the capitation rate faced by the HMO in its county of operation. An AAPCC rate that is one standard deviation above the mean (i.e., about $50) increases the likelihood of entry into a Medicare risk contract by 16 percent. This result has a number of implications. As Adamache and Rossiter (1986) point out, HMOs are more likely to enter high-cost areas where competition is most needed to curb inflationary tendencies. Alternatively, one could argue that HMOs will tend to enter into a capitation agreement only if the potential of a large profit outweighs the risk of serving the elderly. If this profit does not materialize, the HMO may choose to abandon the Medicare market as many have done already.

Conversely, the elderly may not have access to an HMO in lower cost areas. For example, Choice Care in Cincinnati had monthly capitation rates amounting to $165, an amount substantially less than the national average of $200. These low payments, coupled with adverse patient selection, caused this HMO to lose $7 million on its risk contract in 1985. Consequently, Choice Care did not renew its contract with HCFA in 1986 (Ellwood 1986). In an attempt to induce HMOs to maintain their Medicare risk-contracts, the Department of Health and Human Services announced a 13.5 percent increase in payment rates to these organizations. The new payment schedule will be implemented in 1988 (Traska 1987a).

Adamache and Rossiter also pointed out that HMO participation in a risk contract was positively associated with the proportion of area residents over 65 years of age and with federal qualification. The former result is consistent with a priori expectations. A larger concentration of elderly residents increases the likelihood that the Medicare beneficiary will come into contact with an individual who has a Medicare HMO contract, thus allowing the HMO to rely on word-of-mouth advertising. Further, the larger potential market is usually associated with lower unit costs of advertising.

The coefficients of the variables representing market characteristics, organizational characteristics, service use and financial condition were insignificant ($p > .10$). These results suggest that concerns about the disproportionate entry into the Medicare market by inexperienced or financially weak HMOs were unfounded.

In summary, the results reported by Adamache and Rossiter suggest that HMO participation in the Medicare program may be limited to areas with high capitation rates and dense concentrations of the elderly. It is possible that broader participation will occur over time as HMOs learn how to cultivate and manage this market segment and as HMOs become more widely accepted by all segments of society; however, these changes may be painfully slow. Accordingly, if the federal government desires to use HMOs as part of its competitive strategy, it may have to address a tradeoff that apparently exists between broader HMO participation and individual plan cost control, both of which are affected by the level and calculation of capitation payments, a topic we shall address now.

Medicare HMO Capitation Payments

In this section, our focus shifts to Medicare capitation payments, which are linked to the AAPCC and are calculated in three stages. First, the per capita Medicare costs in the United States are projected to the current year. Second, the national rate is adjusted for historical differences between Medicare cost per capita in the county that the HMO serves and the national average. Third, separate actuarial classes for beneficiaries over 65 years of age and disabled beneficiaries are created using age, gender, welfare status (e.g., Medicaid recipients), and institutional status (e.g., resident of a nursing home). These factors are used to calculate a separate premium rate for each of 30 actuarial subclasses.

Although HCFA hoped to develop classes of patients in which expected costs were close to actual medical care expenditures, experience has suggested that this goal has not been achieved. A recent study demonstrated that the variables currently used to define the Medicare HMO subcells collectively explain less than 1 percent of the variation in Medicare payments (Thomas and Lichtenstein 1986b). Supportive evidence is provided by similar results from studies that employed three of the variables (data on welfare status was not available) used to form the AAPCC subcells (Hornbrook 1984; Beebe, Lubitz and Eggers 1985; Anderson, Steinberg, Holloway and Cantor 1986).

The poor predictive power of the AAPCC may create problems similar to those we discussed in our analysis of the reliance on DRGs to establish payment rates for hospital services. The first of these is an incentive to establish a preferential selection policy, which enables the HMO to earn windfall profits by the favorable selection of low-risk enrollees and to avoid losses associated with adverse selection. These related strategies may result in the denial of access to HMO services for many Medicare beneficiaries. If HMOs dominate a local market, this also could result in a serious barrier to care for high-risk individuals. Second, irrespective of how it is established, a capitation rate creates an incentive to reduce the volume of services provided to enrollees. To the extent that fee-for-service physicians provide excessive amounts of services, this incentive is desirable. There is the danger, however, that HMOs may overreact and reduce the volume of services to such a degree that the well-being of enrollees is jeopardized. HMOs whose financial viability is threatened by insufficient capitation rates may have a greater propensity to reduce quality. Finally, if HMOs selectively enroll low-risk patients, a greater percentage of high-risk (and high-cost) patients will be treated by fee-for-service practitioners. This may result in increased outlays by HCFA if the capitation rate remains pegged to 95 percent of adjusted fee-for-service costs.

In recognition of the deficiencies of the current AAPCC formula, efforts have been undertaken to develop and test a new basis for establishing capitation rates for Medicare enrollees in HMOs. Most of the research in this area has emphasized either prior use of services or health status. We will describe these approaches briefly and then evaluate their utility in terms of criteria similar to those used in our assessment of patient classification systems.

Prior Use Capitation Adjusters

Anderson and Knickman (1984) and Beebe, Lubitz and Eggers (1985) have examined the utility of prior use of health services as an adjuster to the AAPCC capitation rate. The ability of prior use to predict future use is documented in a number of studies (Eggers 1980; McCall and Wai 1981; Eggers and Prihoda 1982; Anderson and Knickman 1984; Beebe, Lubitz and Eggers 1985). However, the utility of prior use for setting HMO capitation rates may be mitigated by the regression-to-the-mean, experienced by those who were high (or low) users of medical services in prior periods (Anderson and Knickman 1984; Blumberg 1984; Beebe 1985; Welch 1985c).

Adjusting HMO capitation rates on the basis of prior use has been criticized by a number of analysts. First, this type of adjustment may create an incentive for HMOs to increase use in one period to obtain increased levels of payments in future periods, resulting in inflationary pressures similar to those experienced by hospitals under cost-based reimbursement (Thomas, Lichtenstein, Wyszewianski, and Berki 1983). Second, a prior utilization payment mechanism may reward inefficient providers who are unable to control unnecessary utilization and penalize providers who control utilization effectively (Anderson, Steinberg, Holloway, and Cantor 1986). Similarly, the prior use adjustment factor may create an incentive for physicians to adopt a more elaborate practice style because they will receive a higher capitation rate in the future if they order more tests and services in a prior period (McClure 1984). Ironically, risk-based capitation payments were intended to remove this incentive, which also exists under fee-for-service payment mechanisms.

In response to these criticisms, proponents of the prior utilization approach have suggested modifications that avoid the perverse incentives provided by payments that do not adequately reflect future need of services. McClure (1984) argues that HMO capitation payments should reflect chronic risk for the year, not acute risk factors subject to fluctuations of days or weeks. Although this approach has some conceptual appeal, it has not been tested empirically. Using another approach that is linked to Wennberg's (1984) research on medical practice variations, Anderson et al. (1986) argued that payment adjustments that are based on prior use should exclude admissions precipitated by health problems for which a consensus of physicians believe hospitalization to be highly discretionary (e.g., influenza, sprain, and rheumatoid arthritis). By limiting payment adjustments to services for which treatment patterns are fairly well established, physicians have little opportunity to act on the incentives to "overtreat," which are provided by a prior-use formula.

Anderson et al. (1986) evaluated the utility of a "limited-discretion," prior-use capitation formula by comparing the ability of three capitation models (i.e., AAPCC, traditional prior-use, and limited-discretion prior-use) to explain variation in per capita expenditures among a randomly selected national sample ($n = 189,088$) of Medicare beneficiaries who were alive from 1974 through at least part of 1978. Their "AAPCC model," which included four of five variables (i.e., age, gender, welfare status and Medicare expenditures, but not institutional status) used by HCFA to establish AAPCC payment rates, had the lowest explanatory power ($R^2 = .01$). As expected, the traditional prior-use model, which added to the first equation a variable measuring the total number of times a beneficiary was hospitalized during the two years prior to the year for which expenditures were predicted, had the greatest explanatory power ($R^2 = .04$). A limited-discretion model was formed by replacing the variable for previous number of admissions with two new variables—the number of prior admissions that were for conditions involving (a) limited physician discretion, or (b) moderate physician discretion. The authors reported that the explanatory power ($R^2 = 0.03$) of the limited physician discretion model was only marginally lower than that of the traditional prior-use model. Anderson et al. argued that a slight decrease in explanatory power was a small price to pay for avoiding the incentives created by a system which makes payments without regard for the medical necessity of services.

Functional Health Status Capitation Adjusters

Although prior use capitation adjusters have the advantage of easy and inexpensive data collection for current Medicare beneficiaries, several analysts (McClure 1984, Thomas et al. 1983) are concerned that this type of payment mechanism creates an incentive to provide unnecessary services. Accordingly, they argued that HMO capitation rates should be adjusted on the basis of health status. Thomas et al. (1983) dichotomized possible health status adjusters into perceived health status measures and functional health status indicators. The former refers to the individual's self-rated health. The use of perceived health status as a predictor of health services utilization has been validated in a number of studies (Linn and Linn 1980; Roos and Shapiro 1981); however, since enrollee self-perceptions are subject to provider manipulations, which are not detected easily, perceived health status measures are not likely to be satisfactory capitation adjusters.

Functional health status measures may be a more suitable alternative than perceived health status or prior use for adjusting the AAPCC. The index of Activities of Daily Living (ADL), which we discussed in the section on nursing home patient classification systems (see Chapter 6), is an example of a functional health status measure. ADLs reflect the individual's ability to perform self-care activities (i.e., eating, grooming, bathing, etc.) without assistance. Another functional health status measure is the Instrumental Activities of Daily Living (IADL). These include activities that are more difficult to perform than those included in the ADLs. Functional health status measures were used initially with institutionalized patients and were administered by trained nurses or other interviewers (Katz, Ford, Moskowitz et al. 1963); however, more recent research indicates that instruments measuring functional health status can be completed reliably by a noninstitutionalized population on a self-reported basis (Branch, Jette, Evashwick et al. 1981; Jette and Branch 1981).

Thomas and Lichtenstein (1986a) compared the explanatory power of functional health status with that of a variety of other HMO capitation adjusters, including the current AAPCC variables, perceived health status, and prior use in an analysis of a randomly selected sample ($n = 2,123$) of Medicare beneficiaries in Michigan. Standardized Medicare outlays per beneficiary in 1983 was the factor used as the dependent variable in the regression analysis. As expected, the four AAPCC variables had the lowest explanatory power ($R^2 = .003$) while a prior use measure, the number of Medicare Part B claims filed by the beneficiary in the prior year (i.e., 1982), predicted Medicare outlays the best ($R^2 = .07$).

Perceived health status ($R^2 = .02$) and functional health status ($R^2 = .03$) performed better than the AAPCC model but not nearly as well as the prior-use model.

In a companion study, Thomas and Lichtenstein (1986b) performed regression analysis on their Michigan data base to determine how much variance in Medicare beneficiary outlays was explained by combining variables from different capitation adjustment models. They reported that a model that included age, sex, number of hospital admissions, number of prior year Medicare Part B claims, and functional health status explained 9.2 percent of the variance in Medicare payments per beneficiary.

Evaluation of Medicare HMO Capitation Adjusters

The proposed modifications to the Medicare HMO payment mechanism can be evaluated in terms of criteria similar to those that we used in our assessment of inpatient classification systems in Chapter 5. Specifically, capitation rates should be based on variables that (1) reduce variation between actual and predicted costs (2) are not subject to provider manipulation (3) are easily audited and (4) are inexpensive to collect.

The first criterion, accurate prediction of costs, is similar to the homogeneity criterion used to evaluate patient classification systems. Performance in this dimension can be judged in terms of the percentage of variance explained by the variables in the capitation model. A satisfactory R^2 can be established only by arbitrary methods; however, a review of the explanatory power of other payment mechanisms facilitates comparisons. At the individual level of aggregation, DRGs accounted for 17 percent of the variation in expense per admission of patients hospitalized in Michigan (Calore and Iezzoni 1987). Although officials in the federal government believe that DRGs are sufficiently homogeneous to be used for hospital payments, some analysts (Horn, Horn, and Sharkey 1984) believe that this classification system should be modified to increase its explanatory power. The Resource Utilization Group-II system, which has been used to regulate payment rates of nursing homes in New York, explained 52 percent of the variation in resource consumption (Schneider, Holden, and Fries 1985).

The predictive power of capitation adjusters is much less than that of inpatient classification systems. The AAPCC variables, as a group, explain less than 1 percent of the variance in Medicare expenditures. Regarding the experimental adjusters, even the best predictive model, which uses a combination of AAPCC variables, prior use, and functional health status, had an R^2 of less than .10.

Thomas and Lichtenstein (1986a) suggest that the low values of R^2 reported in research investigations of Medicare HMO capitation adjusters result from a failure to transform data that are skewed. An inspection of the data revealed that most Medicare beneficiaries (70 percent) had no (or low) reimbursable expenses, while a small group of beneficiaries (2.5 percent) had expenditures exceeding $10,000. As a result of the skewness, the regression equations tend to underestimate payments at the high end of the distribution. Since the R^2 reflects the sum of the squared deviations between the actual and predicted payments, the impact of these errors on the R^2 is magnified. Accordingly, it may be appropriate to transform the data so that the normality assumptions required for regression analysis are satisfied.

Thomas and Lichtenstein (1986b) transformed a variety of capitation models by using the logarithm of Medicare payments and found that, in each of the eight regression models they tested, the R^2 of the equation with the logarithmic transformation was more than twice that of its untransformed counterpart. In the transformed equations, the R^2 ranged from .169 to .236. Although the increase in explanatory power is somewhat reassuring to proponents of risk-based capitation payments, transforming the dependent variable does not offer any solace to HMOs, which have beneficiaries that incur extraordinarily high expenditures. Rather, these results highlight the need for special adjustments for this group of beneficiaries.

The solution to the problems caused by the skewed (and unpredictable) distribution of Medicare outlays requires a payment policy that minimizes the risk of excessive losses (i.e., expenditures greater than the capitation rate) and avoids new incentives to overtreat patients. Although the experimental adjusters reduce this problem, the values of R^2 of even the best predictive models suggest that much more work in this area is required. Perhaps the most obvious solution is to include provisions in risk contracts offered to HMOs that authorize additional compensation similar to the outlier payments currently used in the Medicare prospective payment system. Several analysts have pointed out, however, that the Medicare inpatient outlier payments are too low and create incentives for hospitals to implement a preferential admissions policy or to discharge patients prematurely (Lave 1984; Broyles and Rosko 1985); however, these incentives can be reduced by implementing a payment schedule that more accurately reflects the marginal costs of required services.

The second evaluative criterion indicates that the provider should not be able to influence the values of the capitation adjusters in order to obtain a higher payment rate. The third criterion, ease in auditing the adjuster, ensures that violations of the second criteria are detected easily, thereby reducing the incentives to do so.

Since perceptions are subjective and may be transitory, self-reported health status does not score well on either the second or third criterion. Prior use of service can be manipulated by the provider to increase compensation rates; however, retrospective medical audits, which can determine the medical necessity of services provided, may be used to control this type of abuse. Functional health status, if self-reported or measured by the HMO, also is subject to some manipulation. On the other hand, the ADLs or the IADLs have an objective component that is amenable to the auditing process.

The final criterion is that the capitation adjuster should not require data that results in excessive collection costs. Prior-use data is already collected for Medicare beneficiaries; however, obtaining data on the past utilization for those entering the Medicare program will be more problematic and perhaps more costly. Self-reported measures of perceived health status or functional health status could be obtained without much expense. However, the self-reported measures may be less reliable and subject to more manipulation than similar information obtained from trained interviewers or observers hired by the federal government.

Our evaluation suggests that prior use and functional health status are the most promising capitation rate adjusters. Thomas and Lichtenstein (1986a) suggest that both adjusters be used. They reported that the prior-use coefficient is reduced when functional health status variables are added to the regression equation. Thus, if the payment rates are linked to the coefficients of the adjusters, prior use will receive a lower adjustment when it is used in conjunction with functional health status. Since the decision to overtreat is made at the margin, a reduction in marginal revenue (i.e., the per capita rate associated with prior use) will reduce the number of services for which it will be profitable to "overtreat," thereby reducing incentives to order unnecessary services. Ultimately, the decision to adjust capitation rates for prior use or health status or both should be based on better information than is currently available. Accordingly, we conclude this section with some recommendations for future research.

The relatively high predictive power of prior-use variables combined with low data acquisition costs makes them promising candidates for use as HMO adjusters. These advantages are offset by their ability to be manipulated by providers. Thus, we feel that more research should be focused upon the development and testing of prior-use adjusters that are subject to less manipulation. These include chronic conditions as well as services over which physicians have less discretionary power to hospitalize patients; however, acute health problems may be related to future use and should not be ignored. Similarly, although a panel of experts may feel that physicians have a great deal of latitude in their decision to admit a patient to a hospital for treatment, they may also agree that in many instances, hospitalization of patients with "discretionary conditions" is clinically justified. Accordingly, capitation adjustments should not ignore prior use of services for acute or discretionary services. Rather, they should be considered, perhaps, at a lower rate. This, of course, is a complex issue that cannot be resolved without further research.

Finally, possible provider responses to capitation rates have been subject to a great deal of speculation that has not been accompanied by empirical evaluation. Since changes in capitation formulas can have profound effects on beneficiaries, providers, and taxpayers, we suggest that alterations should be implemented on a limited basis and subjected to substantial evaluation before they are adopted on a large-scale basis.

COMPETITIVE EFFECTS OF HMOs

The growth of HMOs is expected to benefit society in two ways: (1) provision of cost-effective services to more enrollees and (2) stimulation of price com-

Figure 11.1
Effect of Entry of New Competitors on Equilibrium Price and Quantity

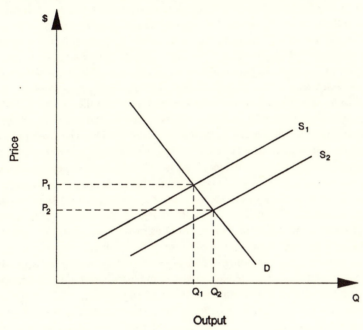

petition among other health care providers and insurers. Although subject to much speculation, little research has been conducted on the competitive effects of HMOs. In this section, we review the existing literature on this topic.

The hypothesized effects of HMO growth are based on the standard economic model shown in Figure 11.1. This model predicts that the entry of new competitors will shift the market supply curve from S_1 to S_2, thereby lowering equilibrium price from P_1 to P_2. This model also predicts an increase in quantity from Q_1 to Q_2 associated with the shift in the supply curve. Total expenditures, however, will be reduced by a decrease in price only in the case of inelastic demand over the relevant price ranges. Thus, advocates of competition embellish this model with the assumption that demand will be restricted by the imposition of utilization controls. Reduction of use, in turn, is expected to reduce HMO costs and premiums.

"Price wars," however, are not the only possible response to increased competition. In contrast to the assumption of perfect competition in which the firm is a price-taker, models of monopolistic competition and differentiated oligopolies—market structures that reflect more closely the conditions in the health care industry—include product differentiation as a possible response to the entry of rivals in the marketplace (Mansfield 1982). Product differentiation, which is used to give monopoly power to the firm, can be achieved by advertising or through product changes such as the addition of new services, changes in the level of amenities, or improvements in convenience factors. Although flawed, Robinson and Luft's (1985) study provides some evidence to support their contention that hospitals have engaged in a "medical arms race" in which competition for physicians and patients is based on the acquisition of new technology. Other evidence suggests that Blue Cross/Blue Shield Plans and other insurers respond to the entry and growth of HMOs by increasing the comprehensiveness of their benefit packages (Goldberg and Greenberg 1980). In the absence of utilization controls, the reduction in out-of-pocket patient expenses is likely to increase demand for health services; however, such a change will increase health insurance premiums, a circumstance that health insurance buyers would like to avoid. Unfortunately, little is known about the response of employers, who purchase 84 percent of private insurance (Farley and Wilensky 1983), to changes in benefits packages. Sapolsky, Altman, Greene, and Moore (1980) reported that employers were concerned more about attracting productive personnel and avoiding strikes than reducing expenditures for benefits; however, recent employer health care cost containment initiatives (Fox, Goldbeck, and Spies 1984), including the growth of employee cost-sharing provisions (Hewitt Associates 1984), suggest that employer policies are changing.

In summary, it is impossible to develop *a priori* expectations about the spillover effects of HMOs on health care expenditures because competitors might respond by engaging in price competition or by demand-inducing product-variation strategies, such as increases in insurance benefits, development of new products, and increases in advertising activities. Further, price competition among insurers and HMOs might be based on strategies to gain favorable selection rather than on actions to increase efficiency (Luft 1981; Jensen, Feldman, and Dowd 1984; Price and Mays 1985).

In the remainder of this section, we restrict our analysis to econometric studies that examined the interrelationships among HMO market share and area-wide health care costs and utilization. A number of case studies (Christianson and McClure 1979; Roghmann, Sorenson, and Wells 1980; Enthoven 1981; Dowd 1986; Luft, Maerki, and Trauner 1986) provide useful background information. We will not include them in the review because the analytical methods employed in a case study fail to control for extraneous factors that might confound the analysis.

Econometric studies have provided conflicting findings for the competitive effect of HMOs. Results from Goldberg and Greenberg (1980) and Merrill and McLaughlin (1986) support the position that indemnity insurers respond to HMO growth by restricting utilization in an effort to control costs; however, Merrill and McLaughlin also reported that the coefficient of the HMO market-share variable in their cost-per-capita equations was positive and significant ($p < .01$), while Hay and Leahy (1984) estimated a positive but insignificant HMO market-share coefficient.

In contrast to the other studies, Hay and Leahy found a positive and significant association between HMO growth and hospital days per capita. The contradictory results are probably due to a variety of methodological problems, which we will discuss in our brief critique of these studies.

Goldberg and Greenberg (1980) estimated several single-equation models using cross-sectional data for 1974 from the Federal Employees Health Benefits Program (FEHBP). In order to test the hypothesis that Blue Cross Plans respond to HMO competition by instituting cost-control programs, the researchers used the state as the level of aggregation and regressed a number of utilization variables pertaining to patient days per 1,000 Blue Cross enrollees in different groups on a number of factors including the market share of HMOs. Negative (and usually significant) coefficients of the HMO market-share variables were estimated, results consistent with the hypothesis that HMOs stimulate cost competition with traditional insurers.

A number of design weaknesses threaten the validity of the results reported by Goldberg and Greenberg. First, the level of aggregation was the state, an area that is inconsistent with the smaller market areas often served by HMOs and Blue Cross Plans. Second, the small sample size ($n = 50$) forced the researchers to conserve degrees of freedom in the regression analyses by using only a limited set of independent variables, including HMO market share, per capita income, and active physicians per 100,000 population. The authors used the last variable as a proxy for geographic region.

It is clear that a number of important demand determinants (see Chapter 3) were omitted, resulting in a specification error. In a footnote, Goldberg and Greenberg present results for a patient day equation in which a regional dummy variable, equal to one for western states, was included. The addition of this variable reduced the value of the HMO market-share coefficient from -17.1 to -11.9, with corresponding reductions in t-ratios from -3.03 ($p < .01$) to -1.71 ($p > .05$). Although the specification of virtually all regression equations is subject to question, a change of this magnitude suggests that the omission of important demand determinants, which are correlated with the western region, caused a serious specification bias. Finally, Goldberg and Greenberg did not assess the impact of HMOs on health system costs. Thus, even if we assume that Blue Cross Plans reduced inpatient utilization, it is possible that savings accrued from this action could have been offset by increased intensity of inpatient services or by an increased use of ambulatory services.

Hay and Leahy (1984), who estimated reduced-form equations for a variety of expense and utilization measures, improved upon Goldberg and Greenberg's methods in the following ways. They used 1978 data from 202 health service areas. In addition to increasing the sample size, the use of the health service area as the level of aggregation is more consistent with the concept of market areas than the use of the entire state. Further, they used a large number of variables that controlled for variations in demographics, and economic and market-supply factors.

Although Hay and Leahy advanced the econometric analysis performed in this area, their study had a number of flaws. The first problem is related to HMO's attraction to high-cost areas (Welch 1984; Adamache and Rossiter 1986). Apparently, HMOs find it easier to compete in high-cost areas because their indemnity rivals must charge higher-than-average premiums. Accordingly, regressing costs against an HMO market-share variable will result in inconsistent estimates arising from the simultaneity relationship of these two variables. The authors recognized this problem but did not pursue its solution.

Second, Hay and Leahy defined market share for Blue Cross Plans and other insurers as the ratio of benefits paid by a particular type of insurance to total personal health expenditures. Both numerator and denominator of Blue Cross and other insurance market-share variables were at the state level of aggregation while the remainder of the variables were aggregated at the health service area level. Furthermore, these variables were defined differently than the HMO market-share variable, which was based on enrollees per 1,000 population. Finally, the authors include the number of HMOs in the area as a second market-share variable. This variable not only lacks theoretical justification but also is likely to be correlated with HMO enrollees per 1,000 population, thus reducing the reliability of the estimates of both coefficients.

Merrill and McLaughlin (1986) estimated cost and utilization equations using data pooled from 25 cross sections during the period 1972–1981. Their explanatory variables controlled demographic and supplier-related factors as well as regulatory environment. In addition, a fixed-effect specification creating a separate intercept for each SMSA was employed, thereby controlling the effects of unmeasured differences between SMSAs.

Although improving on the earlier studies, Merrill and McLaughlin's analysis was not unflawed. First, they used two endogenous factors, beds and HMO market share, as independent variables. Second, their sample mean for HMO market share was 6.2 percent during a period in which the corresponding national average was 3.1 percent, indicating an overrepresentation of SMSAs with large HMOs (Frank and Welch 1985). Since interregional variation in physician utilization dominates intrastate variation (Frank 1981), it may have been preferable to include regional dummy variables, rather than SMSA variables, in their regression analysis. Another indication of the unrepresentativeness of the sample is the insignificant ($p > .05$) regression coefficients for the rate regulation variable in the cost equations. This result is contradicted by many studies (see Chapter 12) conducted during this period, including one which used the SMSA as the level of aggregation (Morrisey, Sloan, and Mitchell 1983).

Finally, it is important to note that each of the studies we reviewed did not analyze data extending beyond 1981. Given the dramatic changes experienced by the health care industry during the 1980s, it is apparent that the applicability of results from these studies to current policy decisions, even if they were valid, would be questionable at best. Accordingly, we end this section with a plea for further research on the competitive effects of alternative delivery systems, which should be expanded beyond HMOs to include PPOs. Such research should incorporate the best features of the studies we reviewed in this section while avoiding their pitfalls. We agree with Frank and Welch (1985) who argued that it is critical to treat area utilization rates and HMO market share as jointly determined. They suggest that this might be accomplished by (1) employing two-stage least-squares, or (2) lagging the endogenous variable (e.g., HMO market share) as well as the dependent variable (e.g., health care costs).

SUMMARY

Although a variety of alternative delivery systems have proliferated during the 1980s, a substantial body of research on performance exists only for HMOs. Due to the confounding influence of a variety of factors affecting HMO research, findings are available to support almost any position that has been put forth regarding the impact of HMOs on the delivery of efficient and effective health care. We have outlined a variety of methodological problems and hope that researchers in the future avoid some of the pitfalls encountered by their predecessors. Although we are uncertain about the impact of HMOs and other alternative delivery systems, it is very clear that they have enjoyed phenomenal growth during the 1980s. Further, HCFA's concern about increases in Medicare Part B expenditures, which averaged over 16 percent during the 1980s, suggests that the federal government will continue to increase its efforts to steer Medicare beneficiaries away from the fee-for-service sector and toward capitated HMOs.

An unequivocal endorsement of the alternative delivery system approach as the principle cost-containment strategy requires valid evaluations of not only the performance of this approach but also that of regulatory interventions. Further, by necessity, evaluations of public policy instruments must be value-laden. Since we have attempted to keep our analysis as value-free as possible, we will defer recommendations regarding future public policy on cost containment until Chapter 13, where we will introduce some of our own values into the analysis. In the next chapter, we review the evidence pertaining to the regulatory cost-containment approaches.

REFERENCES

Abramowitz, K. 1985. *The Future of Health Care Delivery in America*. New York: Sanford C. Bernstein and Co.

Adamache, K. W., and L. F. Rossiter. 1986. The entry of HMOs into the Medicare market: Implications for TEFRA's mandate. *Inquiry* 23(4):349–64.

Anderson, G. F., E. P. Steinberg, J. Holloway, and J. C. Cantor. 1986. Paying for HMO care: Issues and options in setting capitation rates. *The Milbank Quarterly* 64(4):548–65.

Anderson, G., and J. Knickman. 1984. Adverse selection under a voucher system: Grouping medicare recipients by level of expenditure. *Inquiry* 21(2):135–43.

Arnold, R. J., and C. B. Van Vorst. 1985. Supply responses to market and regulatory forces in health care. In J. Meyer, ed., *Incentives vs. Controls in Health Policy: Broadening the Debate*. Washington, DC: American Enterprise Institute.

Arrow, K. 1963. Uncertainty and the welfare economics of medical care. *American Economic Review* 53(4):941–73.

Baker, N., J. McGee, and M. Shadle. 1984. HMO status report 1982–1983. Excelsior, MN: InterStudy.

Bashur, R. L., and C. A. Metzner. 1970. Vulnerability to risk and awareness of dual choice of health insurance plans. *Health Services Research* 5(2):106–13.

Beebe, J. C. 1985. Medicare reimbursement regression to the mean. Health Care Financing Administration, Office of Research, manuscript.

Beebe, J., J. Lubitz, and P. Eggers. 1985. Using prior utilization to determine payments for Medicare enrollees in health maintenance organizations. *Health Care Financing Review* 6(3):27–38.

Berki, S. E., M. Ashcraft, R. Penchansky, and R. S. Fortus 1977. Enrollment choice in a multi-HMO setting: The roles of health risk, financial vulnerability, and access to care. *Medical Care* 15(2):95–114.

Bice, T. W. 1975. Risk vulnerability and enrollment in a prepaid group practice. *Medical Care* 13(8):698–703.

Blumberg, M. S. 1984. At risk for hospitalization: Differences by health insurance coverage and income. In R. M. Scheffler and L. F. Rossiter, eds., *Advances in Health Economics and Health Services Research* 4. Greenwich, CT: JAI Press.

Branch, L., A. Jette, C. Evashwick et al. 1981. Toward understanding elders' health services utilization. *Journal of Community Health* 7(2):80–92.

Brecher, C. 1984. Medicaid comes to Arizona: A first-year report on AHCCCS. *Journal of Health Politics, Policy and Law* 9(3):411–25.

Brook, R. H. 1973. Critical issues in the assessment of quality of care and their relationship to HMOs. *Journal of Medical Education* 48 (4, Part 2):114–34.

Broyles, R. W., and M. D. Rosko. 1985. A qualitative assessment of the medicare prospective payment system. *Social Science and Medicine* 20(11):1185–90.

Buchanan, J. L., and S. Cretin. 1986. Risk selection of families electing HMO membership. *Medical Care* 24(1):39–51.

Calore, K. A., and L. Iezzoni. 1987. Disease staging and PMCs: Can they improve DRGs? *Medical Care* 25(8):724–37.

Cascardo, D. 1982. Factors affecting cost containment in an HMO: A review of the literature. *Journal of Ambulatory Care Management* 5(3):53–63.

Christianson, J. B., and W. McClure. 1979. Competition in the delivery of medical care. *New England Journal of Medicine* 301(15):812–18.

Cunningham, F. C., and J. W. Williamson. 1980. How does the quality of health care in HMOs compare to that in other settings? *Group Health Journal* 1(1):4–25.

de Lissovoy, G., T. Rice, J. Gabel, and H. J. Gelzer. 1987. Preferred provider organizations one year later. *Inquiry* 24(2):127–35.

Diehr, P., D. P. Martin, K. F. Price et al. 1984. Use of ambulatory care services in three provider plans: Interactions between patient characteristics and plans. *American Journal of Public Health* 74(1):47–51.

Donabedian, A. 1966. Evaluating the quality of medical care. *Milbank Memorial Fund Quarterly* 44(3), Part 2:166–203.

Dowd, B. E. 1986. HMOs and twin cities admission rates. *Health Services Research* 21(2):177–88.

Dowd, B. and R. Feldman. 1985. Biased selection in twin cities health plans. In R. M. Schleffer and L. F. Rossiter, eds., *Advances in Health Economics and Health Services Research* 6. Greenwich, CT: JAI Press.

Eggers, P. 1980. Risk differential between Medicare beneficiaries enrolled and not enrolled in an HMO. *Health Care Financing Review* 3 (Winter):91–99.

Eggers, P. W., and R. Prihoda. 1982. Pre-enrollment reimbursement patterns of Medicare beneficiaries enrolled in ''at-risk'' HMOs. *Health Care Financing Review* 4(1):55–73.

Ellis, R. P. 1985. The effect of prior-year health expenditures on health coverage plan choice. In R. M. Scheffler and L. F. Rossiter, eds., *Advances in Health Economics and Health Services Research* 6. Greenwich, CT: JAI Press.

Ellwein, L. K., and D. D. Gregg. 1982. *An Introduction to Preferred Provider Organizations* (PPOs). Excelsior, MN: InterStudy.

Ellwood, D. 1986. Medicare risk contracting. *Health Affairs* 5(1):183–89.

Enthoven, A. 1981. *Health Plan*. Reading, PA: Addison-Wesley.

Farley, P. J. and A. C. Monheit. 1985. Selectivity in the demand for health insurance and health care. In R. M. Scheffler and L. F. Rossiter, eds. *Advances in Health Economics and Health Services Research* 6. Greenwich, CT: JAI Press.

Farley, P. J. and G. R. Wilensky. 1983. Options, incentives, and employment-related health insurance. In R. Scheffler and L. Rossiter, eds., *Advances in Health Economics and Health Services Research* 4. Greenwich, CT: JAI Press.

Feldstein, M. 1971. A new approach to national health insurance. *Public Interest* 23 (Spring):93–105.

Fox, P., W. Goldbeck, and J. Spies. 1984. *Health Care Cost Management: Private Sector Initiatives*. Ann Arbor, MI: Health Administration Press.

Francis, W. 1986. Data Watch: HMO customer service. *Health Affairs* 5(1):173–82.

Frank, R. G. 1981. Pricing and location of physician services in mental health. Ph.D. dissertation, Boston University.

Frank, R. G., and W. P. Welch. 1985. The competitive effects of HMOs: A review of the evidence. *Inquiry* 22(2):148–61.

Freeborn, D., and C. Pope. 1982. Health status, utilization, and satisfaction among enrollees in three types of private health insurance plans. *Group Health Journal* 3(1):4–11.

Freund, D. A., and E. Neuschler. 1986. Overview of Medicaid capitation and case-management initiatives. *Health Care Financing Review* 9(Annual Supp.):21–30.

Gabel, J., D. Ermann, T. Rice, and G. de Lissovoy. 1986. The emergence and future of PPOs. *Journal of Health Politics, Policy and Law* 11(2):305–22.

Galiher, C. B., and M. A. Costa. 1975. Consumer acceptance of HMOs. *Public Health Reports* 90(2):106–12.

Ginsburg, P. B., and G. M. Hackbarth. 1986. Alternative delivery systems and Medicare. *Health Affairs* 5(1):6–22.

Gold, W. E. 1981. Predicting HMO disenrollment behavior: Results of a study of demographic and behavioral characteristics of HMO members. In *Finance and Mar-*

keting in the Nation's Group Practice HMOs, proceedings of the 31st Annual Group Health Institute. Washington, DC, June 14–17, pp. 175–81.

Goldberg, L. G., and W. Greenberg. 1980. The competitive response of Blue Cross to the health maintenance organization. *Economic Inquiry* 18(1):55–68.

Greaney, T. L., and J. L. Sindelar. 1987. An assessment of the anticompetitive effects of preferred provider organizations. *Inquiry* 24(4):384–91.

Greenberg, W. 1985. Demand, supply and information in health care and other industries. In J. Meyer, ed., *Incentives vs. Controls in Health Policy: Broadening the Debate*. Washington, DC: American Enterprise Institute.

Havighurst, C. C. 1983. The contributions of antitrust law to a procompetitive health policy. In J. Meyer, ed., *Market Reforms in Health Care*. Washington, DC: American Enterprise Institute.

Hay, J. W., and M. J. Leahy. 1984. Competition among health plans: Some preliminary evidence. *Southern Economic Journal* 50(3):831–46.

Hennelly, V. D., and S. B. Boxerman. 1983. Disenrollment from a prepaid group plan: A multivariate analysis. *Medical Care* 21(12):1154–67.

Hetherington, R., C. E. Hopkins, and M. I. Roemer. 1975. *Health Insurance Plans: Promise and Performance*. New York: Wiley Interscience.

Hewitt Associates. 1984. Significant benefit changes occurred 1979–1983. *Employee Benefit Plan Review* (April):22–23.

Horn, S. D., R. A. Horn, and P. D. Sharkey. 1984. The Severity of Illness Index as a severity adjustment to diagnosis-related groups. *Health Care Financing Review* (Annual Suppl.):33–45.

Hornbrook, M. C. 1984. Examination of the AAPCC methodology in an HMO prospective payment demographic project. *Group Health Journal* 5(1):13–21.

Hornbrook, M. C., and J. E. Berki. 1985. Practice mode and payment method: Effects on use, costs, quality and access. *Medical Care* 23(5):484–511.

InterStudy. 1983. *National HMO Census–1982*. Excelsior, MN: InterStudy.

InterStudy. 1985. *National HMO Census–1984*. Excelsior, MN: InterStudy.

InterStudy. 1986. *National HMO Ccensus*, June update. Excelsior, MN: InterStudy.

Jensen, G., R. Feldman, and B. Dowd. 1984. Corporate benefit policies and health insurance costs. *Journal of Health Economics* 3(3):275–96.

Jette, A. M., and L. G. Branch. 1981. The Framingham disability study II: Physical disability among the aging. *American Journal of Public Health* 71(11):1211–16.

Juba, D., J. R. Lave, and J. Shaddy. 1980. An analysis of the choice of health benefit plans. *Inquiry* 17(1):62–71.

Katz, S., A. B. Ford, R. W. Moskowitz et al. 1963. Studies of illness in the aged: The index of ADL. *Journal of the American Medical Association* 195(12):194.

Kinnear, T., and J. Taylor. 1979. *Marketing Research: An Applied Approach*. New York: McGraw-Hill.

Langwell, K. M., and J. P. Hadley. 1986. Capitation and the Medicare program: History, issues and evidence. *Health Care Financing Review* 8 (Annual Suppl.):9–20.

Lave, J. R. 1984. Competitive bidding and public insurance programs. *Journal of Health Economics* 3(3):195–98.

Lewis, K. 1984. Comparison of use by enrolled and recently disenrolled populations in health maintenance organizations. *Health Services Research* 19(1):1–22.

Linn, B. S., and M. W. Linn. 1980. Objective and self-assessed health in the old and very old. *Social Science and Medicine* 14A(4):311–15.

Lubitz, J., J. Beebe, and G. Riley. 1985. Improving the Medicare HMO payment formula to deal with biased selection. In R. M. Scheffler and L. F. Rossiter, eds., *Advances in Health Economics and Health Services Research* 6. Greenwich, CT: JAI Press.

Luft, H. S. 1981. *Health Maintenance Organizations: Dimensions of Performance*. New York: John Wiley & Sons.

Luft, H. S. 1985. From policy question to empirical answers. *Journal of Health Economics* 4(4):381–86.

Luft, H. S., J. B. Trauner, and S. C. Maerki, 1985. Adverse selection in a large multiple-option health benefits program: A case study of the California Public Employees' Retirement System. In R. M. Scheffler and L. F. Rossiter, eds., *Advances in Health Economics and Health Services Research* 6. Greenwich, CT: JAI Press.

Luft, H. S., S. C. Maerki, and J. B. Trauner. 1986. The competitive effects of health maintenance organizations: Another look at the evidence from Hawaii, Rochester, and Minneapolis/St. Paul. *Journal of Health Politics, Policy and Law* 10(4):625–58.

McCall, N., and H. S. Wai. 1981. An analysis of the use of Medicare services by the continuously enrolled aged. Stanford Research Institute.

McClure, W. 1981. Structure and incentive problems in economic regulation of medical care. *Milbank Memorial Fund Quarterly* 59(2):107–44.

McClure, W. 1984. On the research status of risk-adjusted capitation rates. *Inquiry* 21(3):205–13.

McGuire, T. B. 1981. Price and membership in a prepaid group medical practice. *Medical Care* 19(2):172–83.

Manning, W. G., A. Leibowitz, G. A. Goldberg, W. H. Rogers, and J. P. Newhouse. 1984. A controlled trial of the effect of a prepaid group practice on use of services. *New England Journal of Medicine* 310(23):1505–10.

Mansfield, E. 1982. *Microeconomics: Theory and Applications, 4th Edition*. New York: W. W. Norton and Company.

Mechanic, D., N. Weiss, and P. D. Cleary. 1983. The growth of HMOs: Issues of enrollment and disenrollment. *Medical Care* 21(3):338–47.

Merrill, J., C. Jackson, and J. Reuter. 1985. Factors that affect the HMO enrollment decision: A tale of two cities. *Inquiry* 22(4):388–95.

Merrill, J., and C. McLaughlin. 1986. Competition versus regulation: Some empirical evidence. *Journal of Health Politics, Policy and Law* 10(4):613–23.

Morrisey, M. A., F. A. Sloan, and S. A. Mitchell. 1983. State rate setting: An analysis of some unresolved issues. *Health Affairs* 2(2):36–47.

Mott, P. D. 1986. Hospital utilization by health maintenance organizations: Separating apples from oranges. *Medical Care* 24(5):398–406.

Moustafa, A., C. E. Hopkins, and B. Klein. 1971. Determinants of choice and change of health insurance plan. *Medical Care* 9(1):32–41.

Pauly, M. 1971. *An Analysis of National Insurance Proposals*. Washington, DC: American Enterprise Institute.

Pauly, M. 1981. Paying the piper and calling the tune: The relationship between public financing and public regulation of health care. In M. Olson, ed., *A New Approach to the Economics of Health Care*. Washington, DC: American Enterprise Institute.

Price, J., and J. Mays. 1985. Biased selection in the Federal Employees Health Benefits Program. *Inquiry* 22(1):67–77.

Price, J. R., J. W. Mays, and G. R. Trapnell. 1983. Stability in the Federal Employees Health Benefits Program. *Journal of Health Economics* 2(3):207–33.

Prottas, J. M., and E. Handler. 1987. The complexities of managed care: Operating a voluntary system. *Journal of Health Politics, Policy and Law* 12(2):253–69.

Robinson, J., and H. Luft. 1985. The impact of hospital market structure on patient volume, average length of stay, and the cost of care. *Journal of Health Economics* 4(4):333–56.

Roghmann, K. J., A. A. Sorenson, and S. M. Wells. 1980. Hospitalizations in three competing HMOs during their first two years. *Group Health Journal* 1(1):26–33.

Roos, N. P., and E. Shapiro. 1981. The Manitoba longitudinal study on aging: Preliminary findings on health care utilization by the elderly. *Medical Care* 19(6):644–57.

Sapolsky, H. M., D. Altman, R. Greene, and J. D. Moore. 1980. Corporate attitudes towards health care costs. *Milbank Memorial Fund Quarterly: Health and Society* 59(4):561–85.

Sauter, V. L., and E. F. X. Hughes. 1983. Surgical utilization statistics: Some methodological considerations. *Medical Care* 21(3):370–77.

Schlesinger, E. S. 1985. Renaissance of the HMO. Boston Consulting Group.

Schneider, D. P., F. Holden, and B. E. Fries. 1985. DRG and RUG Interactions in Resource Allocation. Presented to AHPA/VA Conference, December 1985.

Scitovsky, A., N. McCall, and L. Benham. 1978. Factors affecting the choice between two prepaid plans. *Medical Care* 16(8):660–81.

Seidman, L. 1977. Medical loans and major risk national health insurance. *Health Services Research* 12(2):123–28.

Sorenson, A. A., and R. P. Wersinger. 1981. Factors influencing disenrollment from an HMO. *Medical Care* 19(7):766–73.

Stiefel, M. C., D. A. Gardelius, and D. E. Hayami. 1984. Selection bias: A Comparison of inpatient utilization, demographics, and premiums for HMO "leavers," "stayers," and "joiners." Kaiser Foundation Health Plan of Oregon, manuscript.

Taylor, H., and M. Kagay. 1986. The HMO report card: A closer look. *Health Affairs* 5(1):81–89.

Tessler, R. C., and D. Mechanic. 1975a. Consumer satisfaction with prepaid group practice: A comparative study. *Journal of Health and Social Behavior* 16(1):95–113.

Tessler, R., and D. Mechanic. 1975b. Factors affecting the choice between prepaid group practice and alternative insurance programs. *Milbank Memorial Fund Quarterly* 54(1):149–72.

Thomas, J. W., and R. Lichtenstein. 1986a. Functional health measure for adjusting health maintenance organization capitation rates. *Health Care Financing Review* 7(3):85–95.

Thomas, J. W., and R. Lichtenstein. 1986b. Including health status in Medicare's adjusted average per capita cost capitation formula. *Medical Care* 24(3):259–75.

Thomas, J. W., R. Lichtenstein, L. Wyszewianski, and S. E. Berki. 1983. Increasing Medicare enrollment in HMOs: The need for capitation rates adjusted for health status. *Inquiry* 20(3):227–39.

Traska, M. R. 1987a. Washington Medicaid study challenges HMO care myths. *Hospitals* 61(15):42–44.

Traska, M. R. 1987b. Rate hike: An incomplete fix for Medicare HMOs. *Hospitals* 61(20):44–48.

Vladek, B. 1981. The market vs. regulation: The case for regulation. *Milbank Memorial Fund Quarterly* 59(2):209–23.

Welch, W. P. 1984. HMO enrollment: A study of market forces and regulations. *Journal of Health Politics, Policy and Law* 8(4):743–58.

Welch, W. P. 1985a. Health care utilization in HMOs: Results from two national samples. *Journal of Health Economics* 4(4):293–308.

Welch, W. P. 1985b. Medicare capitation payments to HMOs in light of regression toward the mean in health care costs. In R. M. Scheffler and L. F. Rossiter, eds., *Advances in Health Economics and Health Services Research*, 6. Greenwich, CT: JAI Press.

Welch, W. P. 1985c. Regression toward the mean in medical care costs: Implications for biased selection in health maintenance organizations. *Medical Care* 23(11):1234–41.

Welch, W. P., and R. G. Frank. 1986. The predictors of HMO enrollee populations: Results from a national sample. *Inquiry* 23(1):16–22.

Welch, W. P., and R. G. Frank, and P. Diehr. 1984. Health care costs in health maintenance organizations: Correcting for self-selection. In R. M. Scheffler and L. F. Rossiter, eds., *Advances in Health Economics and Health Services Research* 5. Greenwich, CT: JAI Press.

Wennberg, J. E. 1984. Dealing with medical practice variations: A proposal for action. *Health Affairs* 3(2):6–32.

Wersinger, R. P., and A. A. Sorenson. 1982. Demographic characteristics and prior utilization experience of HMO disenrollees compared with total membership. *Medical Care* 20(12):1188–96.

Wilensky, G. R., and L. R. Rossiter. 1986. Patient self-selection in HMOs. *Health Affairs* 5(1):66–80.

Wintringham, K. 1982. Impact of step-rating and price sensitivity on disenrollment and risk selection. *Group Health Journal* (Summer):15–20.

Wolinsky, F. D. 1980. The performance of HMOs: An analytic review. *Milbank Memorial Fund Quarterly* 58(4):537–87.

Wollstadt, L. J., S. Shapiro, and T. W. Bice. 1978. Disenrollment from a prepaid group practice: An actuarial and demographic description. *Inquiry* 15(2):142–50.

12

REGULATORY APPROACHES TO
HEALTH CARE COST CONTROL

Public and private sector initiatives to contain health care costs are as diverse
as the theories of health care cost inflation that were discussed in Chapter 1.
Governmental authorities have attempted to contain health care expenditures by
(1) regulating revenues, (2) limiting utilization, (3) restricting capital expansion,
and (4) fostering competition and creating market-like incentives. Approaches
that regulate revenues include: prospective payment (PP); the Economic Stabilization Program (ESP); the Carter Administration's Hospital Cost Containment
Act; and the hospital industry's Voluntary Effort (VE). Professional standards
and review organizations and peer review organizations are approaches designed
to control use. Examples of capital controls include the federal review of capital
projects, authorized by Section 1122 of Public Law 92–603 and state certificate
of need programs. The discussion in this chapter will be limited to the first three
federal initiatives and, where relevant, their state and private sector counterparts.

REVENUE REGULATION

The passage of Public Law 98–21 and the implementation of the Medicare pricing system ushered in an era in which prospective payment (PP) has emerged as
the dominant regulatory mechanism for controlling the costs of hospital care. In
addition to the federal program, as of February 1987, prospective payment systems in which the patient and related condition are used to determine rates of compensation for Blue Cross or Medicaid patients were operated in 15 states. As a
consequence, the increased dependence on prospective payment to control the
costs of inpatient care is perhaps the most important change in the financial environment of the American hospital since the introduction of Medicare.

As our review will indicate, available evidence suggests that prospective payment constrained the rate of increase in the costs per day, per case and per

362 COST-CONTAINMENT STRATEGIES

capita. For example, Sloan (1983) who used a national data base for the period 1963–1980 in a multivariate analysis of mature state programs reported that prospective payment restrained the rate of increase in the cost per admission and the cost per day by 4.8 percent and 6.8 percent, respectively.

Although prospective payment is intuitively appealing, several analysts have suggested that rate regulation and the Medicare pricing system in particular induce hospitals to (1) transfer costs from regulated to unregulated patients, thereby reducing the fiscal rigors of prospective payment and the need to control costs; (2) alter admission policies, thereby reducing access to inpatient services; (3) alter the mix of inpatient services consumed after admission, thereby reducing the quality of care; and (4) adopt other similar strategies that result in potentially undesirable outcomes (Lave 1984; Broyles and Rosko 1985); hence, a review of previous findings concerning the desirable and unintended consequences of prospective payment is of importance when viewed from a policy perspective.

In an attempt to limit this chapter to a manageable length, our analysis will focus on recent multivariate studies. Omitted from our review are early studies of individual state rate-setting programs, which were evaluated under the auspices of the Social Security Administration. These studies have been reviewed by Salkever (1979) and Rosko (1982), who reported numerous design problems that severely compromised the validity of the results. Further, except where other data are unavailable, we will not review results from univariate studies, which, by the nature of their research design, confounded the effects of exogenous factors with those attributed to prospective payment programs.

The purpose of this section is twofold. The first is to review previous evaluations of prospective payment in terms of predictions derived from a theoretical model of hospital responses to rate regulation. A congruence between expectations and empirical observations not only enhances the credibility of previous results but also addresses criticisms of recent studies that challenge the methods and findings reported in even the most respected evaluations of prospective payment. For example, Getzen (1985) argues that changes in the rate of increase in costs are attributable more to exogenous factors, such as general economic conditions, than to the fiscal restraints imposed by rate regulation. Dranove and Cone (1985) report evidence that suggests that some of the savings attributed to prospective payment is actually due to a research design problem, termed *regression-to-the-mean* (Cambell and Stanley 1963).

The second objective is to assess prospective payment as a mechanism that is likely to achieve the sometimes conflicting goals of controlling costs and ensuring an equitable distribution of hospital services. Although rate regulation might control the cost per day, the cost per case, or the cost per person, the fiscal incentives created by prospective payment may induce hospitals to implement admission and discharge policies that reduce access to inpatient care and exacerbate inequities in the distribution of service.

Analysts have employed two approaches to identify the possible consequences of prospective payment. The first involves an empirical evaluation of the influence exerted by prospective payment on multiple dimensions of hospital performance. The second employs a set of normative criteria as the basis for assessing the effects of one or more payment mechanisms. In a qualitative evaluation of payment strategies for hospitals, Cleverly (1979) reported that a consensus of the literature (Pauly 1970; Dowling 1974; Lave, Lave, and Silverman 1973) suggests that a payment system should promote efficiency, maintain provider viability, prevent differential pricing or payer cross-subsidization, and require minimal administrative cost. In their qualitative assessment of the Medicare pricing mechanism, Broyles and Rosko (1985) added a fifth criterion and argued that payment systems should prevent behavior that compromises the health status of beneficiaries.

PROSPECTIVE PAYMENT: AN OVERVIEW

Prospective payment is a generic term that refers to financing mechanisms in which rates or levels of compensation are determined prior to a future period and the hospital receives the predetermined amount irrespective of the costs that are incurred. At one extreme is a system in which the approved budget is used to determine the hospital's annual compensation, an amount that is received in periodic installments that are intended to finance operational activity on a current basis. An alternate approach to prospective payment involves the regulation of the rates of payment for identifiable units of output. In particular, the patient and related diagnosis, the patient day, and specific services such as laboratory and surgical care have been used to regulate hospital payments.

In addition to the unit of compensation, prospective payment systems have been characterized in terms of differences in the scope of regulatory authority, utilization controls and sanctions, the process of reviewing payment rates and the factors used to adjust compensation rates. All of these dimensions can influence the effectiveness of prospective payment to control costs.

We will examine the impact of prospective payment on various dimensions of hospital performance in two phases. The first, which is devoted to a review of results derived from studies that relied on the empirical approach, focuses on programs that regulate charges or per diem rates. In addition, this phase also considers empirical studies of payment mechanisms that use case-mix measures to determine prospective prices. Following this discussion is an examination of recent analyses that evaluated prospective payment in terms of one or more normative criteria. The chapter concludes with an examination of the policy implications of previous assessments of prospective payment.

THE REGULATION OF CHARGES AND PER DIEM RATES

Although prospective payment might be characterized in terms of several dimensions, this review is organized in terms of theoretical expectations and empirical findings concerning systems that regulate different units of payment.

As this section will suggest, most of the evidence concerning the effects of prospective payment was derived from evaluations of programs that regulated charges or per diem rates. Further, employing the contemporary criteria for rate regulation suggested by Eby and Cohodes (1985), the emphasis of this section is on previous assessments of state mandated programs for which compliance is compulsory. Voluntary prospective reimbursement mechanisms are omitted from our analysis because they have failed to control costs in most cases (Rosko 1982).

Implemented in 1970, New York operated the only mandatory PP system until seven other states began to regulate hospital rates in either 1975 or 1976 (Dowling 1974; Biles, Schramm, and Atkinson 1980). Appearing in Table 12.1 are the major features that characterize the eight prospective payment systems that have been the focus of empirical research. As suggested by this table, several features were common to these programs. For example, all of the programs had an appeal mechanism; seven of the eight state programs allowed retroactive adjustments to the prospective rate, usually on the basis of unanticipated changes in the prices of inputs or the volume of patients, and reviewed rates at least annually. There were also important differences among the programs. In six states prospective payment applied only to a limited number of payers (usually Blue Cross and Medicaid), while in two states, New Jersey and Maryland, all payers were regulated. In half of the PP states, different units of payment were used for different payers: charges were used as a unit of payment in seven programs, and four programs regulated per diem rates.

Theoretical Expectations

For purposes of exposition, the assessment of findings concerning hospital responses to the regulation of charges or per diem rates is based on expectations derived from the utility-maximizing model initially proposed by Feldstein (1971) and subsequently modified by Cromwell et al. (1976), Sloan and Steinwald (1980) and Rosko (1982, 1984b). Based on normative assumptions concerning the configuration of the product transformation curve and the indifference map depicting the preferences of the hospital, these models (which were reviewed in Chapter 4) suggest several testable hypotheses concerning the response of hospitals to prospective payment systems that regulate per diem rates. Among the most important of these are the following: holding other factors constant, these models posit that the regulation of per diem rates induces the hospital to control or reduce the cost per day and ensure that expenditures per unit are less than or equal to the predetermined rate of compensation. In addition, the regulation of per diem rates also induces the hospital to increase the number of patient days provided during a given period, an outcome that generates revenue directly, increases the number of units to which fixed costs are assigned and thereby reduces average cost per day. Morrisey, Sloan, and Mitchell (1983) derived similar expectations from a physician-exchange model.

In response to revenue restraints imposed by rate regulation, hospitals might adopt several strategies designed to control or reduce the cost per day. For example, an improvement in the efficiency of resource use lowers the amount of factor inputs consumed and, hence, the costs per day. Accordingly, theoretical considerations suggest that hospitals might respond to the imposition of rate regulation by reducing not only the number of full-time equivalents (FTEs) per day but also the per diem cost of consumable supplies. Expenses per day also might be lowered by reducing the prices of factor inputs employed in operational activity. For example, per diem costs might be constrained by resisting demands for higher wages, salaries, and fringe benefits or securing supplies from vendors who offer more favorable terms and lower prices. Also designed to reduce daily costs are decisions to adopt technologies or build facilities that yield cost savings. Further, recognizing that an increase in the intensity of service use tends to increase the cost per day, payment systems that regulate per diem rates induce hospitals to retard the growth in the expansion of the hospital's capacity to provide new components of care. Finally, to the extent that expenditures are sensitive to changes in volume, daily costs might be reduced by lowering the intensity with which ancillary and general support services are provided.

As suggested previously, rate regulation also induces the hospital to increase the number of patient days. As is well recognized, quantity might be expanded by increasing the length of stay and the rate of admissions. The length of stay might be prolonged by extending the patient's period of convalescence in the hospital. Patient days during this period are likely to require a less-than-average amount of resources, resulting in a cost per day that is less than the prospective per diem rate; hence, profits earned during these days might be used to subsidize losses that occur during the earlier, more service-intensive period of the patient's hospital stay. If excess capacity exists after increasing the length of stay, the hospital may attempt to increase the rate of admissions in order to spread fixed costs over more patient days. Since the per diem rates established by regulatory authorities do not reflect costs associated with case-mix differences, hospitals are also induced to admit patients who present conditions that are less complex, and hence less costly to treat.

Systems that regulate the price of each identifiable service, to include daily service charges, are also expected to motivate hospitals to adopt strategies designed to control unit costs and expand volume. Similar to the previous discussion, the regulation of charges induces the hospital to control the cost per unit of each service by improving productivity or acquiring resources at lower prices. In addition, the models proposed previously indicate that the regulation of charges induces the hospital to increase the volume of ancillary and stay-specific services, an outcome that not only generates revenue but also lowers the fixed and average costs per unit of each component of care. As a result, the imposition of systems that regulate charges induces hospitals to expand the volume of stay-specific and ancillary care by increasing the number of admissions, the length of stay, and the intensity of ancillary service use. Table 12.2 provides a summary of expected

Table 12.1
State-Legislated Hospital Cost-Containment Programs

State (year implemented)	Responsible Agency	Payers Covered	Revenue Control Method	Unit of Payment	Frequency of Review	Adjustments	Appeals
Connecticut (1976)	Commission on Hospitals and Health Care	Charge-based	Total revenue	Charges	Annually	Retroactive for volume, unforeseen and significant change in expense	Public hearing before commission
Maryland (1975)	Health Services Cost Review Commission	All payers	Total revenue; departmental revenue, guaranteed revenue per case, or maximum revenue per case	Rate-based charges	As necessary	Inflation, volume, cost beyond control	Public hearing before commission
Massachusetts (1976)	Massachusetts Rate Setting Commission	Charge-based	Total revenue with cost limit	Charges	Annually	Inflation, volume, cost beyond control	Division of Hearing Officers
		Blue Cross	Cost-based	Routine per diem, ancillary charges	Annually	Excess costs may be denied	Courts
		Medicaid	Cost-based with limits	Per diem	Annually	Uncontrollable costs associated with change in government regulations	Division of Hearing Officers
New Jersey (1975)	State Department of Health	Medicaid and Blue Cross	Cost-based	Per diem	Annually	Retroactive for volume, economic factor, pass-through items	Formal appeal before independent hearing officer

366

State (year)	Administering agency	Payers	Rate basis	Payment unit	Frequency	Adjustment	Appeal
New Jersey DRG (1980-1982)	State Department of Health	All payers	Cost-based	Rate per case and controlled charges for outliers	Annually	Regional factor price differentials, retroactive for cost of capital, cost of medical education	Only for errors in rate calculations
New York (1970)	State Department of Health	Medicaid and Blue Cross; Charge-based	Cost-based; Charge increase	Per diem; Charges	Annually; As necessary	Retroactive for actual economic factor and volume; Actual economic factor	Formal appeal before state hearing officer; Appeals board
Rhode Island (1975)	State Budget Office; Blue Cross of Rhode Island	Medicaid and Blue Cross	Total expenses/revenue	Percent of charges	Annually	Retroactive for volume	Binding arbitration before independent mediation
Washington (1975)	Washington State Hospital Commission	Charge-based, including Blue Cross	Total revenue; rates per unit of service by revenue center	Charges	Annually	Volume	Formal hearing before commission or independent hearing officer
Wisconsin (1976)	State Department of Health; Rate Review Committee	Charge-based, including Blue Cross; Medicaid	Total revenue	Charges; Per diem	Prior to any rate change, one a year at most	None	Hearing before independent appeals board

Table 12.2
Expected Changes in Hospital Performance under Alternative Payment Units

	Payment Unit			
	Day	Specific Services	Case (DRG)	Retrospective Costs
Cases treated	+	+	+	+
Average length of stay	+	+	-	+
Efficiency	+	+	+	-
Input prices	-	-	-	+
Intensity of services	-	+	-	+
Complexity of case-mix	-	+	-	+
Growth of new services	-	+	-	+

Key: + indicates increase or decrease less quickly
　　 - indicates decrease or increase less quickly

Source: W. Dowling. 1974. Prospective reimbursement of hospitals. Inquiry 11(3): 166.

responses of hospitals to PP systems relying on the patient day and specific services as the unit of payment. Further, in order to provide a better perspective, this table also includes a summary of expected responses to case-based PP, and traditional retrospective cost-based reimbursement mechanisms.

Although reductions in the cost per unit or increases in the volume of service enable the hospital to avoid deficits, the theoretical model indicates that these outcomes reduce the utility or satisfaction derived by hospital decision makers. Accordingly, if the payment mechanism fails to regulate all sources of patient revenue, the hospital is induced to avoid potential reductions in utility or satisfaction by transferring costs or losses from regulated to unregulated patients or services, a practice that also reduces the fiscal rigors of rate regulation and pressures to control spending.

EMPIRICAL EVIDENCE

Methods

Presented in Table 12.3 is a summary of the research methods and the results derived in recent assessments of prospective payment. As this table indicates, these studies used data pertaining to periods before and after the introduction of prospective payment and compared the costs of hospitals that were subject to rate regulation with the expenditures of institutions included in a control group. Further, the regression models usually included a set of control variables to measure differences in market conditions that influence hospital performance. The regulatory variables, which indicated the presence or absence of prospective payment and other regulatory programs, were defined in categorical terms. Alternate specifications (see Table 12.3) included (1) the percentage of the population enrolled in insurance plans that were subject to rate regulation; (2) percentage of hospital expenditures subject to a new (i.e., less than three-years-old) or mature program; (3) the number of years that a state had operated a prospective payment program; and (4) the effects of a single program in a given year. In the simplest specification, results depict the effects of PP averaged over time and across programs. Consequently, findings may be biased by an ''outlier'' program, which generated results that were significantly different from the group average.

Although the more complex specifications attempted to account for some program differences, none of the national studies estimated individual program effects for separate years. Because of statistical estimation problems (e.g., multicollinearity), his level of specificity is difficult if not impossible to accomplish. Failure to measure differences among PP mechanisms is a serious deficiency since the impact of various rate-setting programs is likely to vary according to their underlying characteristics (Coelen and Sullivan 1981; Cook, Shortell, Conrad, and Morrisey 1983; Morrisey, Conrad, Shortell, and Cook 1984). For example, mature programs constrained costs more successfully than new rate-

Table 12.3
Summary of Recent Multivariate Evaluations of Prospective Payment Programs

Study	Performance Measures	Rate Review Variables	Level of Aggregation	Findings
Coelen and Sullivan, 1981	Δ(expenses/adjusted patient-day) Δ(expenses/adjusted admission) Δ(expenses per capita) Log (expenses/adjusted patient-day) Log (expenses/adjusted admission) Log (expenses per capita)	Separate binary variable for each version of prospective payment in 15 states, of which 8 featured mandatory compliance	Hospitals (expenditures per day and per admission) and counties (expenditures per capita); annual data, 1969–1978	Expenses per adjusted patient-day were contained by nine programs; savings ranged from 1.2 percent to 10.5 percent. Expenses per adjusted admission were contained by seven programs, savings ranged from 1.9 percent to 8.7 percent. Expenses per capita were contained in four programs, savings ranged from 3.1 percent to 7.6 percent. Estimated savings were consistently higher in log equations than in percentage change equations.
Kidder and Sullivan, 1982	Payroll per adjusted patient-day; FTE staff per adjusted patient-day; payroll per FTE staff	Same as Coelen and Sullivan	Hospitals, 1970–1977	Payroll per adjusted patient-day was contained by 10 programs, savings ranged from 3 percent to 11 percent. PP contains FTE staff per adjusted patient-day in six states, ranging from 3.0 percent to 10.0 percent. PP contained payroll per FTE staff in six states, ranging from 2.0 percent to 5.0 percent.

Table 12.3 (continued)

Cromwell and Kanak, 1982	Percentage change in the total number of services classified as: quality-enhancing, complexity-expanding, community-oriented, supportive, competitive, diffusing, peaked, administrative shared services, and clinical shared services	Same as Coelen and Sullivan	Hospitals, 1969–1978	Ambiguous results were obtained. The rate-setting variables were significant ($p < 0.05$) in most equations. No program exerted significant effects in a majority of the equations.
Worthington and Piro, 1982	Admissions per bed; Log (length of stay) Occupancy rate	Same as Coelen and Sullivan	Hospitals, 1969–1978	Increases in admissions per bed, ranging from 2.36 to 5.84, were associated with three rate-setting programs. Increases in length of stay, ranging from 1.0 percent to 8.0 percent, were associated with five programs. A voluntary program in Nebraska caused a 7 percent increase in length of stay. Occupancy rate increases, ranging from 3.0 percent to 7.0 percent, were associated with five programs.
Sloan and Steinwald, 1980	Log (expenses/admission) Log (expenses/adjusted patient-day) Log (labor expenses/adjusted patient-day) Log (labor expenses/admission) Log (RNs/bed) Log (LPNs/bed)	Log (percent population) subject to formula prospective payment (Colorado, Massachusetts, New York)	Hospitals, cluster sample of hospitals located in 33 states and the District of Columbia; annual data, 1969–1975	Ambiguous results. Ordinary-least-squares (OLS) analysis found that formula programs reduced expenses per adjusted patient-day (2.6 percent) and per admission (1.4 percent), and reduced labor expenses per adjusted

371

Table 12.3 (continued)

Study	Performance Measures	Rate Review Variables	Level of Aggregation	Findings
Sloan and Steinwald, 1980 (continued)	Log (other employees/bed) Log (total beds) Log (assets/bed) Log (current nonlabor expenses/bed)	Log (percent population) subject to budget prospective payment (Arizona, Connecticut, Indiana, Kentucky, Maryland, New Jersey, North Carolina, Rhode Island, Wisconsin)		patient-day (1.7 percent) and per admission (0.6 percent). Time series analysis (TSA) found increased costs. Similar results were found for budget programs. Besides expense, significant effects were found only for LPNs per bed, which increased by 19 percent under formula programs.
Sloan, 1981	Cost per admission Cost per adjusted admission Cost per patient-day Cost per adjusted patient-day Total revenue/total cost	Separate variables for the fraction of hospital costs covered by new (in existence two years or less) and old PP programs	State; annual data, 1963-1978	Young PP programs did not have an impact upon hospital costs. Old PP programs reduced cost per day by 6.7 percent and cost per admission by 3.8 percent. Similar results were found for the profitability measure (total revenue/total costs).
Sloan, 1983	Expense/admission Expense/adjusted admission Expense/patient-day Length of stay Total revenue/total expense Δ (expense/adjusted admission) Δ (expense/adjusted patient-day) Δ (adjusted admissions) Δ (adjusted patient-day) Δ (outpatient visits) Δ (length of stay) Δ (total revenue/total expense)	Percentage of hospital revenues regulated by each type of program (six variables): Mandatory regulatory, young Mandatory regulatory, old Voluntary regulatory, young Voluntary regulatory, old Mandatory advisory, young Mandatory advisory, old (Young = first two years of program)	State; annual data, 1963-1978	Mature mandatory PP programs contained cost per admission (4.8 percent) and cost per day (6.8 percent). Neither of these programs nor any of the other programs evaluated, had an impact on any of the other performance measures.

372

Table 12.3 (continued)

Study	Variables	Program measure	Data	Findings
Ashby, 1984	% Δ(total costs per capita) % Δ(average length of stay) % Δ(admissions per capita) % Δ(plant assets) % Δ(beds per capita)	Binary variables for voluntary rate-setting and mandatory PP programs	State; annual data, 1971–1977	The voluntary and mandatory rate-setting variables did not have a significant coefficient ($p<0.10$) in any of the equations. (Note: using Sloan's criteria, most of the rate-setting study periods were new.)
Cromwell and Hewes, 1985	Medicare expenditure and volume statistics including: Log (total reimbursements/beneficiaries) Log (hospital reimbursements) Log (non-hospital reimbursements) Log (hospital inpatient days) Log (physician services) Log (supplier services) Log (home health visits) Log (hospital outpatient visits) Log (skilled nursing facility patient days)	Separate binary variables for each version of prospective payment in 11 states, of which 8 featured mandatory compliance	County, annual data, 1975–1984	Analysis of cumulative effects of state PP programs on Medicare expenditures found reductions in most states ranging from 6.3 percent to 19.6 percent. With the exception of outpatient visits states' PP programs were associated with a decline in the volume of services provided to Medicare patients.
Joskow, 1981	% Δ (total hospital expenses) Log (total hospital expenses) Log (FTE personnel per bed) Log (adjusted inpatient days) Log (average wage of FTE personnel)	Binary variable for mandatory PP programs, and number of years state had a PP program in effect	State; annual data, 1979	PP constrained growth of total hospital expenditures by 2.0 percent per year. No effect was found in the other equations.
Melnick, Wheeler, and Feldstein, 1981	% Δ (total hospital expenses) % Δ (total hospital expenses per admission) % Δ (admissions) % Δ (total hospital expenses per patient-day) % Δ (average length of stay)	Binary variable for mandatory PP programs	State; annual data, 1975–1979	The existence of PP programs was associated with significant reductions in total expenses (1.7 percent), expenses per admission (1.3 percent), expense per patient-day (2.3 percent), and length of stay (0.9 percent).

Table 12.3 (continued)

Study	Performance Measures	Rate Review Variables	Level of Aggregation	Findings
Merrill and McLaughlin, 1986	Level and percent change in: Total hospital expenses per capita (Hospital expenses/patient days) (Hospital expenses/admissions) (Admissions/1,000 population) Average length of stay.	Binary variable (=1) for SMSAs with a mandatory rate review program implemented for 3 or more years.	25 largest SMSAs, annual data, 1971–1981.	Mature PP programs were associated with annual reductions in cost per day (1.2 percent), cost per admission (1.4 percent) and average length of stay (0.1 percent). Insignificant results were found for the other performance measures.
Morrisey, Sloan, and Mitchell, 1983	Log (real expense/population) Log (real revenue/population) Log (real expense/adjusted admission) Log (real expense/adjusted patient-days) Log (total Medicare expense/Part A population) Log (Medicare Part A expense/Part A population) Log (Medicare Part B expense/Part A population)	Binary variables: First two years of program in Massachusetts, Maryland, New Jersey, New York, Washington, Wisconsin Mature New Jersey Mature New York (1972–1975) Refined New York (1976–1981) Mature Massachusetts Mature Maryland Mature Washington Mature Massachusetts or Maryland or Washington Mature Massachusetts or Maryland or New Jersey or New York or Washington	SMSA (34 geographic units were derived from 27 SMSAs by dividing multistate SMSAs into two or more groups); annual data, 1968–1981	State rate-setting had no effect during first two years after implementation. Mature PP programs as a whole reduced expenses per adjusted patient-day (1.6 percent), per adjusted admission (1.7 percent), and per capita (2.0 percent). Insignificant results were found for some states, and significant savings were as high as 3.4 percent per adjusted patient-day, 4.9 percent per adjusted admission, and 5.6 percent per capita.
Romeo, Wagner, and Lee, 1984	Two measures (availability of technology and delay in adoption) were used for each of the following technologies: electronic fetal monitoring volumetric infusion pumps automated factual susceptibility testing centralized energy management systems	Variables for the proportion of patient-days covered by the PP programs in New York, Maryland, and Indiana	Hospitals (in six states), 1980	Significant estimates were found only for the equations for availability of technology. The New York program had a consistent negative effect on the adoption of three cost-raising technologies and a positive effect on one of two cost-reducing technologies. No effect was found in Maryland. Inconsistent results were found in Indiana.

Table 12.3 (continued)

Rosko, 1984a	Cost per admission Cost per patient-day	Binary variables for each year the New Jersey rate-setting program was in effect	Hospitals (in New Jersey and Pennsylvania); annual data, 1971-1978	No effects during first two years of rate-setting. The New Jersey PP program contained annual increases in cost per patient-day (2.7 percent) and cost per admission (2.4 percent).
Rosko, 1984b	Cost per admission FTE personnel per 1,000 patient-days	Binary variable for years in which New Jersey regulated rates.	Hospitals (in New Jersey and Pennsylvania); annual data, 1971-1978	The New Jersey program resulted in savings for cost per admission amounting to $61.48 in inner-city hospitals and $25.19 in hospitals located in other areas. Reductions in personnel per 1,000 patient-days (0.098) were found only in inner-city hospitals.
Rosko and Broyles, 1986	Cost/admission Cost/patient-day Admissions Length of stay	Binary variable for all-payer DRG system	Hospitals (in New Jersey); annual data, 1979-1982	Relative to a two-payer, per diem PP program, the all-payer DRG system caused reductions in cost per admission ($71.16) and length of stay (0.28 days), and an increase in admissions per hospital (1,109.7).
Rosko and Broyles, 1987	Log (cost/admission) Log (cost/patient-day) Log (admissions) Log (length of stay)	Binary variable for all-payer DRG system and two-payer per diem system	Hospitals (in New Jersey and Eastern Pennsylvania); annual data 1975-1982	Relative to hospitals in Eastern Pennsylvania, which were reimbursed retrospectively on a cost basis, the all-payer DRG system caused average annual reductions in cost per admission (4.7 percent), cost per day (3.3 percent), length of stay (2.2 percent), and an increase in admissions per hospital (3.9 percent). Similarly, the two-payer per diem system was associated with average annual reductions in cost per admission (3.2 percent), cost per day (3.0 percent) and an increase in admissions per hospital (2.9 percent). No impact on length of stay was detected.

Table 12.3 (continued)

Study	Performance Measures	Rate Review Variables	Level of Aggregation	Findings
Salkever, Steinwachs, and Rupp, 1986	Log (total inpatient cost) Log (routine cost) Log (ancillary cost) Log (inpatient cost/admission)	Number of months hospital was subject to case-based PP, binary variable for case-based PP, number of months of capped PP's rate was capped, binary variable for capped PP	Hospitals, annual data, 1977–1981	Weak and generally insignificant results were found for the case-based payment program. Significant and negative coefficients were estimated for the more rigorous revenue cap program in which only a few hospitals participated.
Salkever and Steinwachs, 1986	Log (admissions) Log (length of stay) Log (case-mix index)	Same as Salkever et al., 1986	Same as Salkever et al., 1986	Weak and generally insignificant results were found for the case-based payment program. Significant coefficients were estimated for the more rigorous revenue cap program in which only a few hospitals participated. Per case payment was associated with declines in length of stay and the case-mix index and with increases in admissions.
Cromwell, 1987	Δ (net total fixed assets) Δ (buildings and fixed equipment) Δ (gross movable equipment) Δ (beds per hospital) Δ (net total fixed assets/bed) Beds per 1,000 population in county	Number of years a state had a PP program in effect	Hospitals (with exception of beds per 1,000 population in county) 1970–1979	Of 48 coefficients estimated for 8 PP systems, only 6 were negative and significant ($p<.10$). Bed growth per capita was retarded by as much as 7.4%

setting programs (Coelen and Sullivan 1981; Sloan 1981; 1983; Morrisey, Sloan and Mitchell 1983; Rosko 1984a). In addition, rate-setting programs have not been uniformly successful in controlling hospital costs (Coelen and Sullivan 1981; Morrisey, Sloan, and Mitchell 1983; Rosko and Broyles 1986, 1987; Salkever, Steinwachs, and Rupp 1986). The last result suggests that more attention should be devoted to the relationship between program structure and outcomes.

Effects on Cost

Although contradictory results have been reported, the weight of the evidence summarized in Table 12.3 is consistent with and supports the set of expectations concerning the responses of hospitals to rate regulation. Most of these studies concluded that prospective payment has constrained hospital costs. More specifically, rate regulation was found to restrain the rates of increase in the cost per admission by 1.4 to 8.7 percent, in the cost per patient day by 1.2 to 10.5 percent, and in expenditures per capita by 2.0 to 7.6 percent (Coelen and Sullivan 1981; Joskow 1981; Melnick, Wheeler, and Feldstein 1981; Sloan 1981, 1983; Morrisey et al. 1983; Rosko 1984a, 1984b; Merrill and McLaughlin 1986).

Dranove and Cone (1985) examined the possibility that only states with extraordinary hospital costs implemented PP systems, and therefore estimates of cost savings attributable to these programs were biased upward, a methodological problem referred to as *regression to the mean*. Dranove and Cone employed the state as the unit of analysis and used data for the years 1970 and 1982 to assess the effects of prospective payment on the expense per admission, the expense per day, and the expense per capita. Seven independent variables were examined in the study. Six represented factors related to the demand and need for hospital care while the seventh independent variable measured the number of years the PP system had been in operation.

After including a correction factor for regression to the mean in the analysis, the results indicated that the magnitude of overall bias in national studies was small since estimates for cost savings attributable to two state programs (New Jersey and Washington) were understated, while estimates of the savings attributable to the other four programs analyzed in this study (Connecticut, Massachusetts, New York, and Maryland) were overstated. In addition, the findings of the study suggest that the New York program was less effective in controlling costs than the New Jersey program, a result that contradicts the conclusions advanced by Morrisey et al. (1983).

There is concern that some of the savings in hospital costs that have been attributed to state rate-setting programs may have been shifted to nonhospital settings (Eby and Cohodes 1985; Rosko and Broyles 1986). Although this response has not been studied extensively, two studies concluded that, when Medicare Part A (inpatient hospital) expenditures are constrained, Medicare Part B (supplementary medical coverage) expenditures decrease (Morrisey et al. 1983;

Coelen and Yaffe 1983); however, since Medicare Part B expenditures do not represent all nonhospital costs, these results should not be viewed as conclusive.

Effects on Productivity and Factor Prices

Although an extensive body of empirical evidence suggests that state mandated prospective payment systems have constrained the growth of hospital expenditures, there is less evidence documenting how the savings were achieved. Thus, it is not clear whether prospective payment has evoked desirable behavioral responses, such as increased efficiency, or less desirable reactions, such as cost-shifting or reducing the quality of care.

As suggested previously, it is possible that hospitals responded to rate regulation by increasing the efficiency with which resources are used and by restraining increases in factor prices. Among the three major types of resources used by hospitals (i.e., labor, capital, and supplies) employee related costs and labor productivity have received the most attention in previous evaluations of hospital rate regulation. The impact of PP on the costs of consumable supplies has been ignored; however, since supply expenses account for a much smaller percentage of hospital costs than the other two resources, this omission is not serious.

Focusing on 10 individual state PP programs and using data for the period from 1969 to 1978, Kidder and Sullivan (1982) examined the impact of rate regulation on unit labor costs, labor productivity, and payroll per employee. Their analysis suggested that PP reduced the rate of increase in payroll costs per adjusted patient day in eight of ten study states. They also reported that the growth in the number of full-time equivalent employees (FTEs) per adjusted patient day (a measure of labor productivity) and in payroll per FTE staff (a measure of factor price) was reduced in six of ten states featuring PP.

Some corroboration of Kidder and Sullivan's findings are reported in other studies. Adamache and Sloan (1982), who used data pertaining to 1979 collected from 781 hospitals that responded to a mailed questionnaire, reported that PP was associated with a reduction in the compensation paid to entry-level nonunion employees in five of six occupational groups; however, PP failed to exert a significant effect ($p < 0.10$) on the rate of compensation paid to entry-level union employees in any occupational group. Rosko (1984b), who employed multivariate analysis in a study of the New Jersey PP system that regulated per diem rates during the period 1975–1978, reported that the rate of increase in the number of full-time equivalents per patient day was inversely related to the introduction of rate regulation in hospitals that were located in inner-city catchment areas; however, statistically significant effects ($p < 0.10$) were not found for New Jersey hospitals located in other catchment areas.

Effects on Capital Accumulation and the Adoption of Technology

As suggested previously, the fiscal rigors imposed by rate regulation may induce hospitals to adopt capital proposals that yield savings or retard the growth in the capacity to provide new services. As the following indicates, empirical research has focused on the effects of rate regulation on the growth in new services.

Ashby (1984) employed multivariate analysis on a set of pooled time series data for the period from 1971 to 1977. These results suggest that neither mandatory nor voluntary rate setting programs had a significant effect on the percentage change in either hospital plant assets or the number of beds per capita.

Cromwell and Kanak (1982) examined the effects of PP on the adoption of new services. The estimates from their regression equations suggest that only two of fifteen mandatory and voluntary PP programs studied reduced the growth of new hospital services. Romeo, Wagner, and Lee (1984) examined the effects of three PP programs (New York, Indiana, and Maryland) on the availability, extent, and speed of adopting three cost-raising technologies and two cost-reducing technologies. They report that the New York program, which is commonly considered to be the most stringent mandatory PP system, showed consistent negative effects on the adoption of all three cost-raising technologies and a positive effect on the adoption of one of the two cost-reducing technologies. The voluntary Indiana program appeared to stimulate the growth in both cost-reducing and cost-increasing technologies. Statistically significant effects ($p \leq .05$) were not found for any of the technologies in Maryland.

Lee and Waldman (1985), who used the same sample as Romeo et al., used a censored normal estimator to assess the impact of PP on the adoption of five technologies by hospitals. Although they argued that their model, which is a generalization of Mansfield's (1968) delay model of technological innovation, results in more efficient estimates than those obtained by Ordinary Least Squares (OLS) models, none of their PP variables achieved statistical significance ($p \leq 0.05$). This result is at variance with the findings of Romeo et al., but it may be due more to the use of different independent variables than to the relative precision of the estimation techniques employed.

Similar results were reported by Sloan, Valvona, and Perrin (1986) who examined the diffusion of five surgical technologies during the period from 1971 to 1981. They found that mature rate-setting programs often did not have an effect on the diffusion of technology. Even when a significant effect ($p < .05$) was detected, it tended to be inconsequential. For example, they found that PP reduced the probability of hospitals adopting coronary bypass surgery and morbid obesity surgery procedures. Although significant ($p < .05$), the reduction in the probability of adoption was less than 1 percent.

Cromwell (1987) examined the impact of individual PP programs on capital formation. He estimated six regression equations for measures of capital flow (i.e., percentage growth in capital intensity per bed and the growth of beds per hospital) and the level of capital stock (i.e., beds per 1,000 population in the county). With the exception of the capital stock equation, the hospital was the level of analysis. Although an extensive set of independent variables was used, the coefficient of multiple determination for the five capital flow equations ranged from 0.013 to 0.058, suggesting that much of the variation in investment was due to chance and unobserved hospital-specific variables. Although variables were entered for eight mandatory PP systems in each of six equations, resulting in a total of 48 rate-setting variables, only six coefficients were negative and significant ($p < .10$). Among the significant rate-setting coefficients, no consistent pattern among states or measures of capital formation was discernible.

As suggested by these findings, evaluations of the effects of prospective payment on capital accumulation and the adoption of new technology are less conclusive than those that focused on factor prices or the efficiency of resource use. In addition, to the extent that rate regulation affected the accumulation of capital, it is unclear whether reductions in the rate of adopting new services represents a more efficient use of existing resources or whether hospitals are not acquiring capital in which improved technologies are embodied. Accordingly, it is possible that the fiscal rigors imposed by rate regulation exerted potentially adverse effects on the capital mix employed by hospitals, which, in turn, may have reduced the quality of care, an issue that requires investigation.

Effects on Volume

In addition to the incentives that induce hospitals to control the cost per day, improve productivity, and restrain increases in factor prices, models of hospital behavior also suggest that the regulation of per diem rates or charges stimulates an increase in volume that results from an extended length of stay and higher admission rates. Recent studies have examined the effects of rate regulation on these dimensions of performance, and several have reported findings that are consistent with these expectations. In the most comprehensive analysis of the effects of PP on the volume of care to date, Worthington and Piro (1982) report that, in states for which statistically significant results were found, rate regulation increased the length of stay and the number of admissions per bed. Melnick et al. (1981) and Merrill and McLaughlin (1986) reported similar results concerning the effects of PP on the length of stay but found no change in the admission rate. Conversely, Sloan (1981, 1983) concluded that rate regulation failed to exert a significant influence on the admission rate, the length of stay, and the number of patient days; hence, even though the results of previous studies are not conclusive, several analyses report findings that are consistent with expectations derived from the model of hospital responses to programs that regulate per diem rates or charges.

Closely related to the effects of rate regulation on the length of stay and the admission rate is the influence of prospective payment on the hospital-physician relationship and the volume of service prescribed by the medical staff. In a study based on organizational theory, Shortell, Morrisey, and Conrad (1985) concluded that the imposition of rate regulation is positively related to the percentage of pathologists and radiologists who are compensated on a salary basis. As demonstrated by Morrisey et al. (1984), a reliance on salaries to compensate physicians reduces incentives to increase the volume of services that are present in other payment schemes. They also report that the presence of PP is positively related to the length of review of physician credentials for medical staff privileges. Thus, it is possible that, as a result of PP, "greater care will be taken to admit only the most cost-effective and cooperative members to the staff, and hospitals will take a longer time to examine these characteristics" (Shortell, Morrisey, and Conrad 1985, p. 603); however, the length of review of physician credentials could have been affected by a number of other factors not controlled for by their research design, such as a changing liability climate and the emerging surplus of physicians. Although this study may be of interest to those in the field of organizational behavior, it does not address hospital or physician performance measures. Further, the research design, which consists of a multivariate analysis of data pertaining to two years, 1972 and 1981, may result in inferences that reflect trends and are spuriously related to rate regulation, the presence of which also increased from 1972 to 1982.

In general, the findings reviewed in this section indicate that the regulation of charges or per diem rates induced hospitals to increase the number of patient days by extending the length of stay and, to a lesser extent, by increasing the rate of admissions. Further, several studies indicate that prospective payment reduces the cost per day by improving the efficiency of resource use, as evidenced by a reduction in the growth of FTEs per day, and by containing factor prices, in particular, wages and salaries per employee. These findings are consistent with the expectations derived from the model of hospital behavior described previously.

PROSPECTIVE PAYMENT: CASE-BASED SYSTEMS

Perhaps the most dramatic change in the fiscal environment of hospitals is the increased dependence on the patient and the related condition to determine prospective rates of compensation. This section focuses on the properties of the Medicare payment system and the case-based mechanisms that are employed by states and Blue Cross programs.

Medicare Prospective Payment System

Effective October 1, 1983, the provisions of *Public Law* 98–21, the Social Security Amendments of 1983, replaced the traditional retrospective mechanism of financing the use of inpatient care by Medicare beneficiaries with a prospective payment system in which prices were established for each of 467 diagnosis related groups (DRGs). Since the provisions of this law are well known and have been presented elsewhere (Lave 1984; Broyles and Rosko 1985; Manga and Broyles 1986; Guterman and Dobson 1986), only a brief description of the major features of the Medicare PP system is presented here.

Scheduled for implementation during a three-year period, the Medicare prospective pricing system employs the patient and related diagnostic condition as the unit of payment. During each year of the transition period, the payment for each Medicare beneficiary is determined by a composite price consisting of the hospital-specific cost per case and the average federal cost per case. The federal cost per case has regional and national components both of which are computed separately for urban and rural hospitals. The relative importance of the hospital-specific and federal components in determining the prospective prices is scheduled to change during each year of the implementation period; however, the enactment of Public Law 99–272 (the Consolidated Omnibus Budget Reconciliation Act of 1985) extended the transition period by one year. After the implementation process is complete, the role of hospital-specific costs in the determination of prospective rates is to be eliminated, and the price structure will be based solely on rural or urban national averages. The Medicare program will continue to employ the cost-based retrospective system to reimburse the institution for the costs of capital (depreciation, interest, and lease expenses), until an acceptable prospective mechanism is developed.

In addition to these features, the provisions of Public Law 98–21 permit the hospital to retain the net surplus that results from the treatment of those cases for which the prospective price exceeds the corresponding full cost. Conversely, the institution is forced to absorb unfavorable differences between the prospective price and the corresponding full cost. As a consequence, the pricing mechanism enables the hospital to benefit financially from improved management.

State and Blue Cross Plan Prospective Payment Systems

In addition to the Medicare pricing system, prospective payment mechanisms that use the patient and related condition to determine rates of compensation have been implemented in fifteen states. The State of Maryland operated the first case-based payment system in 1976 and, during the period 1980 to 1987, similar mechanisms were adopted in fourteen additional states (see Table 12.4). A more detailed summary of the characteristics of these programs is provided by Hellinger (1985). With the exception of Maryland and California, all of the programs used DRGs to determine payment rates. Further, most programs divide hospitals into separate peer groups for which separate payment rates for each DRG are calculated. Williams, Kominski, Dowd et al. (1984) demonstrated that the use of peer groups in conjunction with DRGs controls interhospital variation in the severity of illness more than the use of DRGs alone. Furthermore, the use of additional peer groups beyond those employed by Medicare (i.e., urban and rural) enables the systems enacted by states and Blue Cross Plans to account for more inter-hospital cost variations that are due to exogenous factors, resulting in a more equitable determination of payments (Rosko 1986).

Although all the programs summarized in Table 12.4 use case-mix to determine rates of compensation, the scope of regulatory authority differs among these payment systems. Among the case-based systems, seven regulated Medicaid payment rates, six regulated Blue Cross payments, and two regulated all-payers. Several analysts contend that all-payer systems prevent the use of differential prices to transfer costs, a practice that reduces the rigors of rate regulation and the pressure to control costs. In addition, it is reasonable to argue that an all-payer system is conducive to the implementation of policies that result in an equitable distribution of the burden of financing the costs of care provided to the medically indigent, a possibility that the architects of the Medicare system failed to consider (Lave 1984; Broyles and Rosko 1985).

Theoretical Framework: Case-Based Systems

The model of hospital responses to a per diem prospective payment system can be modified so as to accommodate PP mechanisms that base the rate or level of compensation on case-mix (e.g., DRGs). Substituting cases treated for patient days in the analysis, the model suggests that prospective payment mechanisms that are based on case-mix induce hospitals to increase the number of patients treated, reduce the cost per case, and lower the level of quality.

As suggested by Rosko and Broyles (1986), the cost per case may be expressed in the general form:

$$FC_k = DC_k + IC_k \tag{12.1}$$

where DC_k represents the direct cost of providing stay-specific and ancillary services to the average case of DRG_k; and IC_k corresponds to the share of all indirect costs that are allocated to each case assigned to DRG_k.

Further, the direct costs per case of DRG_k may be expressed in the form:

$$DC_k = \text{mix of ancillary and stay-specific services/case} \tag{12.2}$$
$$x \text{ mix of resources/service}$$
$$x \text{ set of factor prices.}$$

Equations (12.1) and (12.2) suggest that pricing mechanisms which use DRGs as the unit of payment induce the institution to increase the net surplus or reduce the net loss per case by minimizing DC_k, the components of which combine to determine these direct costs and the indirect costs assigned to each discharge.

Essentially three options might be adopted so as to reduce the first component of direct costs, the mix of ancillary and stay-specific services per case. First, the cost per case might be reduced by compressing the length of stay while

Table 12.4
Case-Based Systems for Setting Hospital Rates

System	Period of Operation	Payers Covered	Rate-Setting Method
Maryland Guaranteed Inpatient Revenue Program	1976–present	All payers	Builds on original rate-setting system; covers 22 of state's 52 acute care hospitals; uses three-or four-digit ICD-9-CM codes, broad patient service categories, or DRGs; bases current year's rate on last year's rate, adjusted for volume and uncompensated care.
New Jersey	1980–present	All payers	Replaced two-payer program, uses DRGs to set rates; rates reflect combination of state and hospital-specific rates according to coefficient of variation of costs in DRG; adjusts for volume and uncompensated care; three-year phase-in period, 1980-1982.
California Medicaid (Medi-Cal)	1980-1982	Medicaid	Payments based on prior year's cost per case not adjusted for case mix; hospitals could appeal rates on grounds that case-mix increased.
Georgia Medicaid	1980-1982	Medicaid	Used cluster analyses on several variables to define 10-12 groups; hospitals paid up to 130 percent of group mean cost per case.
Utah Medicaid	July 1983–present	Medicaid	Uses same system as Medicare, except Medicare's rates are reduced by 20 percent.
Pennsylvania Medicaid	July 1984–present	Medicaid	Uses DRGs; defines eight peer groups based on complex formula that includes teaching status, medical assistance volume, environmental characteristics, and hospital costs; two-year phase-in period.
Ohio Medicaid	October 1984–present	Medicaid	Uses DRGs and 14 peer groups based on area wage rate and teaching status to set rates based on last year's costs; system phased in over two years.

Table 12.4 (continued)

System	Period of Operation	Payers Covered	Rate-Setting Method
Michigan Medicaid	February 1985– present	Medicaid	Rates set using DRGs, several peer groups, and adjustments to rates for area wage level, teaching status, capital costs, and outliers.
Washington State Medicaid	January 1985– present	Medicaid	Uses methodology similar to Medicare PPS; no plans to use peer groups.
Arizona Blue Cross and Blue Shield	November 1983– present	All insureds	Sets rates using DRGs for 10 peer groups of hospitals.
Kansas Blue Cross and Blue Shield	January 1984– present	All insureds	Sets rates using DRGs and five peer groups; billed charges are paid up to 75 percent of DRG rate.
Oklahoma Blue Cross and Blue Shield	January 1984– present	All insureds	Sets rates using DRGs and four peer groups defined using bed size.
Nebraska Blue Cross and Blue Shield	April 1985– present	All insureds	Rates to be set using DRGs; five or six peer groups.
Arkansas Blue Cross and Blue Shield	Feb 1987– present	All insureds	Rates set using DRGs; peer groups not used.
Blue Cross and Blue Shield of Greater Philadelphia	July 1985– present	All insureds	Set rates on basis of cost per case in each hospital adjusted annually by a general inflation factor and for changes in each hospital's case-mix index; peer groups not used.

Sources: Hellinger, F.J. 1985. Recent evidence on case-based systems for setting hospital rates. Inquiry 22(1):78-91.
Rosko, M.D. 1984a. The impact of prospective payment: a multi-dimensional analysis of New Jersey's SHARE program. Journal of Health Politics, Policy and Law 9(1):81-101. Personal communication with Arkansas Blue Cross and Blue Shield and Blue Cross and Blue Shield of Greater Philadelphia.

holding the mix of ancillary services provided during the hospital episode constant. *Ceteris paribus*, implementation of such an approach increases the volume of ancillary services per day and, as a consequence, increases the cost per day, even though the cost per case declines.

Second, the cost per case might be reduced by limiting the volume of ancillary services provided during the hospital episode while holding the length of stay constant. Such a strategy reduces both the volume of ancillary services per day and the cost per day, an outcome that, *ceteris paribus*, decreases the cost per admission.

The third option involves a reduction in both the length of stay and the volume of ancillary care per case. Although this option clearly reduces the cost per case, the potential effects on the cost per day are ambiguous. *Ceteris paribus*, the cost per day will decline if the effects of reducing the volume of service per case exceed those of decreasing the length of stay. The obverse is also possible. Since recent evidence supports the assertion that hospitals respond to a case-based payment system by reducing length of stay (Rosko and Broyles 1986; Guterman and Dobson 1986; Beebe, Callahan and Mariano 1986; Smith and Pickard 1986), it is reasonable to expect only a slight reduction in the cost per day in the absence of substantial increases in efficiency or significant declines in factor prices and the provision of ancillary services.

Finally, *ceteris paribus*, a reduction in length of stay may reduce the occupancy rate, an outcome that forces the hospital to allocate fixed indirect costs to fewer patient days and thereby negates some of the savings resulting from the reduced use of stay-specific services. Therefore, as suggested by the modified model, it is likely that hospitals responded to PP systems based on diagnostic mix by increasing the number of cases treated.

Empirical Results: State All-Payer Systems

Multivariate studies of only two case-based PP systems have been published. Salkever and Steinwachs (1986) compared the performance of hospitals subject to the case and service-based PP systems that operated simultaneously in Maryland. Employing data collected from 46 hospitals during the period 1977 to 1981, the results of this study indicated that the use of case-mix to determine payment rates stimulated admissions, reduced the length of stay, and induced hospitals to treat patients presenting less costly conditions. Further, the analysis suggested that changes in utilization patterns were more pronounced when rates of compensation were established at more stringent levels. In a companion study, Salkever, Steinwachs, and Rupp (1986) examined the effects of the two payment mechanisms on total inpatient costs, routine inpatient costs, ancillary inpatient costs, and the cost per admission. Except for three hospitals that faced very rigorous revenue constraints, the authors reported that the case-based system exerted a weak and generally statistically insignificant impact ($p > .05$) on total costs, a result that they attributed to increases in the number of cases treated.

Rosko and Broyles (1986) compared hospital responses to per diem and DRG-based PP systems that were operated simultaneously by the State of New Jersey. The differential impact of the two PP systems during 1980 to 1982 on the cost per admission, the cost per day, the average length of stay, and cases treated was analyzed. Compared to the per diem PP system, hospitals responded to the DRG program by reducing the cost per admission, compressing the average length of stay and increasing the number of cases treated, results that are consistent with the theoretical model. Insignificant results were found for the cost per day.

Each of these studies relied on methodologies that imposed similar limitations in the interpretation of results. First, by focusing on a relatively short study period, these studies failed to control for trends in hospital performance prior to the implementation of case-based PP systems in Maryland and New Jersey. Second, and perhaps more importantly, the intention of these studies was to compare the relative performance of hospitals under alternative forms of PP, an approach that limits the ability to assess the desirability of basing rate regulation on case-mix. For example, Rosko and Broyles reported that, relative to the experience under per diem PP, the average length of stay declined in hospitals subject to the DRG system in New Jersey; however, the methodology they used prevented an assessment of whether this result was due to reductions in the length of stay under the DRG program or to increases in length of stay under the per diem PP program.

Rosko and Broyles (1987) rectified some of these defects by examining the effects of the two-payment systems in relation to a comparison group of eastern Pennsylvania hospitals that were reimbursed on the basis of costs. In addition, the evaluation period was extended to include the years 1975 to 1982. They reported that, relative to the comparison group, the all-payer DRG system reduced average annual increases in the cost per admission (4.7 percent), the cost per day (3.3 percent), and the length of stay (2.2 percent), but increased the number of admissions per hospital (3.9 percent). One of the most significant findings of this study was that the cumulative impact of the New Jersey DRG system on length of stay during the period 1980 to 1982 was only 6.5 percent, or about 0.5 days, a decrease much less than that attributed to the Medicare PPS.

Similar results were reported by Hsiao and Dunn (1987), who used a longer time-series (i.e., 1971 through 1984) but did not include any independent variables to control the effects of changes in supply and demand conditions. Zuckerman (1987), who restricted his analysis to changes in costs from 1982 to 1983, reported that the case-based systems in Maryland and New Jersey constrained increases in cost per admission and cost per day.

Although these studies examined only two states, two important concerns about PP were raised in each. First, increases in the number of admissions may offset savings in cost per admission. Second, management may respond to PP by reducing the length of stay, an outcome that may exert deleterious effects on the patient's health status. In addition, a reduced length of stay may result in additional expenditures on postdischarge health services.

Thorpe (1987) argues that all-payer systems have broader goals than cost control and, thus, should be evaluated in terms of not only cost increases, but also in terms of changes in hospital financial conditions, access to care by the uninsured, and payment differentials among third-party payers. An excellent conceptual discussion of the possible impact of all-payer systems on these performance measures is available in a recently published book, *Uncompensated Hospital Care: Rights and Responsibilities*, edited by Sloan, Blumstein, and Perrin (1986). Although the use of all-payer systems to address broader problems such as access, uncompensated care, and payment issues has been the subject of much discussion, it has not been the focus of much rigorous empirical research. Accordingly, we will discuss a case study of the New York all-payer system, keeping in mind the usual caveats about this analytical method.

Thorpe (1987) performed tabular analysis using data from New York during the period 1980 to 1985. He assumed that any changes that occurred after January 1, 1983 were due to the all-payer system that was implemented by the New York State Department of Health on that date. Thorpe reported that the implementation of the New York all-payer system was associated with (1) a small increase in the access to care by the uninsured, whose share of patient days increased by .7 percent; (2) a reduction in the number of hospitals with a deficit, from 131 to 90, as well as a reduction of the total losses (amounting to $308 million) incurred by hospitals; and (3) a reduction in payment differentials (i.e., gross charge discounts and gross charge markups) by about 20 percent. These outcomes occurred during a period in which cost increases in New York hospitals were slightly below the national average. Similar outcomes were attributed to the New Jersey all-payer system by Rosko (1988), who examined data for the period 1976 to 1985.

Empirical Results: Medicare Pricing System

The paucity of available data prevents an econometric assessment of the influence exerted by the Medicare PP system on costs or utilization behavior; however, in recognition of the importance of this payment system, the following (with the exception of the studies by DesHarnais, Kobrinski, Chesney, Long et al. [1987] and Hogan, Chesney, Wroblewski, and Fleming [1987]) focuses on the results reported in univariate analyses of the short-term effects of the payment system. The limitations of univariate analyses, which allow exogenous factors to confound results, are severe. DesHarnais and associates examined a cohort ($n = 729$) of short-term hospitals from nonwaivered states and improved upon the simple univariate analysis by using data from the third quarter of each year of the period from 1980 to 1983 to predict values of performance measures for the third quarter of 1984. They compared actual with forecasted values for Medicare and non-Medicare patients. The use of a reference group provides some assurance that the analysis controls, albeit weakly, for system-wide changes that might confound the data for Medicare patients. As the researchers point out, however, the absence of a randomized design and a control group made it difficult to separate historical trends from the effects of the Medicare prospective pricing mechanism.

Hogan, Chesney, Wroblewski, and Fleming (1987) examined the impact of the Medicare PP system on the technical efficiency of a national sample ($n = 300$) of hospitals. Data envelopment analysis (see Chapter 7) was used to construct an index of technical efficiency that was used as the dependent variable. The set of independent variables included a binary variable for prospective payment as well as variables for hospital characteristics thought to effect efficiency. Given the limitations of data envelopment analysis, the reliance upon only two years of data (i.e., 1983 and 1984), and a possible underspecification bias caused by the omission of market supply and demand variables, the results reported by Hogan et al. should be accepted with caution. Accordingly, the implications of the following results should be viewed as suggestive and not definitive.

Employing data from the Medicare Statistical System, Guterman and Dobson (1986) analyzed the impact of the Medicare pricing mechanism on hospitals during its first year, fiscal year 1984. As anticipated, hospitals responded to case-based payment rates by reducing length of stay from 10.0 days in fiscal year 1983 to 9.1 days in fiscal year 1984. This trend continued in fiscal year 1985 when average length of stay fell to 8.4 days (Beebe, Callahan, and Mariano 1986). As expected, the decline in length of stay was accompanied by an increased reliance upon the services of home health care agencies and skilled nursing homes. In a cohort of hospitals followed from 1980 to 1984, discharges of Medicare patients to the care of home health agencies in the third quarter of 1984 were about 45 percent higher than the amount predicted by historical trends. Similarly, discharges to skilled nursing facilities were about 16 percent more than expected (DesHarnais et al. 1987).

Responses to the payment mechanism have raised concerns that the quality of patient care may have been compromised. Long, Chesney, Ament et al. (1987a, 1987b) report that hospitals responded to the Medicare PPS in 1984 by providing Medicare patients with fewer diagnostic tests, laboratory tests, and Xrays; however, the use of these tests returned to their pre-PPS levels in 1985, suggesting that the changes observed in 1984 were of a "one-time" nature. A preliminary report by the General Accounting Office (1985) concluded that Medicare patients are being discharged from hospitals with a lower health status as a result of the incentives provided by the Medicare prospective pricing mechanism. These conclusions are supported by the preliminary findings reported by Coe, Patterson, and Wilkinson (1985), who suggest that, because of a reduced length of stay, Medicare patients were discharged with a higher level of dependence in activities of daily living. In contrast to these results, DesHarnais,

Kobrinski, Chesney et al. (1987) reported that the Medicare PPS had no short-term impact on several measures of quality such as consultation rates, rate of inhospital deaths, and readmission rates.

The apparently paradoxical findings that hospitals provided fewer services without adversely affecting quality can be explained by an increase in the level of clinical effectiveness or efficiency. Hogan et al. (1987) report that in the first year after PP, the technical efficiency of a national sample ($n = 300$) of hospitals increased by 2.5 percent. The results of this study should be viewed with caution because the findings are subject not only to limitations of data envelopment analysis but also may be biased by DRG-upcoding and unmeasured changes in quality. Further, Wyszewianski, Thomas, and Friedman (1987) argue that the development of management control systems, one cost-containing response to the imposition of PP, can also improve the quality of care. For example, quality will improve by the elimination of unnecessary services since such services almost always impose at least a minimal risk on the patient.

The discharge of beneficiaries with greater health needs is not necessarily undesirable if patients are provided with appropriate modalities of care; however, the discharge of beneficiaries with increased needs or a greater dependence in the performance of activities of daily living may increase the costs of posthospital care. Indeed, Guterman and Dobson (1986) report that the rate of increase of Medicare expenditures (deflated by the Consumer Price Index) for skilled nursing care and home health care increased by 4.2 percent and 17.8 percent, respectively, from fiscal year 1983 to fiscal year 1984. In contrast, the average annual changes in (deflated) Medicare expenditures on skilled nursing care and home health services were $-.3$ percent and 16.4 percent, respectively, during the period from 1973 to 1982. These findings suggest that the incentives to reduce the length of stay shifted the focus of spending from hospitals to long term-care facilities, an outcome that reduces the potential for controlling the costs of the health industry.

Contrary to expectations derived from the theoretical model and those expressed by many policy analysts, as well as the experience of case-based pricing mechanisms in New Jersey (Hsiao, Sapolsky, Dunn, and Weiner 1986; Rosko and Broyles 1987) and Maryland (Salkever and Steinwachs 1986), Guterman and Dobson reported that the number of Medicare admissions per thousand enrollees declined by 3.5 percent from fiscal year 1983 to fiscal year 1984. The decline in admissions may emanate from a desire to avoid the fiscal risks that result from the provision of inpatient service when payment rates are determined on the basis of case-mix. For example, Ozatalay and Broyles (1987) examined the interrelationship between net return, fiscal risk, as measured by the variance in cost, and the diagnostic mix of beneficiaries. The analysis focused on twelve Major Diagnostic Categories (MDCs) that collectively represented 83 percent of the total operating costs assigned to Medicare patients during fiscal year 1983. The results indicated that, among the twelve diagnostic groups, six were statistically dominated (i.e., exhibited lower net returns and higher variances in cost than other MDCs). In addition, of the remaining MDCs, the results indicated that a profit maximizing hospital is induced to treat only those elderly patients presenting MDC-2 (Diseases of the Eye) and deny admission to all other beneficiaries; hence, the provisions of Public Law 98–21 may have induced administrators to minimize the fiscal risks to which their institutions were exposed by implementing admission policies that reduce the number of Medicare inpatients.

It is also possible that the decline in the number of Medicare admissions may be attributable to increases in the cost-sharing arrangements in the Medicare program or to changes affecting the entire health care system. Support for the latter contention is provided by the experience of Blue Cross admissions, which declined concurrently with the implementation of the Medicare PP system (Scheffler and Gibbs 1985).

Technological advances, which have changed the locus of care provided to the elderly, have also reduced the number of Medicare admissions. For example, DesHarnais, Chesney, and Fleming (1987), who examined a national cohort of hospitals during the period 1980 to 1985, reported that Medicare admissions for DRG 039 (lens procedure) dropped from a total of 15,121 cases in 1983 to 11,197 in 1984 to 2,109 in 1985. The shift in lens procedures from the inpatient to outpatient settings accounted for 54 percent of the decrease in Medicare admissions to the study hospitals between 1984 and 1985.

As a result of reductions in the length of stay and the number of admissions, the number of patient days per thousand Medicare enrollees declined by 14.2 percent from fiscal year 1983 to fiscal year 1984. The decline in the volume of patient days consumed by beneficiaries has interacted with fixed payment rates to reduce the rate of increase in Medicare payments to hospitals. From fiscal year 1983 to fiscal year 1984, "real" Medicare payments (i.e., deflated by the Consumer Price Index) increased by 3.8 percent, an amount that is substantially less than the real average annual increase of 10.0 percent that occurred during the period 1973 to 1982 (Guterman and Dobson 1986). More recent data suggest that the savings persisted beyond the first year. For example, from calendar year 1985 through 1986, real Medicare expenditures for hospital services increased by 2.9 percent (Arnett, Freeland, McKusick, and Waldo 1987). Although the Medicare PP system has constrained expenditures in the short-term, initially savings were not at the expense of profits. An audit by the Inspector General of the Department of Health and Human Services showed that average Medicare margins (i.e., revenue minus expense) earned by hospitals amounted to 14.4 percent in 1985 and 9.56 percent in 1986. ProPac predicts margins will fall to 2 percent in 1987 and will turn negative in 1988. The downward trend has been attributed to increased costs and inadequate payment adjustments (Kimball 1988).

Finally, Carter and Ginsburg (1985) reported that the Medicare pricing system induced changes in hospital coding practices that resulted in a 2.8 percent increase in the Medicare case-mix index (MCMI), a measure that reflects the costliness of a hospital's Medicare patient mix, during fiscal year 1984. Unfortunately, this study was unable to decompose the change in the MCMI into changes due to thoroughness in documentation or to "gaming" the system. The methodology employed in this study also precluded an assessment of whether these changes were a one-time response to the new prospective pricing mechanisms, or if future increases in the MCMI might be attributed to coding changes.

NORMATIVE EVALUATIONS

Thus far, the discussion has considered findings derived from studies that used the empirical approach to the assessment of prospective payment. With this section, the focus shifts and examines the effects of prospective payment from a normative perspective, such as the one developed by Cleverly (1979) or Broyles and Rosko (1985). In addition to controlling costs by improving efficiency, or acquiring resources at lower prices, the normative criteria employed previously suggest that any payment mechanism should (1) preserve the fiscal viability of providers, (2) result in equitable payments from multiple purchasers, and (3) ensure that the use of service is determined by health needs rather than fiscal incentives that are specific to the patient or the provider. The following section evaluates prospective payment in terms of these criteria.

Fiscal Viability

As suggested above, one objective of any financing mechanism is to ensure the fiscal viability and welfare of efficient providers. In this regard, rates of compensation must be established at levels that are commensurate with the conflicting goals of controlling costs and preserving the fiscal welfare of participating hospitals. The nexus of the conflict might be identified by observing that, if rates of payment are "too high," the payment system creates little, if any, incentive to control costs. Conversely, if rates are "too low," the fiscal viability and long-term survival of the hospital may be jeopardized; hence, in order to achieve the goal of preserving the fiscal welfare of providers, payment rates must be established at levels that satisfy the financial requirements of hospitals. Unfortunately, the fiscal needs of American hospitals are normatively determined, a feature that complicates the dual tasks of data collection and operational measurement. In the absence of commonly accepted measures of fiscal need, indicators of profitability have been used to assess the influence of prospective payment on the economic welfare of hospitals.

Employing regression analysis, Sloan (1981, 1983) used the ratio of revenue to total cost as a measure of institutional viability. In both studies, Sloan concluded that PP did not affect profitability. Similar results are reported by Morrisey et al. (1983) who compared the impact of PP on revenue and costs during the period from 1968 to 1981. They concluded that, since costs were reduced more than revenue, hospital profits were not adversely affected by rate regulation.

Employing a sample of 48 hospitals subject to rate regulation and a comparison group of 223 nonregulated hospitals, Cleverly (1986) examined the impact of PP on five financial ratios: current ratio, operating margin ratio, return on total assets, average age of plant, and viability index. The source of data was the Financial Analysis Service of the Hospital Financial Association. The evaluation period consisted of the years 1978, 1979, and 1980. A repeated measures analysis of variance method was used to test for significant effects of rate regulation.

Cleverly reported that hospitals subject to rate regulation had less favorable values ($p < .05$) for all five financial ratios than their nonregulated counterparts; however, these results should be viewed as inconclusive for two reasons. First, there was no "pretest" period in the research design, and the less favorable financial position of regulated hospitals that existed in 1978, the first year of this study, may have been due to factors other than PP. Second, the results of this study indicate that the financial position of regulated hospitals did not deteriorate vis-à-vis nonregulated hospitals during the study period, a result one would expect if PP exerted a deleterious effect on the financial position of hospitals.

Applying tabular analysis to a set of data pertaining to standard financial ratios and encompassing the years 1975 to 1979, Rosko and Broyles (1984) concluded that the New Jersey PP system, which regulated per diem rates for Medicaid and Blue Cross Plan patients, had a slight affect upon the financial status of the average New Jersey hospital. When the data were disaggregated, however, findings suggested that PP resulted in a serious deterioration of the financial position of teaching hospitals as well as hospitals located in inner city areas. In contrast, PP exerted little impact on nonteaching hospitals and hospitals located in suburban areas. The differential effects on the fiscal position of hospitals located in inner cities is probably attributable to the relative inability of these institutions to escape the rigors of prospective payment by adopting differential pricing policies to transfer costs from regulated to unregulated patients or services and to a heavier uncompensated care burden. Rosko (1988) reported that the implementation of the all-payer DRG system was accompanied by a redistribution of operating surplus margins among New Jersey hospitals. During the period (i.e., 1980 to 1983) in which New Jersey hospitals were adjusting to the DRG payment mechanism, profitability was erratic. In contrast, after hospitals were able to complete adjustments, the average inner-city hospital not only earned unprecedented profits (i.e., positive operating margins) in 1984 and 1985, but also narrowed the differential in the average value of the operating margin ratio that existed between suburban and inner-city hospitals when the partial-payer system was in effect. Corroborating evidence is provided by Hsiao et al. (1986), who analyzed data from 1978 to 1983 and reported hospitals that suffered operating losses in 1978 tended to earn a surplus in the post-DRG period (i.e., after 1980), while other hospitals tended to have slightly smaller but positive operating margins in 1983 (Hsiao et al. 1986).

Bentkover, Schroeder, and Lee (1985) applied tabular analysis to a set of standard financial ratios collected from the New York Division of Reimbursement for the period 1974 to 1980. They concluded that the New York State PP system caused a significant deterioration of the financial position of hospitals. The impact of rate regulation was more pronounced in hospitals located in "downstate New York" (i.e., metropolitan New York City area) than in upstate New York. Similar to results reported by Rosko and Broyles, the adverse effects of prospective payment on the economic welfare of institutions located in the New York City area may be attributable to the relative inability of inner-city hospitals to rely on differential prices to avoid the fiscal pressures of rate regulation.

Equitable Prices

As suggested by Cleverly (1979), all purchasers should pay the same price for a given service, and the profit margins of all services should be uniform. Conversely, Broyles and Rosko (1985) argued that a partial-payer system such as the Medicare pricing mechanism creates an incentive that induces hospitals to employ differential prices to transfer costs or losses from beneficiaries to unregulated patients or services, thus forcing one group to finance the use of care by others. To the extent that hospitals succeed in transferring costs and using unregulated patients to subsidize losses resulting from the provision of care to Medicare recipients, the fiscal rigors of rate regulation and incentives to improve efficiency are reduced.

Although a paucity of data prevents an assessment of the impact of the Medicare system on the use of differential prices to transfer costs, a limited amount of information concerning cost shifting among state prospective payment programs exists. For example, Worthington, Cromwell, and Kamens (1979) examined the prospective payment system operating in New Jersey during the period from 1976 to 1979 and concluded that unregulated charge-based purchasers paid as much as 25 percent more per patient day than regulated purchasers. As suggested by Hadley and Feder (1985), however, the application of markups of this magnitude to services financed by commercial insurers is common in states without PP. In a study of the two-payer SHARE Program in New Jersey, Rosko (1984b) indirectly examined the relationship between PP and cost-shifting. It was expected that PP exerted a greater impact on the costs of inner-city hospitals than suburban hospitals since the members of the latter group typically treat more patients who could be used for cross-subsidization purposes, thereby allowing them to avoid the rigors of PP. Applying regression analysis to a set of data for the period from 1971 to 1978, Rosko found that PP reduced the level of increase in the cost per admission, amounting to $61.48 in inner-city hospitals and $25.19 in suburban hospitals. Of course, these results may be confounded by factors not controlled in the regression analysis. In a more recent analysis, Rosko (1988) concluded that, consistent with a priori expectations, payment differentials (e.g., mark-up ratios) were reduced substantially after New Jersey implemented an all-payer rate-regulation program.

Since most of the state prospective payment programs did not regulate Medicare payment rates, federal officials were concerned that, prior to the implementation of Public Law 98–21, the Medicare program may have been used to cross-subsidize regulated patients. Cromwell and Hewes (1985) examined this issue by applying multivariate estimation procedures to a set of Medicare beneficiary-based data that was compiled from a sample of approximately 1,300 counties in states with and without PP systems for the period from 1974 to 1978. They examined performance measures for inpatient and outpatient expenditures and volumes of care (see Table 12.3). Contrary to the concerns expressed by policy analysts, the Medicare program was not a victim of cost shifting; rather, it may have benefited from the incentives to contain costs embodied in the state-mandated PP systems, even in those states in which Medicare payments were not regulated. In the 11 states with PP systems that were studied, 6 coefficients were significant ($p < 0.10$) and negative in the equation in which hospital expenditures per Medicare beneficiary became the dependent variable. Results reported in this study indicate that cumulative savings accruing to the Medicare program ranged from 0.1 percent to 22.84 percent. Only the coefficient of the variable representing New Jersey was positive and significant ($p < 0.10$). This coefficient indicates that the introduction of prospective payment in New Jersey motivated hospitals to transfer costs, a practice that resulted in increases in Medicare expenditures amounting to 32.9 percent during the study period. This conclusion corroborates the studies of cost-shifting in New Jersey by Worthington, Cromwell, and Kamens (1979) and Rosko (1984b).

Outpatient services, which were not regulated by most state PP systems, represent another area that hospitals might use to subsidize the costs of care provided to regulated inpatients. Focusing on nonhospital expenditures for Medicare beneficiaries, results reported by Cromwell and Hewes suggested a pattern similar to the one for inpatient expenditures. When nonhospital expenditures per beneficiary became the dependent variable, coefficients representing 7 states with PP were negative and significant ($p < 0.10$), suggesting cumulative cost savings ranging from 3.3 percent to 12.9 percent accrued to the Medicare program. Only the coefficient for the program in Western Pennsylvania was positive and significant ($p < 0.10$). This result suggested that increases in nonhospital expenditures per Medicare beneficiary amounted to 4.7 percent during the years 1977 and 1978.

Cromwell and Hewes also examined the extent to which prospective payment systems mandated by states induced hospitals to increase the volume of inpatient and outpatient services provided to Medicare patients who were not regulated. Regarding inpatient services, the days of care provided to beneficiaries may have increased in response to the New Jersey PP program by as much as 20 to 25 percent during the period 1975 to 1978; however, in the other states where a statistically significant coefficient for the rate-setting variable was estimated, Medicare patient days declined by 7.7 to 12.8 percent. Estimated increases in Medicare outpatient visits amounting to 55 percent in New Jersey and 13 percent in New York were reported. Only the Wisconsin program was associated with

a decline (10 percent) in outpatient visits; however, with the exception of physician services in New York and Massachusetts, as well as the number of patient
days provided by skilled nursing facilities in New York, state regulation programs
either had a negative effect or exerted no influence on the volume of services
provided by physicians, home health agencies, and skilled nursing facilities.

In summary, the results reported by Cromwell and Hewes suggest that, during
the period from 1974 to 1978, the Medicare program was not used to cross-
subsidize losses incurred in the provision of services to patients whose payments
were regulated by state rate-setting programs. Rather, it appears that the Medicare
program benefitted from some of the responses elicited from these payment
mechanisms. Unfortunately, there is a paucity of rigorous empirical evidence
pertaining to the use of other payers for cross-subsidization purposes. For example, commercial insurers, who control a smaller market share, have less power
than the Medicare program or Blue Cross plans to prevent cross-subsidization;
however, a recent empirical study by Hadley and Feder (1985) suggests that
consumer sensitivity to prices, which has increased in response to recent changes
in insurance cost-sharing provisions, as well as the growth of Preferred Provider
Arrangements (PPA), have discouraged hospitals from practicing cost-shifting.
This result confirms expectations derived from the economic model of cost-
shifting behavior developed by Foster (1985).

Distribution of Service

As suggested by Anderson (1978), access to medical care is equitable if the
use of service is determined by health needs rather than the fiscal incentives that
are specific to the provider or the patient. Accordingly, it is reasonable to argue
that payment systems that induce hospitals to alter the admission rate, the length
of stay, and the use of ancillary services may result in an incongruence between
health needs and the consumption of service, thus exacerbating inequities in
access.

As indicated previously, the Medicare pricing system and other payment mechanisms based on inadequate measures of case-mix induce hospitals to reduce the
proportion of inpatients presenting not only conditions for which a net loss is
anticipated but also diagnoses associated with fiscal risks, as measured by the
variance in cost, that are excessive in relation to expected net returns. When
combined with the growth of alternate delivery mechanisms, such as HMOs,
these factors have probably contributed to the decline in Medicare admissions
and a reduced access to inpatient care. On the other hand, systems that regulate
charges or per diem rates have induced the institutions to increase the rate of
admissions (Worthington and Piro 1982), an outcome that may have resulted in
unnecessary or inappropriate hospital stays.

Similarly, payment mechanisms that base rates of compensation on DRGs
induce hospitals to reduce the length of stay and the consumption of ancillary
services per case. Further, the dramatic reduction in the length of stay experienced

by Medicare beneficiaries has prompted concerns that earlier discharges may be due more to a reduction in the provision of needed services than to improvements in the efficiency of patient management (Staff Report, U.S. Senate 1985; Walker, Broyles, and Rosko 1985). When combined with observed declines in the number of admissions and increases in the level of dependence of Medicare beneficiaries upon discharge from the hospital, previous findings suggest that the reliance on case-mix to determine prospective prices appears to have increased the dependence of utilization behavior on fiscal incentives that are specific to the hospital, while reducing the dependence of utilization behavior on health status.

SUMMARY OF HOSPITAL RESPONSES TO PROSPECTIVE PAYMENT

Several conclusions concerning the influence of prospective payment on hospital performance emerge from this review. Among the most striking of these is that hospitals are adept at responding to the different incentives created by alternate forms of rate regulation. For example, available evidence suggests that hospitals responded to the regulation of per diem rates or charges by reducing daily costs, increasing the length of stay, and, to a lesser extent, stimulating admissions. Conversely, responses to case-based payment mechanisms were dominated by the adoption of policies that resulted in reductions in the cost per discharge and the length of stay. In addition, it also appears that the fiscal pressures of rate regulation induced hospitals to improve the efficiency of resource use, as evidenced by reported declines in the number of FTEs per day, and to resist pressures to increase wages or salaries.

Although the weight of evidence is consistent with theoretical expectations concerning the containment of unit costs and volume adjustments, findings pertaining to other potential responses are less conclusive. In particular, we found that the expected effects of rate regulation on capital formation and the adoption of new services have not been verified empirically. The mixed results concerning these dimensions of performance may be attributable to imprecise measures of hospital capital or to data deficiencies, resulting in findings that fail to capture the long-term process of capital adjustment.

Concerning the normative criteria, the influence of prospective payment on the economic welfare of hospitals and the pricing policies adopted by management depends on the structural characteristics of the payment mechanism, as well as on factors that are exogenous to rate regulation. For example, the fiscal arrangements that finance uncompensated care and provide an infusion of working capital to inner-city hospitals were political compromises that insured the passage of legislation that created the basis for the all-payer DRG program in New Jersey. Accordingly, the financial position of inner-city hospitals improved dramatically after 1980, when the DRG system replaced the SHARE program that regulated per diem rates and applied to two payers. Similarly, incentives to adopt differential pricing policies are reduced by all-payer systems, subsidies for uncompensated care, and countervailing pressures exerted by consumers who are subject to higher deductibles and coinsurance rates, or by corporations that establish programs such as PPAs to control expenditures on employee health benefits. Given the mixed findings summarized in this review, however, the prevalence and extent of cost shifting remain controversial issues.

Furthermore, we are concerned that rate regulation exacerbates inequities in the distribution and use of service. Although fragmentary, available evidence seems to suggest that mechanisms that fail to adjust rates of compensation for case severity or finance the costs of care provided to the indigent induce hospitals to avoid treating patients in these categories. Finally, a recommendation to expand a particular cost-control mechanism such as prospective payment should be based on other considerations, such as the potential efficacy of other strategies (e.g., increased competition), the performance of PP in other sectors of the health care industry, and political and social values. Accordingly, our final word on prospective payment will be written in the next (and last) chapter.

PROSPECTIVE PAYMENT OF NURSING HOMES

The cost of nursing home care has increased from $10.1 billion in 1975 to $35.2 billion in 1985, an average annual rate (22.6 percent) that exceeded the growth rate of expenditures in all other sectors of the health care industry (Waldo, Levit, and Lazenby 1986). In response to these increases, Medicaid programs, which financed about 42 percent of nursing home expenditures in 1985 (Waldo et al. 1986), have implemented a variety of payment mechanisms designed to contain program outlays. The variety of nursing home payment mechanisms is at least as diverse as the set of hospital payment mechanisms that we discussed in the previous sections of this chapter. An excellent brief summary of the major dimensions of nursing home payment systems is provided by Holahan and Cohen (1987).

Compared to the large body of evidence on hospital rate-setting, relatively little is known about the impact of prospective payment on nursing homes. The research that has been conducted in this area has focused upon prospective payment mechanisms developed by state Medicaid programs.

Using the state as the level of aggregation, Harrington and Swan (1984) tested the hypothesis that the form of reimbursement had an impact upon Medicaid payment rates per day. Regression analysis was performed on a data set that included the years 1979 to 1982. The analysis contrasted the rate of increase in Medicaid payment rates to nursing homes under retrospective reimbursement with three types of alternate payment systems: prospective/facility-specific, prospective/class (i.e., a group rate), and a combination of prospective and retrospective methods. The alternate payment systems were analyzed as a group and as individual types of systems. The authors reported that states with alternative payment systems in general, and facility-specific payment systems in particular, showed significantly lower increases in Medicaid payment rates for skilled nursing facilities (SNFs) than states that maintained retrospective payment systems; however, no similar differences were found for rates set for intermediate care facilities (ICFs).

Buchanan (1983), who performed tabular analysis, also found support for the contention that prospective payment is associated with lower Medicaid payment rates for nursing homes. He reported that between 1975 and 1982 the average rate paid to SNFs rose by 89.9 percent and 120 percent in prospective and retrospective payment systems, respectively. Similar trends were found for ICFs during the same period; however, when the influence of retrospective and prospective payment on differences in payment rate per patient day in individual years was considered, statistically significant ($p < 0.05$) results were found for SNFs in only one year, 1982. The analysis of ICFs found significant results in 1976 and 1982.

Buchanan also reported that, compared to states with retrospective payment systems, states with prospective payment mechanisms had significantly greater ratios of Medicaid patients per 1,000 elderly population, Medicaid patient days per 1,000 elderly population, and Medicaid certified beds per 1,000 population. Thus, he concludes that the application of prospective payment by Medicaid authorities resulted in a reduction of Medicaid expenditures without having adverse consequences on the elderly's access to nursing home services. Although Buchanan's conclusions appear to be at variance with the conventional wisdom that low Medicaid payment rates to nursing homes result in reduced access for Medicaid patients, these positions are not necessarily at variance. For example, the decision to implement a preferential admissions policy is likely to be based on perceptions of potential profits and losses. Payment methods per se do not affect profits, however. Rather, it is the rigor with which rates are set that affects profits. Thus, it is conceivable that Buchanan's results may have been due to the comparison of nursing homes in states that set relatively generous prospective rates with nursing homes in states that retrospectively pay on the basis of a very restrictive definition of allowable costs. Since most states face pressures to contain costs in their Medicaid programs, this scenario is not implausible.

The results of the studies conducted by Buchanan (1983) and Harrington and Swan (1984) should be accepted with caution because of two serious methodological difficulties. First, both studies used the Medicaid payment rate as the dependent variable. Although Medicaid reimbursement levels may be related to costs, it is well known that they are lower than payments made by Medicare or private sources (Nyman 1985). Thus, if the real intent of the research is to evaluate the efficacy of prospective payment as an instrument that controls all costs, it would have been preferable to use expenditures per unit of service as the performance measure. Second, neither study controlled for interstate differences in factors that affect costs. This is an especially serious deficiency since the evidence reported by Harrington and Swan (1984) suggested that among states with retrospective reimbursement systems those with lower Medicaid payment rates in a given year were more likely to subsequently change to a prospective payment system. Accordingly, it is impossible to determine whether results of these studies are due to prospective payment or to interstate differences that were not adequately controlled.

Holahan's study (1985) of nursing home responses to reimbursement mechanisms attempted to rectify some of the weaknesses of earlier studies as described above. Unfortunately, by limiting the study to only 10 states, Holahan reduced the extent to which the results of the study can be generalized. Holahan used the percentage change in total nursing home costs from 1978 to 1980 as the dependent variable in his regression analysis. Independent variables were used to control for the effects of changes in area wage levels, capacity utilization, and case-mix. In addition, two separate specifications of binary variables were used to estimate the impact of payment policy on nursing home costs.

In one set of equations, a binary variable was entered for states with retrospective payment methods, and another binary variable was entered for states with a prospective payment formula that incorporated an adjustment for projected inflation plus approved base-year costs. The reference category in this equation was states with a flat-rate prospective payment system in which rates were set at the projected median costs for each group, with facilities grouped by geographic area, size, and level of care. In the second specification, a binary variable was entered for each state, except one that served as the reference category. The results from this equation were analyzed by comparing the coefficients of the state variables that were grouped into the three types of reimbursement systems. This facilitated analysis of the disparate performance that occurred in the different states. The results suggest that, in general, the two forms of prospective payment were associated with smaller percentage changes in nursing home costs from 1978 to 1980. The results of this study, however, should not be viewed as definitive because of the small number of states that were represented and because only one variable, changes in area wages, was used to control for interstate differences that might affect nursing home costs.

Harrington and Swan (1987) examined nursing home expenditures and utilization in 42 states during the period 1978 to 1983. They improved upon their earlier study (1984) by examining independent variables that accounted for the effects of state Medicaid policies as well as supply and demand conditions. Harrington and Swan (1987) reported that ICF reimbursement rate had a positive and significant effect ($p \leq .05$) on Medicaid nursing home expenditures, while utilization controls appeared to be ineffective.

Although expenditure control is of interest to many, we feel that increased emphasis on other outcomes is needed. Rosko, Broyles, and Aaronson (1987) analyzed a number of structural differences between the hospital and the nursing home industries, and concluded that the problems facing long-term care providers are the converse of those confronting hospitals. They argued that, unlike the Medicare pricing mechanism which was implemented to control costs and the financial obligations of the federal government, reform of nursing home payment mechanisms should be designed to emphasize improvements in access, quality assurance, capacity expansion, and inducements for appropriate resource utilization. Accordingly, we conclude our discussion of nursing home payment mechanisms with a plea for more experiments (e.g., see Thorburn and Meiners 1986) and/or program changes (with subsequent evaluations) to deal with the "real" problems confronting the nursing home industry.

ECONOMIC STABILIZATION PROGRAM

The Nixon administration's Economic Stabilization Program (ESP) was developed to limit inflation by controlling prices in all sectors of the economy. The program was in effect from August 15, 1971, until April 30, 1974. The regulations enforced by the program were changed several times. Initially, during Phase I, wages and prices were frozen throughout the economy for 90 days. During this period, separate regulations were developed for different sectors of the economy. Because of the unique characteristics and problems of the health care industry, separate wage and price controls were developed by the Committee on the Health Services Industry for institutional and noninstitutional providers of health services (Ginsburg 1978). Following the recommendations of the committee, a 6 percent ceiling on the annual rates of increase in total hospital charges was imposed by the Price Commission of the ESP. Wage rate increases were limited to 5.5 percent per year and nonlabor cost increases were restricted to 2.5 percent per year.

Multivariate studies of the impact of the ESP wage and price controls on hospital behavior reported conflicting findings. Ginsburg (1978) reported a statistically insignificant impact of the program on hospital costs. Sloan and Steinwald (1980) found similar results when using ordinary-least-square regressions; however, statistically significant results were found in two studies that concluded that ESP exerted a small negative effect on hospital costs, ranging from 0.5 percent to 3.3 percent (Sloan and Steinwald 1980; Sloan 1981).

Several explanations of ineffectiveness of ESP in the hospital sector have been offered. First, hospital executives may have perceived that their current performance may have been used to determine future cost ceilings. Thus, an incentive to overspend the budget in one year of the cost control program in order to receive a higher level of reimbursement in the future may have existed. Second, it was difficult for hospitals to comply with a set of regulations that were very ambiguous. Finally, many hospital administrators believed that the controls would not be seriously enforced (Ginsburg 1978).

THE VOLUNTARY EFFORT

The Carter administration's proposed Hospital Cost Containment Act of 1977 (S. 1391 and H.R. 6575) contained provisions that would restrict the rate of increase in inpatient hospital revenues to 8.7 percent in 1978 (Dunn and Lefkowitz 1978). Although this proposal was never enacted, the threat of increased government regulation induced the hospital industry to form the "Voluntary Effort." This program was created jointly by the American Hospital Association, the Federation of American Hospitals, and the American Medical Association in November 1977. The Voluntary Effort proposed three major goals: (1) a 2 percent reduction in hospital costs in 1978 and 1979, (2) no net increase in hospital beds in 1978, and (3) a reduction in the amount of total capital expenditures by 20 percent of the average hospital capital investment made during the period from 1975 to 1977. Cost-containment committees were developed by the hospital industry in each of the 50 states to help achieve the cost-containment goals (Abernathy and Pearson 1979).

Although the Voluntary Effort lasted only one year, it appears to have succeeded not only in postponing federal cost-containment efforts (albeit temporarily) but also in reducing the rate of increase in hospital cost per admission and cost per patient day by about 2.8 to 4.9 percent, depending upon specification of the regression equation (Sloan 1981). Since this program was in effect for only one year, however, it was impossible to use time-series analysis to confirm that these results were actually due to the Voluntary Effort and not to some anomaly that may have occurred in the economy in 1978.

UTILIZATION REVIEW

Hospitals have been subject to utilization review requirements, mandated by the federal government, since 1966. Concerned about the potential abuse of benefits provided under the Medicare, Medicaid, and Maternal and Child Care programs (respectively, Title XVIII, XXIX, and V of the Social Security Amendments of 1965) the Social Security Administration developed utilization review (UR) requirements for hospitals participating in these programs. The federal government required that each hospital must have a UR committee that assessed admissions, the duration of the stay, and professional services from the perspective of medical necessity and for the purpose of promoting the most efficient use of available health facilities and services (Myers 1970). The Senate Sub-Committee Staff on Medicare/Medicaid (U.S. Senate 1970) concluded that UR failed to act as an effective cost-control mechanism because of inadequate regulations and poor administrative control mechanisms.

Under the authority of Public Law 92–603, Professional Standards Review Organizations (PSROs) were established in 1972 with the goal of reviewing hospital utilization for quality and appropriateness. Review was limited to hospital use that was financed by the Medicare, Medicaid and Maternal and Child Care programs (Blumstein 1978). As a result of a political compromise, local physicians could establish and control the PSROs and delegate much of the actual utilization review work to hospitals.

Implementation of the PSRO program was slow. As of 1977, 108 conditional PSROs were established, but none were fully operational. By 1980, only two-thirds of the hospitals in the United States were under PSRO review. From 1979 to 1983, the PSRO program received diminished support. Enacted in 1982, Public Law 97–248 repealed existing PSRO regulations and replaced them with provisions that created peer review organizations (PRO). PROs are performance-judged organizations that compete for government contracts rather than receive grants (Webber and Goldbeck 1984). The recent implementation of PROs has precluded rigorous empirical assessment of their impact on hospital performance.

Two factors make an evaluation of the PSRO program difficult. First, the program had two mandates (i.e., cost containment and quality assurance) that may have been in conflict. Second, there was a wide variation in the performance of individual PSROs (Luft 1985; Deacon, Lubitz, Gornick et al. 1979).

Evaluations of the effects of the PSRO program can be grouped into two categories: studies that focused on PSROs, and studies that examined other regulatory programs but which statistically controlled and estimated the effects of PSROs. The research design for the latter group of studies is the same as that described earlier in this chapter.

Mixed results were found in the former group of studies. The Department of Health, Education, and Welfare Office of Planning, Evaluation, and Legislation (OPEL) study (1979) found that PSROs had no demonstrable effect on utilization; however, the evaluation of the PSRO program sponsored by the Health Care Financing Administration (U.S. Department of HEW, HCFA 1980) found that PSROs significantly reduced utilization rates in hospitals for Medicare beneficiaries. This study, limited to Medicare beneficiaries, found that PSROs had a benefit-to-cost ratio ranging from 1.035 to 1.504, depending on the assumptions used.

As summarized in Table 12.5, the ability of PSROs to contain costs has not been supported by most national studies that focused primarily on hospital rate regulation. Worthington and Piro (1982) reported that PSROs resulted in a slight decrease in average length of stay that was offset by an increase in admissions per bed, resulting in a higher hospital occupancy rate. Other studies (Coelen and Sullivan 1981; Sloan 1983; Merrill and McLaughlin 1986) found that PSROs were associated with positive and insignificant levels ($p < .05$) of hospital expenditures and utilization. In contrast to the bulk of the evidence, Ashby (1984) reported that PSROs were associated with lower per capita costs and lower admissions per capita.

Most studies suggest that the PSRO program failed to contain hospital costs. The ineffectiveness of this program can be attributed to many factors. First, PSROs relied on peer review, which required the cooperation of physicians; however, the American Medical Association and many local medical societies opposed them. Second, governmental financial support never matched operating needs (Webber and Goldbeck 1984). Third, PSROs did not attempt to address all dimensions of patient management that affect costs. Utilization review conducted by PSROs focused on unnecessary hospitalizations and excessive lengths of stay, but it did not attempt to control the performance of unnecessary diagnostic and therapeutic procedures on hospitalized patients. Finally, PSROs emphasized

Table 12.5

Summary of Recent Multivariate Evaluations of Professional Standards and Review Organizations

Study	Performance Measure	Impact of PSROs on Performance
Coelen and Sullivan (1981)	Cost per day Cost per capita Cost per admission	+ + n.s.
Worthington and Piro (1982)	Length of stay Admissions per bed Occupancy rate	- + +
Sloan (1983)	Length of stay Cost per day Cost per admission	n.s. + +
Ashby (1984)	Cost per capita Length of stay Admissions per capita	- n.s. -
Merrill and McLaughlin (1986)	Length of stay Cost per day Cost per admission Cost per capita	n.s.[1] n.s. n.s. n.s.

Key: At p ≤ .05 level of statistical significance the association between PSROs and hospital performance can be positive (+), negative (-), or insignificantly different from zero (n.s.).

[1] Although the coefficient of PSRO variable was insignificant in an annual change equation, it was significant when the dependent variable was specified at its level in a given year.

control of unnecessary services, rather than the promotion of more cost-effective patient management strategies (Blumstein 1978).

REGULATION OF CAPITAL FORMATION

Beginning in the mid–1960s, states and the federal government implemented various forms of capital formation regulation. Although there is a great amount of diversity among these programs, they can be dichotomized as exerting direct or indirect controls (Salkever and Bice 1979). Direct controls are exercised typically under the authority of state certificate-of-need (CON) laws, which specify legal means to prohibit organizations from carrying out disapproved projects. Direct sanctions include the denial or suspension of operating licenses. Indirect controls use economic sanctions whereby third-party payers may refuse to compensate providers for costs associated with investment projects or service changes that fail to receive prior approval from designated agencies (Lewin & Associates, Inc. 1975).

The first CON law was enacted by the State of New York in 1964. By 1974, 24 states operated some type of CON program (Salkever and Bice 1979). Two laws have provided federal support for capital controls. Section 1122 of Public Law 92–603, the Social Security Amendments of 1972, authorized support for indirect control of capital formation. This section allowed states to designate agencies to review plans for facility or service expansion for projects that cost more than $100,000. Reimbursement for the costs of unapproved capital projects can be withheld by federal payers (i.e., Medicare, Medicaid, and Maternal and Child Care programs); however, hospitals are able to recover these lost payments from other sources, including other third-party payers that do not have a "conformance" clause in their reimbursement contracts. This clause links reimbursement for capital costs to project review and approval by designated agencies. As of July 1979, about one-half of the 72 Blue Cross plans had hospital contracts containing conformance clauses (Salkever and Bice 1979).

Additional federal support for CON controls was provided by Public Law 93–641, the National Health Planning and Resources Development Act of 1974. This law mandated states to enact CON legislation by 1980 or become ineligible for federal subsidies to support regional health planning. Only three states failed to enact CON legislation by 1980. Although popular in the 1970s, reliance on controls to restrict capital formation has diminished during the 1980s. An AHA survey indicates that in light of waning congressional support for Section 1122, review programs, and the subsequent repeal of the CON provisions of Public Law 93–641, legislators in eleven states (as of August 1987) abandoned CON and Section 1122 review programs (AHA 1987).

The methods used to estimate the effects of programs to control capital expansion on hospital performance were similar to those used in the prospective payment evaluations. In general, binary variables are used to represent the presence, comprehensiveness, and maturity of programs designed to regulate capital formation. Sloan (1981) included separate binary variables for young and mature CON programs. In addition to maturity, Sloan and Steinwald (1980) used variables for CON programs that were comprehensive (i.e., reviews capital projects costing less than $100,000) and noncomprehensive (i.e., reviews only capital projects that cost more than $100,000). Joskow (1981) used two specifications: a binary variable and a variable depicting the number of years the CON program had been in operation.

Before presenting the empirical results, it is important to note that although some attempt was made by a few researchers to reflect the diversity of regulatory programs, a true depiction of their diversity was not accomplished. For example, although dimensions of maturity and comprehensiveness were included in some of the model specifications, no attempts were made to reflect differences in the criteria used to evaluate capital proposals or the willingness of courts to reverse

CON decisions. Therefore, it is possible that the effects of individual programs may be radically different from the average regression coefficients reported in the studies.

Virtually all of the empirical studies to date report that CON and Section 1122 reviews exerted no impact on hospital expenditures (Policy Analysis, Inc. 1980; Sloan and Steinwald 1980; Melnick, Wheeler, and Feldstein 1981; Sloan 1981; Joskow 1981; Coelen and Sullivan 1981; Ashby 1984; Merrill and McLaughlin 1986). One exception with a statistically significant result found that noncomprehensive CON programs were associated with increased hospital expenditures (Sloan and Steinwald 1980). Other analyses suggest that controls on capital formation had no impact on total assets or the diffusion of services (Hellinger 1976; Salkever and Bice 1979; Cromwell and Kanak 1982). Salkever and Bice (1979) suggest that when regulation of capital succeeded in constraining the growth of numbers of beds, hospitals substituted investment in new services for beds. Sloan and Steinwald (1980) corroborated these findings and also reported that Section 1122 review is positively associated with increases in the ratio of registered nurses per bed and licensed practical nurses per bed.

A likely explanation for the lack of success in controlling hospital investment is industry capture. Noll (1975) points out several ways in which Health Systems Agencies (HSA) could fall prey to industry capture while carrying out their CON function. First, because of the high cost of acquiring specialized information, the regulator may rely on industry members for data, and thus may become vulnerable to distorted information. Second, members of the industry are usually more concerned about the regulatory agencies' decisions than any individual member of the general public. Thus, the industry is more prone to sue the agency than is the general public, and the threat of legal action may create a proindustry bias on the part of the agency. Third, the legislation that created HSAs, Public Law 93–641, also charged them to ensure that the general public has access to health facilities. Thus, the HSA charter implicitly requires the organization to ensure the industry's health. A final force for industry capture is that the regulator's decisions can possess a life-or-death quality. For example, if physicians argue that certain equipment is necessary for the preservation of life, the regulatory agency will find it difficult to deny approval for installation of that equipment.

SUMMARY

Prospective payment of hospitals has been the only regulatory intervention in the United States for which a substantial body of evidence, documenting cost control, exists. Even though hospital rate regulation has succeeded in reducing the rate of increase in hospital expenditures, the efficacy of rate regulation is in doubt because of its possible adverse consequences. Empirical studies have associated the introduction of prospective payment with consumer cross-subsidization, deterioration in the financial position of hospitals located in urban areas, and a greater level of dependence of patients upon discharge. Although these consequences have not been studied as extensively as hospital costs, the available evidence suggests that further study and comparisons with other cost-containment mechanisms are required before prospective payment can be endorsed unequivocally. The merits of regulatory intervention, among other topics, are discussed in the next chapter.

REFERENCES

Abernathy, D. S., and D. A. Pearson. 1979. *Regulating Hospital Costs: The Development of Public Policy*. Ann Arbor, MI: AUPHA Press.

Adamache, K., and F. Sloan. 1982. Unions and hospitals: Some unresolved issues. *Journal of Health Economics* 1(1):81–102.

American Hospital Association. 1987. More states deregulate capital expenditures. Anonymous letter in *AHA News* 23(36):3.

American Hospital Association. 1988. PPS margins are down, hospital costs are up. *AHA News* 24(5):1.

Anderson, R. 1978. Health status indices and access to medical care. *American Journal of Public Health* 68(5):458–63.

Arnett, R. H., M. Freeland, D. McKusick, and D. Waldo. 1987. National health expenditures, 1986–2000. *Health Care Financing Review* 8(4):1–36.

Ashby, J. 1984. The impact of hospital regulatory programs on per capita costs, utilization, and capital investment. *Inquiry* 21(1):45–60.

Beebe, K., W. Callahan, and A. Mariano. 1986. Medicare short-stay hospital length of stay, fiscal years 1981–85. *Health Care Financing Review* 7(3):119–25.

Bentkover, J. D., R. E. Schroeder, and A. J. Lee. 1985. Effects of rate review on the financial viability of New York hospitals: A retrospective assessment. *Hospital & Health Services Administration* 39(3):94–105.

Biles, B., C. J. Schramm, and G. J. Atkinson. 1980. Hospital cost inflation under state rate-setting programs. *New England Journal of Medicine* 303:664–68.

Blumstein, J. F. 1978. The role of PSROs in hospital cost containment. In M. Zubkoff, I. Raskin, and R. S. Hanft, eds., *Hospital Cost Containment*. New York: Prodist.

Broyles, R. W., and M. D. Rosko. 1985. A qualitative assessment of the medicare prospective payment system. *Social Science and Medicine* 10:1185–1190.

Buchanan, R. J. 1983. Medicaid cost containment: Prospective reimbursement for longterm care. *Inquiry* 20(4):334–342.

Cambell, D., and J. Stanley. 1963. *Experimental and Quasi-Experimental Designs for Research*. Chicago, IL: Rand McNally and Company.

Carter, G., and P. Ginsburg. 1985. *The Medicare Case-Mix Index Increase: Medical Practice Changes, Aging, and DRG Creep*. Santa Monica, CA: Rand Corporation.

Cleverly, W. O. 1979. Evaluation of alternative payment strategies for hospitals: A conceptual approach. *Inquiry* 16(2):108–18.

Cleverly, W. O. 1986. Hospital financial condition under state rate regulatory programs. *Hospital & Health Services Administration* 31(2):135–47.

Coe, M., P. Patterson, and A. Wilkinson. 1985. Impact of DRG payment system on the discharge status of medicare patients. Paper presented at 113th Annual APHA Conference, Washington, DC.

Coelen, C., and D. Sullivan. 1981. An analysis of the effects of prospective reimbursement programs on hospital expenditures. *Health Care Financing Review* 2(1):1–40.

Coelen, C., and R. Yaffe. 1983. The national hospital rate-setting study: Summary of current findings on the effects of hospital prospective payment systems. Paper presented to the Labor-Management Health Care Cost Containment Conference, Atlantic City.

Cook, K. S., S. M. Shortell, D. A. Conrad, and M. A. Morrisey. 1983. A theory of organizational response to regulation: The case of hospitals. *Academy of Management Review* 8(2):193–205.

Cromwell, J. 1987. Impact of state hospital rate setting on capital formation. *Health Care Financing Review* 8(3):69–82.

Cromwell, J., and H. Hewes. 1985. Medicare expenditures under state hospital rate setting. *Health Care Financing Review* 7(1):97–109.

Cromwell, J., and J. R. Kanak. 1982. The effects of prospective reimbursement programs on hospital adoption and service sharing. *Health Care Financing Review* 4(2):67–88.

Cromwell, J., C. Coelen, E. Lefson, et al. 1976. Analysis of prospective payment systems for upstate New York: Summary. Final report, HEW–05–74–261, Cambridge, MA: Abt Associates.

Deacon, R., J. Lubitz, M. Gornick et al. 1979. Analysis of variations in hospital use by Medicare patients in PSRO areas, 1974–1977. *Health Care Financing Review* 1(1):79–98.

DesHarnais, S., E. Kobrinski, J. Chesney, M. Long et al. 1987. The early effects of the prospective payment system on inpatient utilization and the quality of care. *Inquiry* 24(3):7–16.

DesHarnais, S., J. Chesney, and S. Fleming. 1987. The impact of the prospective payment system on hospital utilization and the quality of care: Trends and regional variations in the first two years. Paper presented to the American Public Health Association Annual Meeting, New Orleans.

Dowling, W. 1974. Prospective reimbursement of hospitals. *Inquiry* 11(3):160–80.

Dranove, D., and K. Cone. 1985. Do state rate-setting regulations really lower hospital expenses? *Journal of Health Economics* 4(2):159–76.

Dunn, W., and B. Lefkowitz. 1978. Hospital Cost Containment Act of 1977: An analysis of the administration's proposal. In M. Zubkoff, I. Raskin, and R. S. Hanft, eds., *Hospital Cost Containment*. New York: Prodist.

Eby, C. L., and D. R. Cohodes. 1985. What do we know about rate-setting? *Journal of Health Politics, Policy and Law* 10(2):299–327.

Feldstein, M. 1971. Hospital cost inflation: A study of nonprofit price dynamics. *American Economic Review* 61(5):853–72.

Foster, R. W. 1985. Cost-shifting under cost reimbursement and prospective payment. *Journal of Health Economics* 4(3):261–71.

General Accounting Office. 1985. Information requirements for evaluating the impacts of medicare prospective payment on post-hospital long-term care services: Preliminary report. Gaithersburg, MD: General Accounting Office.

Getzen, T. E. 1985. Time series analysis of income and health expenditures: Is regulation endogenous? Paper presented to the American Public Health Association Annual Meeting, Washington, DC.

Ginsburg, P. B. 1978. Impact of the Economic Stabilization Program on hospitals: An analysis with aggregate data. In M. Zubkoff, I. Raskin, and R. S. Hanft, eds., *Hospital Cost Containment*. New York: Prodist.

Guterman, S., and A. Dobson. 1986. Impact of the Medicare prospective payment system for hospitals. *Health Care Financing Review* 7(3):97–114.

Hadley, J., and J. Feder. 1985. Hospital cost shifting and care for the uninsured. *Health Affairs* 4(3):67–80.

Harrington, C., and J. H. Swan. 1984. Medicaid nursing home reimbursement policies, rates, and expenditures. *Health Care Financing Review* 6(1):39–49.

Harrington, C., and J. H. Swan. 1987. The impact of state Medicaid nursing home policies on utilization and expenditures. *Inquiry* 24(2):157–72.

Hellinger, F. J. 1976. Prospective reimbursement through budget review: New Jersey, Rhode Island, and Western Pennsylvania. *Inquiry* 13(3):309–20.

Hellinger, F. J. 1985. Recent evidence on case-based systems for setting hospital rates. *Inquiry* 22(1):78–91.

Hogan, A. J., J. Chesney, R. Wroblewski, and S. Fleming. 1987. The impact of the medicare prospective payment system on hospital efficiency: A data envelopment analysis. Paper presented to the American Economic Association Annual Meeting, Chicago.

Holahan, J. 1985. State rate-setting and its effects on the cost of nursing home care. *Journal of Health Politics, Policy and Law* 9(4):647–67.

Holahan, J., and J. Cohen. 1987. Nursing home reimbursement: Implications for cost containment, access, and quality. *The Milbank Quarterly* 65(1):112–47.

Hsiao, W., and D. Dunn. 1987. The impact of DRG payment on New Jersey hospitals. *Inquiry* 24(3):203–11.

Hsiao, W. C., H. M. Sapolsky, D. L. Dunn, and S. L. Weiner. 1986. Lessons of the New Jersey DRG payment system. *Health Affairs* 5(2):32–45.

Joskow, P. L. 1981. *Controlling Hospital Costs: The Role of Government Regulation*. Cambridge, MA: MIT Press.

Kidder, D., and D. Sullivan. 1982. Hospital payroll costs productivity and employment under prospective reimbursement. *Health Care Financing Review* 4(2):89–115.

Kimball, M. C. 1988. Hospital Medicare profits collapsing. *HealthWeek* 2(3):1, 36.

Lave, J. 1984. Hospital reimbursement under Medicare. *Health and Society* 62(2):251–65.

Lave, J., L. Lave, and L. Silverman. 1973. A proposal for incentive reimbursement for hospitals. *Medical Care* 11(1):79–89.

Lee, R. H., and D. M. Waldman. 1985. The diffusion of innovations in hospitals. *Journal of Health Economics* 4(4):373–80.

Lewin & Associates, Inc. 1975. An analysis of state and regional health regulation. Final report submitted to the Health Care Financing Administration, Contract No. HEW–05–73–212. Washington, DC.

Long, M. J., J. D. Chesney, R. P. Ament, S. I. DesHarnais et al. 1987a. The effect of PPS on hospital product and productivity. *Medical Care* 25(6):528–38.

Long, M. J., J. D. Chesney, R. P. Ament, S. I. DesHarnais et al. 1987b. The continued effect of PPS on the hospital product and productivity. Paper presented to the American Public Health Association Annual Meeting, New Orleans.

Luft, H. S. 1985. Competition and regulation. *Medical Care* 23(5):383–400.

Manga, P., and R. Broyles. 1986. Evaluating and explaining U.S.–Canada health policy.

In S. Nagel, ed., *Public Policy Analysis and Management* 4. Greenwich, CT: JAI Press.

Mansfield, E. 1968. *Industrial Research and Technological Innovation*. New York: Norton.

Melnick, G. A., J. Wheeler, and P. J. Feldstein. 1981. Effects of rate regulation on selected components of hospital expenses. *Inquiry* 18(3):240–46.

Merrill, J., and C. McLaughlin. 1986. Competition versus regulation: Some empirical evidence. *Journal of Health Politics, Policy and Law* 10(4):613–23.

Morrisey, M. A., F. A. Sloan, and S. A. Mitchell. 1983. State rate setting: An analysis of some unresolved issues. *Health Affairs* 2(1):36–47.

Morrisey, M. A., D. A. Conrad, S. M. Shortell, and K. S. Cook. 1984. Hospital rate review: A theory and an empirical review. *Journal of Health Economics* 3(1):25–47.

Myers, R. J. 1970. *Medicare*. Homewood, IL: Richard D. Irwin.

Noll, R. 1975. The consequences of public utility regulation of hospitals. In R. Hanft, and P. Rettig, eds. *Controls on Health Care*. Washington, DC: National Academy of Science.

Nyman, J. A. 1985. Prospective and 'cost-plus' medicaid reimbursement, excess medicaid demand, and the quality of nursing home care. *Journal of Health Economics* 4(3):237–60.

Ozatalay, S., and R. W. Broyles. 1987. Net returns, fiscal risks and the optimal patient mix for a profit maximizing hospital. *Journal of Medical Systems* 11(5):33–47.

Pauly, M. 1970. Efficiency, incentives and reimbursement for health care. *Inquiry* 7(1):114–31.

Policy Analysis, Inc. 1980. Evaluation of the effects of certificate-of-need programs. Report to DHEW under contract no. HRA–230–7F–0165. Washington, DC.

Romeo, A., J. Wagner, and H. Lee. 1984. Prospective reimbursement and the diffusion of new technologies in hospitals. *Journal of Health Economics* 3(1):1–28.

Rosko, M. D. 1982. *Hospital responses to prospective rate setting*. Unpublished doctoral dissertation, Temple University.

Rosko, M. D. 1984a. The impact of prospective payment: A multidimensional analysis of New Jersey's SHARE Program. *Journal of Health Politics, Policy and Law* 9(1):81–101.

Rosko, M. D. 1984b. Differential impact of prospective payment on hospitals located in different catchment areas. *Journal of Health and Human Resources Administration* 7(1):61–83.

Rosko, M. D. 1986. Hospital rate regulation and market incentives: Complementary approaches to cost containment. *Journal of Health and Human Resources Administration* 8(4):320–38.

Rosko, M. D. 1988. The efficacy of all-payer rate-regulation: The New Jersey experience. Paper presented to the Atlantic Economic Society Annual Meeting, Philadelphia.

Rosko. M. D., and R. W. Broyles. 1984. Unintended consequences of prospective payment: Erosion of hospital financial position and cost-shifting. *Health Care Management Review* 9(3):35–43.

Rosko, M. D., and R. W. Broyles. 1986. Impact of the New Jersey all-payer DRG system. *Inquiry* 23(1):65–73.

Rosko, M. D., R. W. Broyles. 1987. Short-term responses of hospitals to the prospective pricing mechanism in New Jersey. *Medical Care* 25(2):88–99.

Rosko, M. D., R. W. Broyles, and W. E. Aaronson. 1987. Prospective payment based on case-mix: Will it work in nursing homes? *Journal of Health Politics, Policy and Law* 12(4):683–702.

Salkever, D. S. 1979. *Hospital-Sector Inflation.* Lexington, MA: D.C. Heath and Company.

Salkever, D. S., and T. W. Bice. 1979. *Hospital Certificate-of-Need Controls: Impact on Investment, Costs, and Use.* Washington, DC: American Enterprise Institute.

Salkever, D. S., and D. M. Steinwachs. 1986. *Hospital Admissions, Length of Stay, and Case-mix Impacts of Per Case Payment: The Maryland Experience.* Cambridge, MA: National Bureau of Economic Research.

Salkever, D. S., D. M. Steinwachs, and A. Rupp. 1986. Hospital cost and efficiency under per service and per case payment in Maryland: A tale of the carrot and the stick. *Inquiry* 23(1):56–65.

Scheffler, R. M., and J. Gibbs. 1985. *Blue Cross Utilization Rates: Before and After Prospective Payment.* Berkeley: University of California.

Shortell, S. M., M. A. Morrisey, and D. A. Conrad. 1985. Economic regulation and hospital behavior: The effects on medical staff organization and hospital-physician relationships. *Health Services Research* 20(5):597–628.

Sloan, F. A. 1981. Regulation and the rising cost of hospital care. *The Review of Economics and Statistics* 63:479–87.

Sloan, F. A. 1983. Rate regulation as a strategy for cost control: Evidence from the last decade. *Health and Society* 61(2):195–207.

Sloan, F. A., and B. Steinwald. 1980. Effects of regulation on hospital costs and input use. *Journal of Law and Economics* 23(1):81–109.

Sloan, F. A., J. F. Blumstein, and J. M. Perrin, eds. 1986. *Uncompensated Hospital Care: Rights and Responsibilities.* Baltimore, MD: Johns Hopkins University Press.

Sloan, F. A., J. Valvona, and J. M. Perrin. 1986. Diffusion of surgical technology: An exploratory study. *Journal of Health Economics* 5(1):31–61.

Smith, D. B., and R. Pickard. 1986. Evaluation of the impact of Medicare and Medicaid prospective payment on utilization of Philadelphia area hospitals. *Health Services Research* 21(4):529–46.

Staff Report. 1985. Impact of Medicare prospective payment system on the quality of care received by medicare beneficiaries. Special Committee on Aging, U.S. Senate, John Heinz, Chairman.

Thorburn, P., and M. R. Meiners. 1986. Nursing home patient outcomes: The results of an incentive reimbursement experiment. Long-Term Care Studies Program Research Report, Department of Health and Human Services Pub. No. (PHS) 86–3400. Rockville, MD: National Center for Health Services Research and Health Care Technology Assessment.

Thorpe, K. 1987. Does all-payer rate setting work? The case of the New York prospective hospital reimbursement methodology. *Journal of Health Politics, Policy and Law* 12(3):391–408.

U.S. Department of Health, Education and Welfare, Health Care Financing Administration. 1980. Professional Standards Review Organization. Health Care Financing Research Report No. 0–311–168/418. Office of Research Demonstration and Statistics. Washington, DC.

U.S. Department of Health, Education and Welfare, Health Service Administration. 1979.

An evaluation of Professional Standards Review Organization 1979 program evaluation. Office of Planning, Evaluation and Legislation, Washington, DC.

U.S. Senate. 1970. Medicare and Medicaid: Problems, issues and alternatives. Report
of the staff to the Committee on Finance. Washington, DC.

Waldo, D., K. Levit, and H. Lazenby. 1986. National health expenditures, 1985. *Health
Care Financing Review* 8(3):1–21.

Walker, L., R. Broyles, and M. Rosko. 1985. Consequences of the DRG payment system
on hospitalization for the elderly: The elderly at risk. Paper presented to the
American Public Health Association Annual Meeting, Washington, DC.

Webber, A., and W. B. Goldbeck. 1984. Utilization review. In P. D. Fox, W. B. Goldbeck, and J. J. Spies, eds. *Health Care Cost Management*. Ann Arbor, MI: Health
Administration Press.

Williams, S. V., G. F. Kominski, B. E. Dowd et al. 1984. Methodological limitations
in case-mix hospital reimbursement, with a proposal for change. *Inquiry* 21(1):17–
31.

Worthington, N. L., J. Cromwell, and G. Kamens. 1979. Prospective payment in New
Jersey. *Topics in Health Care Financing* 6(1):82–98.

Worthington, N. L., and K. A. Piro. 1982. The effects of hospital rate setting programs
on volumes of hospital services: A preliminary analysis. *Health Care Financing
Review* 4(2):47–67.

Wyszewianski, L., J. W. Thomas, and B. A. Friedman. 1987. Case-based payment and
the control of quality and efficiency in hospitals. *Inquiry* 24(3):17–25.

Zuckerman, S. 1987. Rate setting and cost-containment: All payer versus partial-payer
approaches. *Health Services Research* 22(3):307–26.

13

EPILOGUE: THE LONG AND WINDING ROAD

Apparently it has become de rigueur to refer to Lewis Carroll in the last chapter of a health economics book. Since imitation is the sincerest form of flattery, we pay homage to Sy Berki and Bob Evans by agreeing—yes, the way we go does matter. It is also important, however, to understand where we are and how we got here. Despite significant government and private efforts, access and cost containment continue to be the dominant concerns of health care analysts in the United States.

ACCESS TO HEALTH SERVICES

Access to health care services has been limited by the ability to pay and the availability of providers. Our review of health insurance in Chapter 2 found that more than 30 million Americans may be without health insurance and many others have inadequate protection against the risks of accident and illness. Further, the specter of a widespread AIDS epidemic, as well as other factors such as the emergence of for-profit health care enterprises, has caused policy analysts to reconsider the need for national health insurance. Clearly, we need to examine strategies that will ensure more equitable access to health services without simultaneously creating inflationary pressures.

In Chapters 9 and 10, we reviewed research that indicated that, in spite of an emerging surplus of physicians, some areas and specialties have a shortage of physicians. We are encouraged by a few studies that suggest that market mechanisms may be automatically redressing perceived imbalances in the physician services market; that is, more physicians are locating their practices in less populated areas, which historically have been subject to physician shortages. Similarly, economic pressures may be influencing medical students to choose specialties that are in short supply.

Although less conclusive evidence is available, it appears that the surplus has caused the physicians services market to turn from a "seller's market" to more of a "buyer's market." As the relative supply increased, more physicians have competed for patients on the basis of convenience, a trend that should improve access. Some experts argue that the physician surplus has reduced the resistance of practitioners to HMOs and other alternate delivery systems. This change in physician attitudes enhances the feasibility of competitive strategies, including Medicaid-sponsored case management systems—delivery modalities that have the potential to improve the quality and accessibility of services used by the poor.

RISING HEALTH CARE COSTS

As discussed in Chapter 1, increases in health care expenditures have been due to the interactions of demand-side and supply-side factors. As a response to the rapid increases in expenditures for health services during the last twenty years, a number of cost-containment mechanisms have been implemented or proposed. As our analyses in Chapters 11 and 12 indicated, prospective payment and competition among alternate delivery systems appear to have the most promise of containing costs while maintaining access. All of the policy initiatives have some flaws, however, and the information available is insufficient to make an unequivocal recommendation about future policy directions. Great strides have been made nevertheless in reducing the information gap.

Perhaps the most important advance has been the explicit recognition of the multiproduct nature of health care providers, a subject discussed in Chapter 4. This recognition has led to the development of more precise measures of output (Chapters 5 and 6). These advances have facilitated some very sophisticated research on the structure of production and the determinants of costs (Chapters 7 and 8). Further, the implementation of payment mechanisms, adjusted for patient-mix, has mandated the compilation of more detailed data pertaining to output and costs. Thus, we look forward to more sophisticated research in a variety of sub-sectors (i.e., hospitals, nursing homes, ambulatory care) as data becomes available to support the requirements of more rigorous theoretical models. These developments will place researchers in a better position to analyze policy options, and consequently, legislators will be able to make more informed decisions.

POLICY DIRECTIONS

Now that we know where we are, it is appropriate to determine the path we should take. As Evans (1984) pointed out, the role of economic analysis is to clarify the implications of different institutional frameworks and policy choices; it cannot serve as a source of social objectives or values—though economists frequently try to do so. Thus, we feel it incumbent to point out that our discussion of future policy directions is determined in part by economic analysis and in part by our own personal beliefs. The values and social objectives that we present are also tempered by the cultural and political realities of the United States. For example, some might agree that in order to achieve socially desirable goals, it is necessary to impose insurance systems similar to those used in the United Kingdom or Canada. We are constrained by the fact that Americans have different values and political processes than the British or Canadians.

Before discussing policy options it is necessary to establish goals and appropriate ways of achieving them. We agree with Berki (1972, p. 227), that the "long-run objective should be the establishment of an environment that fosters and maintains physical, mental, and social health where disease is a geriatric, genetic, and stochastic residue." Further, we believe that in order to achieve the long-range goal, the following short-run objectives should be addressed:

1. Access to medically useful treatment should be increased.
2. Health services should be produced as efficiently as possible.
3. Care consistent with accepted standards of quality should be assured.
4. Innovations in better technology, organizational forms, delivery modes, and financing mechanisms should be encouraged.
5. A financial base, adequate to achieve the first four goals, should be available.

In considering what policy directions should be taken, we first sought guidance from the discipline of welfare economics, the subdiscipline that considers the nature of policy recommendations that the economist is entitled to make. As suggested by Baumol (1972), a number of options have been proposed. Some suggest we must do the following:

Accept the status quo;

Only recommend policies that hurt no one;

Recommend policies for which there is a net gain in the utility of everyone involved; or,

Accept the arbitrary judgment of some authority or groups of authorities (e.g., Congress or the public as a whole as indicated by a referendum).

None of these approaches is completely satisfactory. For example, consider the policy options of recommending alternatives that harm no one or proposing strategies that increase the utility of everyone. Recognizing that the needs of the many may outweigh the needs of the few, Great Britain rations certain life-saving services such as renal dialysis on the basis of cost-benefit analysis. Although this is a rational way of maximizing benefits, little solace is offered to those who are denied access to care and thus are condemned to premature death.

Although we feel constrained by political realities, a reliance on the electorate or their representatives can result in suboptimal choices. Legislators may make decisions on the basis of political debts rather than on the public good. Public referendums may be decided by an uninformed electorate, influenced by slick hyperbole rather than sound logic.

These examples illustrate the harsh reality of the policy issues confronting those who must decide how health care services will be financed or delivered in the United States. Given the vested interests in maintaining the status quo, it is probably more fruitful to consider the best acceptable alternative rather than the "best" technical course of action.

In the United States, the policy debate has focused on "competitive" versus "regulatory" strategies. As discussed in Chapters 11 and 12, neither approach is monolithic. At one extreme is a totally free market system; and the other is a system that is owned and sponsored by the government. The existence of substantial consumer ignorance about medicine and an unequal distribution of income preclude a serious consideration of the "free enterprise approach." On the other hand, socialized medicine, as exemplified by the British National Health System, is not congruent with the values of many Americans. Such an approach is not a realistic policy option unless the fabric of American society is altered radically. A number of intermediate options, discussed in Chapters 11 and 12, are more feasible. It is beyond the scope of this book to give a complete social and political evaluation of these options. Instead, we will discuss briefly and in general terms the requirements of sound health policy.

As we discussed in Chapter 1, the inflationary spiral that has plagued the health care industry for over two decades is due to a complex interaction of supply-side and demand-side factors. Accordingly, it is not surprising that piecemeal programs that have only dealt with one aspect of the problems facing the industry have failed to exert a significant impact. The Medicare prospective payment system can be used to illustrate the inadequacies of a piecemeal approach. Although this payment mechanism may have reduced federal outlays, some of the savings may have been achieved at the expense of other payers who have suffered from "cost-shifting." Other reported savings may have been due to transferring costs either vertically (e.g., to nursing homes and home care agencies) or horizontally (e.g., free-standing surgi-centers) in the production process. In sum, the effects of the Medicare prospective payment system may be likened to squeezing a balloon. Costs are contracted in some areas but are expanded in others.

It is clear that in order to contain costs and to assure access, the government must squeeze the entire balloon and address financing and cost-containment issues in a comprehensive manner. However, pressure can be applied in a number of ways. Conceptually, the simplest structure would be a national health insurance system that guaranteed equitable access while providing incentives for the production and use of effective and efficient services.

Moving from concept to practice, however, entails a great leap, perhaps over the insurmountable opposition experienced by those who prefer to maintain the status quo. The political power of various interest groups, such as physicians, hospitals, health insurers and others is substantial and will undoubtedly require compromise. On the other hand, a number of trends suggest that, in the 1990s, a climate more favorably disposed towards national health insurance might exist. For example, recent election results suggest that the political pendulum has been reversed and that liberal causes will enjoy a resurgence. The AIDS epidemic has sensitized many about the devastating effects of catastrophic insurance. Similarly, the high rates of unemployment during the ''Reagan recession'' have revealed the fragility of employer-sponsored insurance arrangements. The realities of the international marketplace have demonstrated the need for employers to contain health care benefits. Finally, the changing character of the health care industry (i.e., a stronger orientation towards profits) requires more government involvement in areas traditionally handled by private organizations.

Although the implementation of a comprehensive national health system is unlikely in the near future, we are hopeful that a compromise solution will be developed. It is more realistic to expect a comprehensive system for the poor and the unemployed, with a comprehensive safety net of catastrophic insurance for the employed and the elderly. Although such a system requires a greater reliance on the government as a source of financing in order to ensure access, cost containment can be addressed in a number of ways. A direct approach would rely on government regulations. Alternatively, incentives for cost containment might be applied in a competitive approach in which market pressures induce health care systems to compete for patients (or government or industry contracts) on the basis of price, quality, access, and other salient attributes of health care. Hopefully, this book will stimulate research that will help us to take the best path.

REFERENCES

Baumol, W. J. 1972. *Economic Theory and Operations Analysis*, 3rd ed. Englewood Cliffs, NJ: Prentice-Hall.
Berki, S. E. 1972. *Hospital Economics*. Lexington, MA: D. C. Heath and Co.
Evans, R. G. 1984. *Strained Mercy: The Economics of Canadian Health Care*. Toronto: Butterworth.

ABBREVIATIONS

AAPCC: adjusted average per capita cost
ADL: activities of daily living
ADRG: alternate diagnosis related group
ADS: alternative delivery systems
AHA: American Hospital Association
AID: automatic interaction detector
ALOS: average length of stay
AMA: American Medical Association
AMI: acute myocardial infarction
ANOVA: analysis of variance
AVG: ambulatory visit groups
CES: constant elasticity of substitution production function
CHC: community health center
CMI: case-mix index
CMP: competitive medical plan
CON: certificate of need
COTH: Council of Teaching Hospitals
CPHA: Commission on Professional and Hospital Activities
CSI: computerized severity index
CV: coefficient of variation
DEA: data envelopment analysis
DHEW: U.S. Department of Health, Education, and Welfare

DHHS: U.S. Department of Health and Human Services

DMU: decision-making units

DRG: diagnosis related group

ESP: Economic Stabilization Program

FEHBP: Federal Employees Health Benefits Program

FERISA: Federal Employee Retirement Income Security Act

FTE: full-time equivalent

GAO: General Accounting Office

GMENAC: Graduate Medical Education National Advisory Committee

HCFA: Health Care Financing Administration

HIES: Health Insurance Employer Survey

HIO: health insuring organization

HIS: Health Interview Survey

HMO: health maintenance organization

HSA: health systems agencies

IADL: instrumental activities of daily living

ICD: International Classification of Diseases

ICD–9–CM: International Classification of Diseases, 9th Revision, Clinical Modifications

ICDA–7: International Classification of Diseases - Adapted - 7th Revision

ICDA–8: International Classification of Diseases - Adapted - 8th Revision

ICF: intermediate care facility

ICU: intensive care unit

IPA: individual practice association

JCAH: Joint Commission on the Accreditation of Hospitals

LAC: long-run average cost

LTC: long-term care

MAC: major ambulatory category

MADC: major ambulatory diagnostic category

MCAT: medical college admission test

MCMI: Medicare case-mix index

MDC: major diagnostic category

MEDISGRPS: Medical Illness Severity Grouping System

MHS: multihospital system

NAMCS: National Ambulatory Medical Care Survey

NBME: National Board of Medical Examiners

NCHSR: National Center for Health Services Research

NLRA: National Labor Relations Act

NMCES: National Medical Care Expenditure Survey

NMCEUS: National Medical Care Expenditure and Utilization Survey

OB/GYN: obstetrics and gynecology

ODE: Office of Demonstrations and Evaluation

ORD: Office of Research and Demonstrations

OT: occupational therapy

OTA: Office of Technology Assessment

PGP: prepaid group practice

PIR: prospective individualized reimbursement model

PMC: patient management category

PP: prospective payment

PPA: preferred provider arrangements

PPO: preferred provider organization

PRO: peer review organization

ProPAC: Prospective Payment Assessment Commission

PSRO: Professional Standards and Review Organizations

PT: physical therapy

RN: registered nurse

RNI: resource need index

RUG: resource utilization group

SDC: staged disease category

SES: socioeconomic status

SII: severity of illness index

SMSA: Standard Metropolitan Statistical Area

SNF: skilled nursing facility

SSA: Social Security Administration

TEFRA: Tax Equity and Fiscal Responsibility Act of 1982

UHDDS: Uniform Hospital Discharge Data Set

UMW: United Mine Workers of America

UR: utilization review

VA: Veterans Administration

VE: voluntary effort of hospital industry

VNA: visiting nurse agency

NAME INDEX

SUBJECT INDEX

ABOUT THE AUTHORS

MICHAEL D. ROSKO is Acting Director of and an Associate Professor in the Graduate Program in Health and Medical Services Administration at Widener University. He is the coauthor, with Robert W. Broyles, of *Financial Planning and Internal Control Under Prospective Payment*. His numerous articles have been published in the *Journal of Health, Politics, Policy and Law*, *Journal of Health Care Marketing*, *Handbook on Health Services Administration*, *Journal of Hospital Marketing*, and many other journals.

ROBERT W. BROYLES is a Professor in the Graduate Program in Health and Medical Services Administration at Widener University. He is the author of *Hospital Accounting Practice: Volume II, Managerial Accounting, Hospital Accounting Practice: Volume I, Financial Accounting*, and *Management of Working Capital in Hospitals*, and the coauthor of four other books in the field of health administration. His articles have appeared in *Hospital and Health Services Administration*, *Journal of Medical Systems*, *Health Care Management Review*, and *Medical Care*, among others.